Nourish for Menopause

Rachel Graham, the Menopause Nutritionist, is a practising nutritional therapist and medicinal chef with over 25 years of experience. She works predominantly in women's health with an emphasis on menopause, and is an accredited menopause educator from The Menopause Charity.

'This is an excellent book, and I am very impressed with the research and detail that Rachel has put in. It is so important that we translate science into our everyday lives, and what better way to do this than by educating us on how to cook healthy food for the menopause that looks after bone, brain and heart health with these delicious, nutritious ingredients. Women going through menopause will relish all the wonderful information here that will empower generations of women to come.' **Mary Ryan**

'*Nourish for Menopause* provides a nutrient-dense and plant-forward approach to supporting better health during menopause. I absolutely love Rachel's food-first and positive approach to feeling good. This is a great book to recommend, and a great reminder of what women need to consider in terms of nutrition.'
Domini Kemp

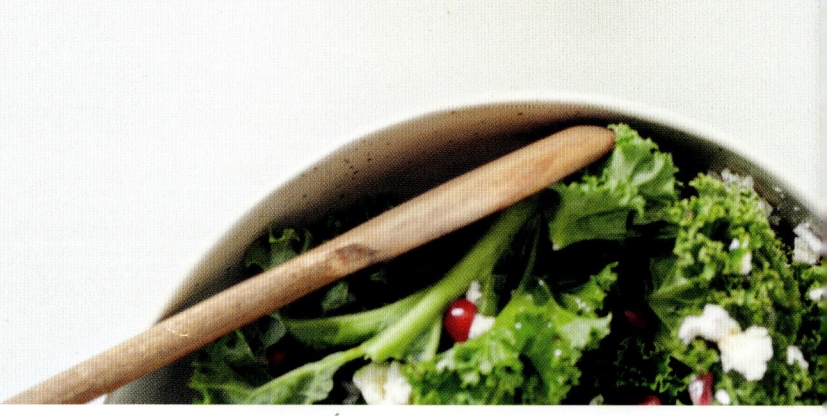

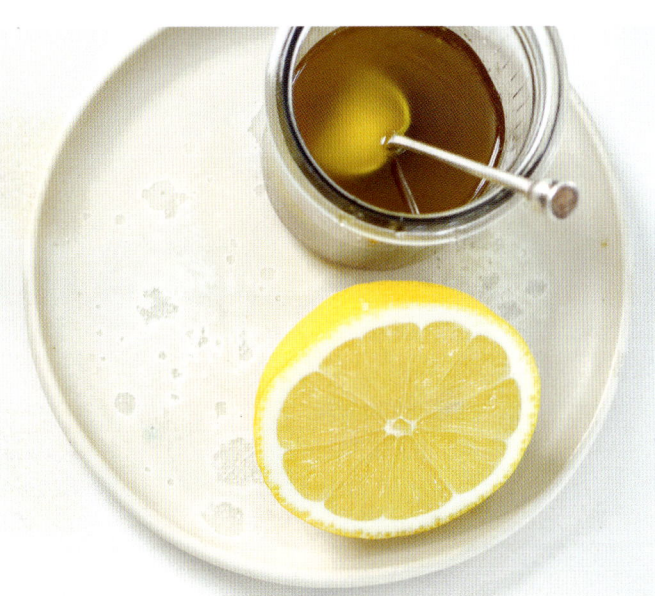

Nourish for Menopause

TRANSFORM YOUR MENOPAUSE WITH GREAT NUTRITION

RACHEL GRAHAM

GILL BOOKS

Gill Books
Hume Avenue
Park West
Dublin 12
www.gillbooks.ie

Gill Books is an imprint of M.H. Gill and Co.

© Rachel Graham 2024

This is Rachel Graham's first book, originally published under a different title and now reprinted as Nourish for Menopause.

978 18045 8311 1

Designed by Graham Thew
Photography by Joanne Murphy
Food styling by Orla Neligan
Illustrated by Andrii Yankovskyi and Lydia Moran
Edited by Sands Publishing Solutions
Proofread by Alicia McAuley
Printed by L.E.G.O. SpA, Italy
This book is typeset in 10.5pt Calluna

The paper used in this book comes from the wood pulp of sustainably managed forests.

All rights reserved.
No part of this publication may be copied, reproduced or transmitted in any form or by any means, without written permission of the publishers.

A CIP catalogue record for this book is available from the British Library.

5 4 3 2 1

This book is not intended as a substitute for the medical advice of a physician. The reader should consult a doctor or mental health professional if they feel it necessary.

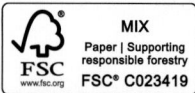

To all the women taking action in the kitchen to future-proof their health ... This book is for you! xx

Contents

Part one: Understanding menopause viii
Introduction 1
The Big Four – how to reduce your risk 7

Part two: Future-proofing your health 10
Bone health: The importance of strong and healthy bones 11
Brain health: The omega-3 non-negotiable ... 13
Digestive health and detoxification: The power of fibre 18
Heart health: The elephant in the room 20
The truth about sugar 23
The meno-middle: Why am I gaining weight? 29
Designing a healthy diet and how to use this book 33

Part three: The Meno 8 38
1. Phytoestrogens 39
2. Fibre 43
3. Omega-3 49
4. Calcium and magnesium 53
5. Antioxidants 57
6. Protein 64
7. Probiotics 68
8. Brassicas 71

Part four: Recipes 78
1. Phytoestrogens 79
Tofu scramble 80
Crispy tofu Thai red curry 83
Roasted aubergine involtini 85
Ramen bowl 88
Sweet potato, lentil, shitake, tofu and lemongrass curry 90
Edamame bean hummus 91
Edamame and sesame rainbow slaw 92
Organic soy golden milk 95
Chicory and smashed avo 96
Falafels 99

2. Fibre 101
Porridge bread 102
Spirulina, lime and mint overnight oats 104
Oat and flaxseed porridge with blueberry compote 105
Pecan cinnamon granola 107
Oat and hemp seed porridge 108
Sweet potato and apple breakfast cookies ... 110
Vegan power bowl 113
Apple doughnuts 114
Roasted carrot and yellow pepper hummus .. 117
Sage and date hummus 118
Avonaise 120
Beetroot ketchup 121
Savoury granola 122
Date and ginger caramel 124
Pear tart with date and ginger caramel 125
Rhubarb, pear and apple compote 128
Carrot cake squares 129

3. Omega-3 133
Lime chia pudding 134
The nutrient powerhouse smoothie bowl ... 137
Mediterranean seafood bouillabaisse 138
Harissa charred salmon 140
Flaxseed crackers 143
Balsamic dressing 144
Smoked mackerel pâté 146
Mackerel niçoise salad 149
Summer rolls 150
Salmon kedgeree 154

4. Calcium and magnesium 157
The recovery-boosting salad in a jar 158
Minestrone bean stew 161
Red lentil, turmeric and kale hotpot 162

Kale quinoa wraps 163
Grilled baby gem Casear salad 164
Spinach, pea and mint risotto with roasted
    asparagus and prawns 167
Nori seaweed hand roll 169
Almond butter 170
Almond milk 173
Chocolate tahini bliss balls 174
Hazelnut butter brownies 177

5. Antioxidants **179**
Beetroot, ginger and fennel juice 180
Carrot, red pepper, orange and ginger juice .. 183
Life-giving green juice 184
Sweet potato toast 186
Mango, turmeric and hemp seed smoothie .. 189
The lit-from-within chicken salad 190
Tomato, chilli and fennel soup 192
Parsley gremolata 195
Basil pesto 196
Roasted Mediterranean vegetables 197
Carrot, ginger and celery soup 199
The glow bowl 200
The fountain-of-youth smoothie bowl 202
Sweet potato gnocchi 204
Roasted Med veg lasagne 207
Porcini mushroom risotto 211
Banana nice-cream 215

6. Protein **217**
Roasted Med veg frittata 218
Courgette rolls 219
Shakshuka 220
Courgette tortillas 222
Falafel wrap 223
Moroccan spiced chicken tagine 225
Moroccan quinoa 226

Lentil and mushroom burgers 228
Mushroom and lentil Bolognese 231
Mushroom and lentil shepherd's pie 232
Chicken bone broth 235
Bircher muesli 237
Mocha chia protein overnight oats 238
Pear-a-misu 240
Turmeric roasted chicken breast 243
Daily dahl 244
Thrive protein balls 247

7. Probiotics **249**
Sauerkraut with fennel and apple 250
Coconut yoghurt 253
Apple cider vinegar 255
Four-seed rye sourdough bread 256
Probiotic lime green smoothie 259
Frozen yoghurt bark 260

8. Brassicas **263**
Steamed cauliflower rice 264
Roasted cauliflower, chickpea and sweet
    potato salad 265
Cauliflower pea mash 266
Rocket, pine nut and Parmesan salad 268
Balsamic roasted Brussels sprouts 270
Flash-cooked tender stem broccoli 271
Balsamic roasted cabbage steaks 273
Cauliflower chickpea lemon curry 274
Kale salad 276
Cheesy kale chips 279

Resources 280
Acknowledgements 282
Endnotes 283
Index 285

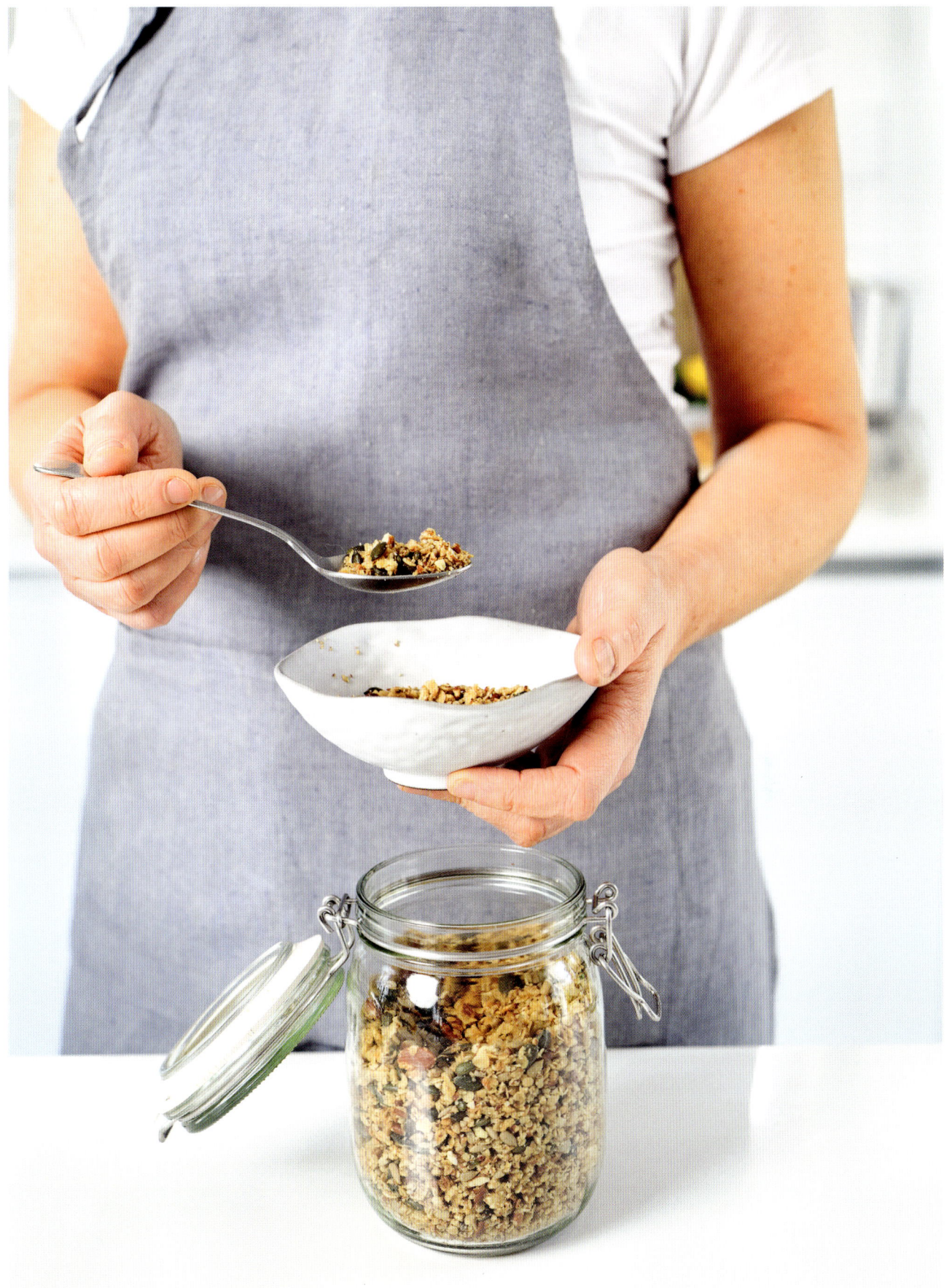

Part one: Understanding menopause

Introduction

They say that health is something you only appreciate once you get sick – and I am inclined to agree.

Ten years ago, out of the blue, my menopause hit me. I was 43 years old and it seemed like my health was changing for the worse from one day to the next. Now that I look back, I realise that several symptoms had actually been affecting me for a while – a few years, probably – but I didn't connect the dots and understand that this was, in fact, menopause.

At the time, these symptoms seemed unrelated. Frequent waking in the night, hot flushes, joint aches, brain fog, lack of concentration, feeling anxious and more emotional than usual. I now know that these 'unrelated' issues were all classic menopause symptoms.

Everyone's experience of menopause is different. Some really struggle, while others seem to sail through this life stage. Menopause is such an individual journey, and that's part of why it's so important to educate yourself early on: you need to know what to expect. Many women, however, arrive at this life stage unprepared.

Why? Because menopause has been shrouded in secrecy and taboo for decades – despite the fact that it directly affects 50 per cent of the population (and indirectly affects the other 50 per cent). Women can be in denial about what's happening to them, but there's nothing to be ashamed of; it is a natural part of life, as much so as puberty and pregnancy.

FACT: IF YOU WERE BORN FEMALE, YOU WILL EXPERIENCE MENOPAUSE. IF YOU HAVEN'T YET, IT'S IN THE POST!

A good diet will lay the foundations for greatly improved menopause symptom management. Optimised nutrition is also fundamental to future-proofing your health and reducing known risk factors for chronic disease. How you nourish your body at this life stage will directly affect both the frequency and severity of your menopause symptoms. If ever you needed a good reason to prioritise your nutrition, this is it.

This is my life stage too, and I want many of the same things that you do – more energy, better-quality sleep, better memory and concentration and to maintain a healthy weight. But trying to figure all of this out on your own is not easy; there is a lot of conflicting information out there. A reliable source of evidence-based information, explaining the nutrients to optimise now and paired with delicious-tasting recipes containing an effective dose of those beneficial nutrients – this kind of practical resource is the missing piece of the menopause puzzle. So many of my clients were coming to me with symptoms similar to my own but were unaware of what they needed to eat to effectively nourish themselves. Despite the recent increased awareness around menopause, there was still no menopause-specific medicinal cookbook for Irish women – and that's the reason that I wrote this one!

As a practising nutritional therapist and medicinal chef – certified in lifestyle medicine, plant-based nutrition, fermentation and raw-food mastery – tasty, healthy food is my passion. I understand how great nutrition can completely transform your health. In my online nutrition clinic, I focus predominantly on women's health with an emphasis on menopause. I'm an accredited menopause educator from the Menopause Charity, qualified to advise women on the various treatment options available to manage the symptoms of menopause. I offer practical cooking demos to help women take action in the kitchen to future-proof their health.

Menopause is a time in women's lives when we are often freer to explore more of what *we* want to do: learn a new skill, start a new career, travel more ... the Chinese call this the 'second spring'. I love this take on menopause because it epitomises a new, exciting and positive life that is just beginning for us! Now is the time to look after yourself and prioritise your health, so that you can add quality of life to this next stage.

How to use this book

My goal in writing this cookbook and nutritional manual was to provide tasty, medicinal recipes that nourish your body and transform your mid-life health. I have included lots of variety and fresh flavour combinations to inspire you and get you into the kitchen. There are over 100 delicious health-focused recipes, optimised in eight categories.

I call these categories my **Meno 8**, and they are:
1. Phytoestrogens
2. Fibre
3. Omega-3
4. Calcium and magnesium
5. Antioxidants
6. Protein
7. Probiotics
8. Brassicas

Each section of the book is dedicated to one of these eight categories and explains why they are a crucial part of your healthy menopause diet, including referenced health claims and the recommended daily amount (RDA). The recipes have been designed to provide benefits beyond basic nutrition – to help you balance your hormones, feel energised and maintain a healthy weight. Each recipe is packed full of nutrients and active properties that help to strengthen your bones, support your liver detoxification processes, enhance your energy levels, balance your hormones and improve your digestion.

The recipes have all been analysed using professional software to track 16 important nutrients. Highlighting the RDA and milligram/gram weight of each nutrient, this information is displayed as an easy-to-read bar chart at the bottom of every recipe. This will enable you to achieve your RDA of each nutrient and to balance your hormones.

As I've already mentioned, menopause is often the stage of our lives when we start to develop niggling health issues. It's when the years of wear and tear on our body become apparent, and unless we take action, at best we may not feel like ourselves, and at worst we can get sick. Either outcome will impact our quality of life. My goal is to show you how to include all the important nutrients daily, in effective doses. Simply put, I want to help you to use food as your pharmacy.

The Meno 8 RDAs – your daily goals

300mg
Phytoestrogens

35g
Fibre

400mg
Omega-3

1,200mg Calcium
>300mg Magnesium

6,000 ORAC units
Antioxidants

0.8–1.2g per kg of body weight
Protein

2 servings
Probiotics

2 servings
Brassicas

Support your menopausal body – don't punish it

As women, our well-being is somewhat dependent on our hormones. When oestrogen starts to decline, it can trigger a cascade of seemingly unrelated symptoms that can really affect our quality of life. Making decisions about our health is an ongoing process. What is working for us now may not work so well down the line, so we need to be open to making changes to our health plan as we progress through this life stage.

In fact, the key to this life stage is our capacity to adapt in the face of hormonal fluctuations and life stressors. It can be challenging, but it *is* possible to thrive. With this cookbook and the medicinal recipes contained in it, you are well equipped to make that a reality.

Why is it that, despite living in an era with so much information at our fingertips, so many of us are still confused about what to eat, when to eat and how best to nourish our bodies? In my experience, women going through menopause seem to be struggling with this issue the most. The fact is that menopause is so unsettling that it can be hard to know what food we need to prioritise for health, energy and symptom reduction.

Menopause can hit us hard, with multiple (seemingly unrelated) health issues, all requiring our attention. One of the main sources of frustration is the annoying weight gain. Compounding this is the loss of energy, which often prevents us from exercising. Our aching joints play a role, too. Together these symptoms can result in us ending up quite sedentary, at a time in our lives when we need to prioritise exercise and movement, and not just for weight loss. This is the time to take preventative action to promote healthy ageing and disease prevention.

Many of my mid-life clients arrive at Clinic feeling unhealthy, bloated and tired. They haven't yet joined the dots between these symptoms and the multitude of other menopause symptoms they may be experiencing – from sore joints and aching muscles to sluggish digestion, mood swings and chronic fatigue.

In fact, most women usually put up with all these symptoms, not even mentioning them in any great detail, assuming this is their lot now that they are in menopause. However, feeling unhealthy, bloated and tired is not a normal part of ageing – and you don't have to put up with it.

You may also have noticed that everything that was working up until now to tackle the annoying weight gain no longer does. No matter what you do, you just can't shift it …

To solve this puzzle, you need to keep in mind that your biological landscape has changed and the goalposts have been cruelly moved. You need to work with your body, not against it. You need a different approach – a more health-focused approach. Once you take the focus off weight loss and turn your attention instead to all the ways you can support your body (using nutrition, exercise, relaxation and meditation, as well as making time for social connections), your body will come back into balance and may even start to relinquish those extra pounds. This is a multipronged approach that also has multiple benefits to your overall health, beyond just weight loss.

By using this approach, you will:

- Reduce the chronic inflammation that may have been there for years. The fact is, inflammation is often the root cause of aching joints, weight gain, fluctuating blood glucose and much more.
- Improve your digestion and the detoxification processes that are integral to increasing your metabolism and energy levels, not to mention disease prevention.
- Create a personalised nutrition 'template' that will future-proof your well-being, improve your mid-life health and reset your hormones.

It's time to clean up your diet and optimise the Meno 8. It's time to thrive.

My eight building blocks

So, to help you focus on your intake of these eight categories, I have eight building blocks for you to consider when trying to improve your diet.

1 Eat the rainbow

Eat lots and lots of fruit and vegetables every day. The best antioxidant-rich foods have the strongest colours. Aim to include something green, yellow, blue, purple, red and orange every day to achieve 6,000 ORAC (oxygen radical absorbency capacity) units – the daily recommended amount of antioxidants to maintain your health. You'll learn more about antioxidants in part three of the book.

2 Control your blood glucose

Controlling your blood glucose is necessary for maintaining energy levels, reducing cravings, improving cognitive ability, preventing arterial damage and reducing cholesterol. Sugar and refined carbohydrates – for example, white bread, white rice and white pasta – are known as high glycaemic foods. When you consume these foods, they cause a blood-sugar spike, followed by a rapid drop. With every glucose spike, insulin is released, and this constant triggering of insulin has many negative effects on the body. Over time, these fluctuations lead to exhaustion and weight gain, not to mention an increased risk of heart disease.

You can control your blood glucose with correct dietary choices – for example, by adopting a low-GL diet. You will learn more about this in part two, in the sections on heart health and sugar.

3 Reduce meat

All animal proteins – from meat to cow's milk dairy – contain a fatty acid known as arachidonic acid. This is a pro-inflammatory compound, and while some dietary intake is important for normal health, an unbalanced ratio of omega-6 to omega-3 fatty acids can promote inflammation in the body by triggering an immune response when consumed. This ratio can be caused by high animal-protein consumption, so it's important to include healthy sources of omega-6 fatty acids in your diet, such as nuts, seeds and plant oils.

Inflammation is only intended as a temporary defence mechanism – for example, for healing an acute illness or rushing to the site of infection by releasing immune cells. Causing the immune system to be in a constant state of defence weakens it over time. This could also be a contributing factor to the immune-related allergies and sensitivities that are so typical at this life stage.

Finally, several studies confirm that the higher your intake of meat and other animal products, the higher your risk of heart disease and cancer[1]. In 2015, based on evidence from epidemiology studies, the World Health Organization (WHO) classified processed meats (bacon, sausages, ham and the likes) in the same category as cigarettes (category 1): 'carcinogenic to humans'. It also classified red meat in category 2A ('probably carcinogenic to humans') in association with colorectal cancers.

4 Eat more plants

Plants provide the broadest range of nutrients, phytochemicals, antioxidants and minerals of any food type, and they should play a major part in your diet now. I recommend including 8–10 portions of fruits and vegetables every day. This might sound like a lot, but it's easier than you think:

→ Add greens and other veg (minimum three types) to a breakfast smoothie or have a selection – such as tomatoes, spinach and mushrooms – with eggs.
→ Have a large salad or soup for lunch (minimum four types of veg).
→ Fill half your plate with vegetables for dinner (minimum three types).
→ Snack on veggies, nuts, seeds and whole fruits to optimise your intake.

Also crucial for your menopause health are plant proteins, which are found in beans, grains, lentils, legumes, tofu and tempeh. Rich in fibre, B vitamins and phytoestrogens, plant proteins have low to no saturated fats, and they are heart-healthy, anti-inflammatory and cancer-protective.

5 Eat quality fats

The type of fat you consume is key. The typical western diet contains too many omega-6 fats (found in meat) and hydrogenated vegetable oils (also known as trans fats) – for example, soy and corn oil. The goal is to decrease your intake of these poor-quality fats and increase your intake of heart-healthy, monounsaturated fats – that is, olive oil, oily fish, flaxseeds and chia seeds.

6 Eat more fibre

All nutrients are important, but if I had to pick a favourite, it would be fibre. Despite being found in carbohydrate-rich foods such as fruits, vegetables, nuts and wholegrains, fibre does not contribute any carbohydrates to our diet. It is a critical food source for our beneficial gut bacteria; without it, they will starve and die off. Eating enough fibre keeps these gut bugs thriving and multiplying, rewarding us with improved mood, memory and concentration and, of course, improved digestion and elimination.

7 Reduce your exposure to chemicals

We are all exposed to toxins and chemicals on an ongoing basis: in our food, our environment and our beauty and personal-care products. Our bodies have a tough time trying to expel these toxins, which end up being stored in our fat cells and can lead to hormone-dependent cancers. Chemicals such as BPAs, PCBs and phthalates also contribute to our oxidative load, as do the antibiotics and hormones in factory-farmed meat.

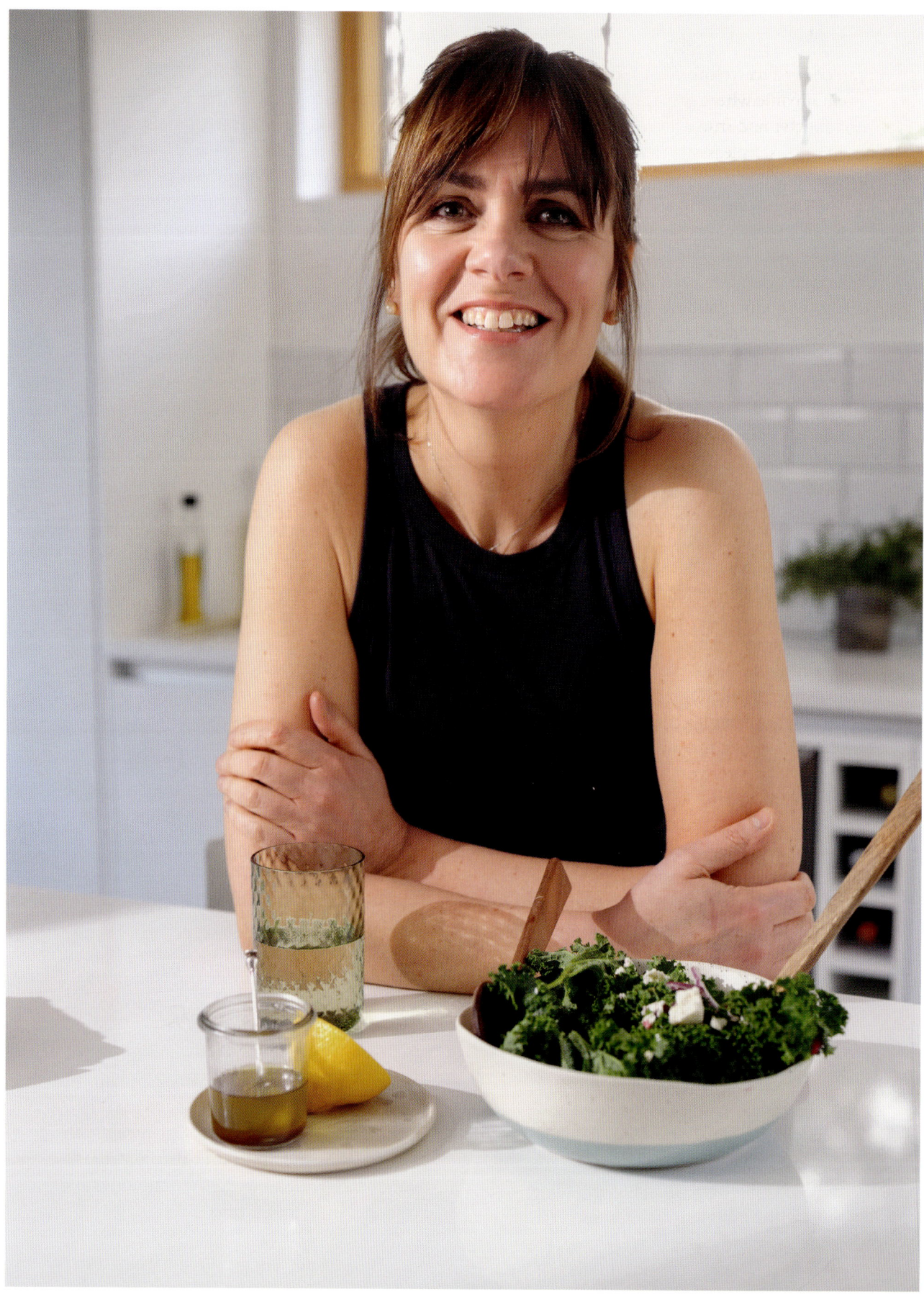

You can reduce your oxidative load by trying to eat organic where possible (including milk, eggs, butter and fruit and veg). Opt for glass, ceramic or stainless-steel food storage and buy locally grown produce that is in season; this is when it is at its best, both nutritionally and in terms of taste. Switch to natural household cleaning products (which have the added benefit of being refillable) and rethink your self-care products such as skincare, shampoo, toothpaste and deodorant. My rule of thumb is that if I wouldn't put it in my mouth, I don't put it on my skin.

8 Stay well hydrated

Drink a minimum of two litres of hydrating fluids every day. If you are doing high-intensity training, add an extra half-litre for every 30 minutes of exercise. Water is important for many reasons, including supporting our liver's detoxification processes, helping to transport nutrients around our bodies and regulating bowel movements for effective daily elimination. Drinking water also helps to reduce water retention and puffiness. It may seem counterintuitive, but the more water you drink (up to a maximum of three litres per day), the less water you will store – your body is retaining water because it needs it.

The Big Four – how to reduce your risk

The transition to menopause can be a bumpy one, and many women focus on the more overwhelming symptoms, such as hot flushes, night sweats, mood swings, anxiety and problems with memory and concentration.

However, during this life stage, we also find ourselves at an increased risk for conditions that cannot be ignored.

1. **Cardiovascular disease**
2. **Type 2 diabetes**
3. **Osteoporosis**
4. **Alzheimer's disease and dementia**

I call these the Big Four, because they are serious, chronic health conditions that have the potential to shorten our life.

Having said that, they are all lifestyle-related diseases. This means that we have some control over them – we can make effective changes to reduce our risk. Good nutrition is the foundation of this. Nothing will positively impact our long-term health and well-being more than a really good diet.

Cardiovascular disease

The elephant in the menopause room is cardiovascular disease. Why? Because the risk of heart attacks is five times higher after menopause than before, and heart disease is the leading cause of death for females over the age of 70.

We really need to protect our heart health during this life stage. You can read more about this in the heart health section in part two.

Type 2 diabetes

At this life stage, women are also at an increased risk for type 2 diabetes – and this carries with it a greater risk of cardiovascular disease, so the two are intrinsically linked. Type 2 diabetes is a condition of blood sugar dysregulation and carbohydrate metabolism – an issue that is common in menopausal women. This is because the way we metabolise carbohydrates changes, with our body not responding to the insulin that is being produced – insulin is effectively broken.

How does insulin work?
Insulin's job is to remove glucose (from the food we have just eaten) from the bloodstream and deliver it to the cells to create energy. When our body is no longer responding effectively to the insulin that is being produced, it can be likened to a spluttering car, out of fuel, struggling to get going. No wonder we often feel tired at this life stage: we can't get glucose into our cells.

High-GL foods
When we regularly consume high-GL foods – that is, refined carbohydrates, sugar and starch – we can become insulin-insensitive or pre-diabetic over time.

This means that insulin no longer works properly, and we will likely experience multiple daily glucose spikes. These continuous glucose spikes can damage our arteries, as well as our good cholesterol – a process known as glycosylation. Damaged cholesterol leads to elevated LDL cholesterol (the bad type), and our kidney function can become impaired, raising blood pressure.

A change in diet can be very effective in increasing our insulin sensitivity, and it can even reverse this pre-diabetic condition. A survey[2] carried out at the Harvard School of Public Health in 2006 showed that a high-GL diet (that is, a diet high in refined carbohydrates, sugar and starch) doubles the risk of heart disease in comparison to a low-GL diet (or a diet rich in whole foods or fibre-rich foods).

You can learn more about the benefits of a low-GL diet in part two, but here are some simple steps that I would recommend to reduce your intake of high-GL foods:
→ Aim to become more aware of both the quality and the quantity of carbohydrates that are being consumed.
→ Switching from refined white carbohydrates to complex whole carbohydrates (wholegrain or whole wheat) is a good place to start for more balanced blood sugars.
→ Reducing overall carbohydrate consumption is recommended – even complex carbohydrates will still convert to glucose.

Osteoporosis

Irrespective of diet, lifestyle or environmental factors, our risk for osteoporosis naturally increases during menopause, as a result of our loss of oestrogen. This risk is often underestimated by women and even healthcare professionals.

Osteoporosis means an increased risk of bone fractures or breaks. It might not be life-threatening, but a hip fracture or a broken bone (followed by months of recovery and rehab) would have a massive impact on our independence – now and 10 years from now. We all want to remain active and mobile in our 50s, 60s, 70s and beyond, so strengthening our bones has to be a priority now.

The new WHO guidelines for osteoporosis prevention recommend a two-pronged approach:
→ Adding calcium-rich foods and other important minerals (such as magnesium) to our diet, and optimising our vitamin D intake to increase calcium absorption.

→ Regular weight-bearing exercise.

You can learn more about this in the bone health section in part two.

Alzheimer's disease and dementia

Multiple studies have shown that oestrogen is very important for brain function. Without oestrogen, the female brain functions sub-optimally. This would certainly explain why, around the time of menopause, we often suffer from poor memory and concentration, anxiety and depression, as well as a whole host of other nervous-system issues.

Leading neuroscientist Dr Lisa Mosconi explains the fundamental differences in how the female brain ages in comparison to the male brain in her book *The XX Brain*. Women have a greater risk of stroke and depression than men, for example, and are also twice as likely as men to develop Alzheimer's disease, which Mosconi suggests may be due in part to differences in hormones. Bearing these differences in mind, we must use *all* the tools at our disposal to reduce our risk of Alzheimer's disease and dementia.

What can we do?

A key intervention in the fight against dementia is the quality of our diet. Research[3] tells us that a diet rich in antioxidants can improve our cognitive function. We also know that blood-sugar control and improving insulin sensitivity are important steps in the prevention of Alzheimer's disease. In fact, Alzheimer's is sometimes referred to as type 3 diabetes because of its close association with blood-sugar dysregulation.

As we age, we can struggle to digest and absorb animal proteins, leading to nutrient deficiencies. These nutrient deficiencies (for example, B vitamins and trace minerals such as zinc) have been linked to Alzheimer's disease. One thing that we can make an effort to eat more of is turmeric, nature's most potent anti-inflammatory! Anecdotal evidence shows that an elderly population in rural India eating large amounts of turmeric had 4.4 times less incidence of Alzheimer's disease than Americans of similar age.

Brain health

→ Elevated cortisol (the stress hormone) causes poor cognitive function – that is, poor memory, concentration and focus – independent of life events.

→ Being apple-shaped or having a concentration of fat around the middle (known as central adiposity) increases inflammation in the body, predisposing women to insulin resistance and Alzheimer's disease.

→ Balancing blood glucose is key to preventing cognitive impairment.

→ A study of 2,000 women in Denmark found that the risk for developing cognitive dysfunction was 44 per cent higher in those with impaired fasting glucose[4].

Part two:
Future-proofing your health

Bone health: The importance of strong and healthy bones

One of the four chronic health conditions I refer to in part one, osteoporosis, is defined as the loss of bone mass, leading to fragility and an increased risk of fractures.

The risk factors for osteoporosis include:
- Being postmenopausal
- Early menopause or surgical menopause
- An absence of periods related to menopause
- Low body weight and eating disorders
- Lack of physical activity (weight-bearing exercise)
- Smoking
- Excessive alcohol intake
- Coeliac disease
- Prolonged use of some medications (asthma, thyroid, seizure)
- Poor diet and dietary insufficiencies

The window of time to be concerned about is the few years before and the few years after our last period – usually from age 48 to 54. During this time, women may experience their most rapid decline in bone density and their greatest increase in osteoporosis risk (after the age of 70, women experience a natural decline in bone density and their risk of osteoporosis may further increase).

Hip fractures are very common in postmenopausal women. This is because the neck of the thigh bone increases in size as we age, which in turn increases the likelihood that our thigh bone will buckle and misplace. Weight gain (which is also very common at this life stage) can further compound the problem by increasing the load on our bones, at a time when our bones are losing strength.

Recovery from a hip fracture can be slow, and this affects our physical health, with a loss of independence and mobility (some women may have to convalesce in a nursing home, either temporarily or long term), but it can also lead to a decline in our mental health.

Let's do some myth-busting about bones and our calcium intake.

MYTH	FACT
To prevent osteoporosis, we need to increase our calcium intake – specifically from cow's milk dairy.	Cow's milk dairy is not the only or even the best dietary source of calcium. Some plant sources contain more calcium than cow's milk dairy products.
Our bones are static body parts that simply hold us upright.	Bone does much more than provide structure to our bodies. It is living tissue that stores minerals, nutrients and fat. It also produces red blood cells and platelets.

As a result of microscopic damage from daily physical activity, our bones also go through a continuous renewal process known as bone turnover. Think of it as an ongoing house renovation, with both the demolition team and the builders in at the same time. Bone turnover involves breaking down and replacing areas of damage, followed by removal and the process of forming new bone. This work is carried out by our osteoclast and osteoblast cells.

Usually, for women up to the age of 30, the re-formation of bone outweighs the breaking-down process. However, in menopause, the opposite is true. Bone loss is accelerated, and we can lose as much as 20 per cent of our bone mass. This can manifest as bone loss in other areas of the body – such as deterioration in our jaw, contributing to problems with our teeth.

How do you find out if your bones are okay?

Get a DEXA scan (a type of X-ray) to confirm how much bone tissue you have. Your DEXA results are issued as a T-score, comparing your bones to those of a young healthy person.

- **+1 to -1** means your bone health is in the normal range
- **-1 to -2.5** means your bone health is below the normal range (usually classified as osteopenia)
- **-2.5 and below** means you are in the osteoporosis range

Consider a diagnosis of osteopenia a yellow card: it is a warning to make changes and to place more emphasis on a healthy diet and lifestyle to strengthen your bones. Osteoporosis can be a real blow to our health and quality of life, so it's worth doing all you can to minimise the risk and prevent it.

What you can do

- **Eat quality protein every day.** Work out the right amount (0.8g to 1.2g of protein per kilogram of body weight) and ensure you consume this daily, spreading it evenly over three meals.
- **Take a vitamin D supplement** – but get your vitamin D levels checked first! You may have adequate levels that just need maintaining with a low dose, or you may already have elevated levels, in which case adding an extra dose could quickly lead to toxicity. Vitamin D increases the uptake of calcium, so it plays a key role in maintaining your bone tissue.
- **Eat calcium-rich foods daily.** I've put together a chapter of my favourite calcium-containing recipes on p157.
- **Exercise.** Focus on weight-bearing exercise – such as yoga, Pilates and weight training – to strengthen your bones.
- **Keep an eye on your calcium intake.** You are aiming for 1,200mg of calcium per day, ideally from plant-based sources. This simple but effective tool from the International Osteoporosis Foundation – www.osteoporosis.foundation/educational-hub/topic/calcium-calculator – is an effective way to check your intake.

What we need to know about cow's milk dairy

When thinking about calcium to support bone health, most people immediately think of cow's milk dairy products. Decades of marketing messages from the dairy industry about the importance of dairy for strengthening our bones are firmly etched into our consciousness. While milk and other dairy products are certainly good sources of calcium, they aren't the only options – many plant-based foods also provide high levels of calcium.

The problem with cow's milk is that it includes a sulphur-containing amino acid that acidifies our blood. This excess acidity has to be neutralised by the body, which in the process causes the bone to dissolve and be excreted in our urine. Animal proteins like cow's milk have two to five times more of these sulphur-containing amino acids than plant-based sources of calcium.

An article[5] in *The New England Journal of Medicine* summarises the evidence for the benefits and possible risks associated with the consumption of cow's milk. The authors describe the relationship between milk consumption and the risks of fracture, obesity, cardiovascular disease, allergies and various cancers. Ultimately, they

Foods rich in calcium

DAILY GOAL = 1,200MG

569mg/90g
Sardines (47% RDA)

300mg/240ml
Cow's milk (25% RDA)

488mg/245g
Yoghurt or kefir (41% RDA)

202mg/30g
Cheese (17% RDA)

350mg/125g
Kale, cooked (29% RDA)

244mg/225g
Spinach, cooked (20% RDA)

81mg/100g
Okra (7% RDA)

74mg/70g
Bok choi (6% RDA)

73.9mg/30g
Almonds (6% RDA)

42.8mg/90g
Broccoli (4% RDA)

suggest that the moderate consumption of cow's milk can provide important nutrients and may have some health benefits, but that excessive consumption should be avoided to minimise the risk of negative health outcomes.

The most health-beneficial dietary sources of calcium are actually green leafy vegetables and legumes, or 'greens and beans'. They have several advantages over cow's milk dairy products, including that they are: antioxidant-rich; a source of complex carbohydrates, fibre and iron; very low in fat; and cholesterol-free.

To summarise

If you want to reduce your osteoporosis risk in order to remain independent, mobile and active in your later years, now is the time to optimise your diet and focus on healthy lifestyle choices. Make a conscious effort to increase your daily calcium intake from dietary sources and remember that vitamin D increases the uptake and absorption of calcium, so get your cardio outdoors in nature for the double win – weight-bearing exercise and vitamin D!

Brain health: The omega-3 non-negotiable

At this life stage, we really start to notice the decline of our cognitive functions: our memory, concentration and focus.

It can be quite scary as we struggle to remember people's names or our PINs. We might find ourselves losing our train of thought mid-conversation, or maybe we can't formulate the right words. What's happening? Can we really blame it all on our declining hormones?

Lifestyle factors also play a key role, and stress has been identified as a major player in our cognitive decline as we age. Modern life is very taxing on our brains. We are juggling the demands of work, running a household and possibly looking after elderly parents and/or grandchildren. We're constantly required to multitask, remember things, concentrate and communicate. We are submitted to a barrage of stimulation from multiple sources – from our phones and social media to radio and television.

Add to this mix the psychological symptoms of menopause (which are more prevalent than the physical ones), and it's no surprise we are experiencing chronic anxiety, stress and progressive cognitive decline. In some cases, it can even lead to depression.

So, how can we support our brain and keep it in top condition for healthy ageing? Simply put, we have to make our nutrition a priority. A healthy, balanced diet is essential for a nourished brain and nervous system.

Memory and concentration

The part of our brain that plays a major part in memory is the cerebral cortex. Its normal function is dependent on multiple factors, many of which are influenced by nutritional intake.

Neurotransmitters are the chemicals that help our nerve cells communicate. They are reliant on nutrients like choline, amino acids and B vitamins.

In addition, the neurotransmitter cell membrane (essentially the structure of the nerve cell itself) requires healthy fats – omega-3s and phospholipids – to effectively communicate with other neurotransmitters. This is what I refer to as your brain firing on all cylinders.

We know instantly when we are *not* firing on all cylinders – we might be unable to concentrate or struggling for words. Time to nourish our cell membranes with healthy fats!

Eat to feed your brain

Our brain requires two specific ingredients to function optimally. I call it the 'lock and key' recipe:

1. Amino acids (the lock)
2. Co-factor nutrients (the keys)

Amino acids are the building blocks of protein – organic compounds that our body uses to make proteins. 'Complete proteins' contain all nine essential amino acids: the ones we can't produce ourselves and *need* to get from our diet. Foods that contain complete proteins are typically high in protein – such as eggs, soy foods (tempeh, tofu), spirulina, poultry, dairy, fish and seeds (pumpkin and sesame).

I recommend trying to include more plant-based protein (for example, spirulina, organic soy, quinoa, seeds, beans and grains) than animal protein. Apart from the nutrients, you will get the added benefit of fibre (prebiotics) to feed your beneficial gut bacteria and help them to multiply (turn to p18 to learn more about this in my section on digestive health).

Co-factor nutrients are the keys that convert the amino acids into usable neurotransmitters. They are:

- All the B vitamins and folate (think green leafy veg)
- Vitamin C (yellow peppers, citrus, kiwi, strawberries, broccoli, sprouts, kale and salad greens)
- Zinc (green leafy veg, pumpkin and sesame seeds, almonds, tofu)
- Copper (soy, oysters, shitake mushrooms, sesame and sunflower seeds, Brazil nuts, cashews and hazelnuts)

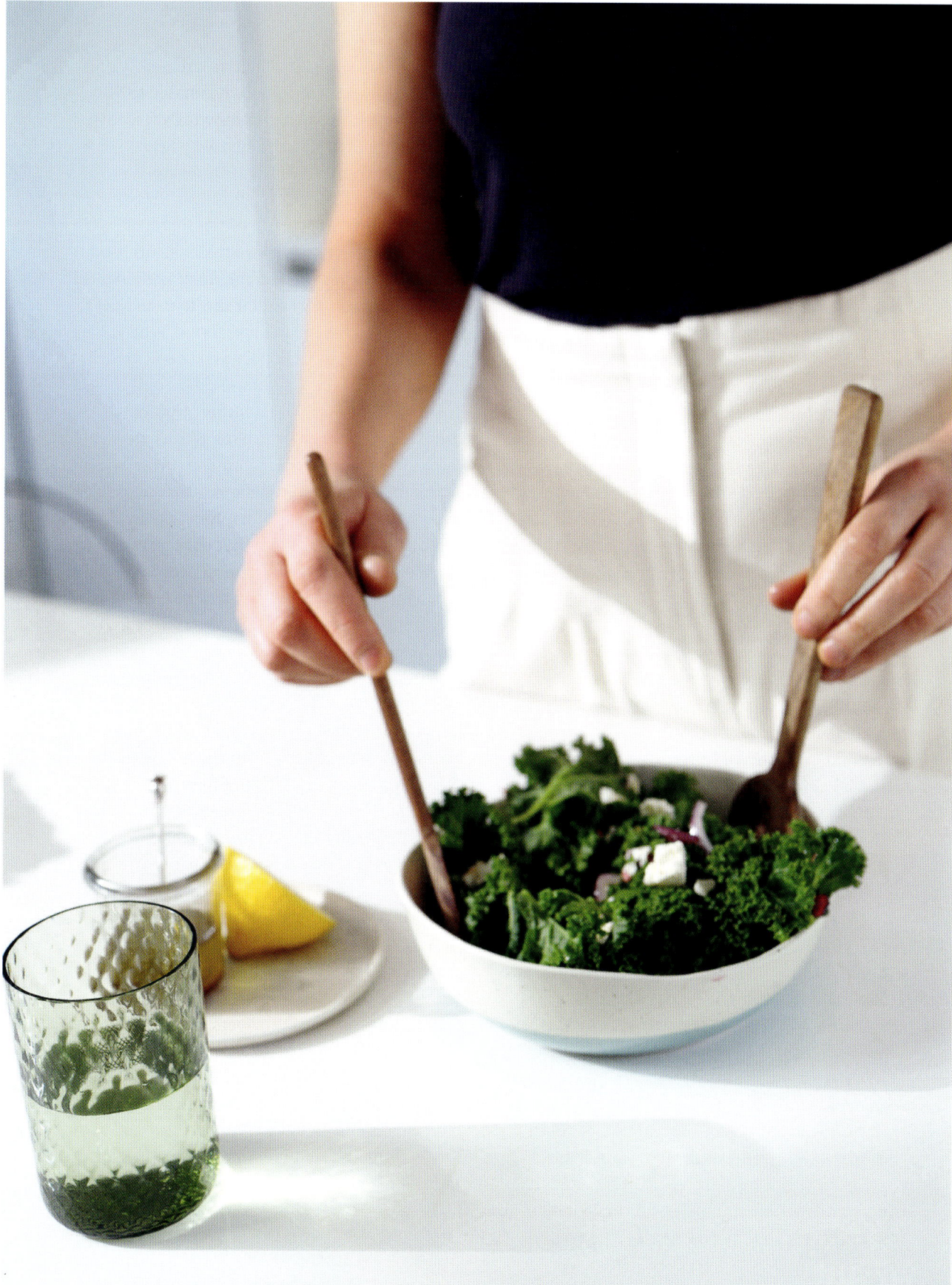

Neuroplasticity

A brand-new and exciting area of brain science, neuroplasticity looks at how our brain is constantly growing and changing – making new brain cells, as well as forming better neural connections – based on the food we eat.

The fact that we can make new brain cells is really exciting – who couldn't do with a few new brain cells, after all? All of these amazing possibilities revolve around a single molecule called BDNF (brain-derived neurotrophic factor). BDNF is a growth factor for your brain; it acts like a fertiliser, playing a big role in the prevention of neurodegenerative diseases like Alzheimer's and dementia.

BDNF naturally declines as we age; however, we know from research studies[6] that nutrition plays a key role in increasing levels of BDNF concentrations in humans – another reminder to eat healthily!

Poor memory is very unsettling, and it can spiral into chronic anxiety and depression. In my experience, cognitive function is the one area in which many of us want to see improvements, so here are my recommendations for optimising your diet with key nutrients for your brain to remain mentally sharp in your mid-life years.

Seven nutrients that are great for your brain

1 Healthy fats

Found in oily fish (salmon, mackerel, sardines, kippers, herring) and in plant-based sources such as chia seeds and flaxseeds, omega-3 fats can help you maintain healthy blood pressure, reduce inflammation and cholesterol, and support heart health. Getting plenty of them in your diet is critical for your overall health. Research[7] tells us that getting adequate omega-3 fats in your diet can also boost your BDNF levels.

We can't discuss healthy fats without mentioning extra virgin olive oil, the benefits of which are numerous. For starters, it is high in monounsaturated fatty acids (MUFAs), the most crucial molecules in determining your brain's ability to perform and think clearly. Our brain is mostly made of fat (nearly 60 per cent), and olive oil is considered a **brain food that improves focus and memory** and that may help fight age-related cognitive decline.

Olive oil also regulates our mood. One 2011 study found a link between the intake of monounsaturated (MUFA) and polyunsaturated (PUFA) fats and a reduced risk of depression. The findings also suggest that cardiovascular disease and depression may share some common nutritional determinants related to the types of fat we consume.

We also know that there is a direct link between trans-fat intake and depression – in other words, the higher the rate of trans-fat consumption (and the lower the rate of PUFA and MUFA intake), the greater your chances of battling mood disorders such as **depression**.

2 Antioxidants

Think in colour and eat the rainbow – every colour represents a phytonutrient that is important for our health. Plants contain phytonutrients that sing to our DNA; our bodies recognise them as optimum fuel and can instantly utilise them. These phytonutrients, contained in antioxidant-rich foods, are also beneficial for our gut bacteria and microbiome, which is important because it determines our brain health. Good antioxidant status, along with good blood circulation, is vital for optimal brain function.

Polyphenols are powerful antioxidants that are naturally found in plants. Superfoods like berries, olives, cocoa, peppermint and flaxseeds are all rich in polyphenols, which can raise our BDNF levels.

3 Curcumin (turmeric)

Curcumin is the active property contained in the spice turmeric. Animal studies indicate the neuroprotective effects of curcumin in activating and increasing BDNF in the brain, with antidepressant-like effects.

Turmeric is also one of nature's most potent anti-inflammatories. I recommend including it in your daily diet by adding it to smoothies, soups and hot drinks like my Organic Soy Golden Milk (see p95).

4 Magnesium

Magnesium is required mostly by the brain to aid mood and sleep. It also helps to reduce anxiety and brain fog, and it is integral for neurotransmitter function. Animal studies[8] have confirmed the antidepressant activity of magnesium and how it can significantly increase levels of BDNF.

Chronic stress depletes magnesium stores, as a result of poor gut health, and most symptoms of magnesium deficiency are very similar to menopause symptoms.

Magnesium-rich foods include seaweed, coriander, pumpkin seeds, flaxseeds, cacao and almond butter.

5 Prebiotics

Prebiotics are specific types of indigestible dietary fibre that feed and support the friendly bacteria in our gut. This can lead to changes in how the gut interacts with our brain – via our immune system, vagus nerve and neurotransmitters – which could lead to potential changes in how we think and feel.

If you haven't considered the connection between your gut and your brain before, think about when you feel nervous about an exam or a presentation: you may feel butterflies in your stomach or need to run to the loo. This is because. buried deep in our gut, is a very thin layer called the enteric system, which is made up of the same cells and neurons that make up our brain.

There are more than 100 million neurons in the gut. This 'second brain' communicates with our brain via the vagus nerve (the microbe superhighway), and it is responsible for what we call our 'gut instinct'.

It's no surprise, then, that maintaining a healthy gut can boost your mood, increase your brain activity, eliminate feelings of anxiety and help you sleep. More and more research is confirming how our gut microbiome has a profound impact on our nervous system.

Prebiotics include foods such as garlic, leeks, asparagus and artichokes.

6 Vitamin B12

There is some evidence that vitamin B12 might be an important co-factor nutrient involved in the production of BDNF[9]. Good sources of B12 include fish and shellfish, eggs and fortified foods such as cereals, plant milks and nutritional yeast; look out for some B12-rich recipes in the omega-3 section of this cookbook (p133).

Some people have a genetic (usually autoimmune-related) mutation and lack the protein called intrinsic factor, which is located in the gut and enables you to absorb vitamin B12. Without intrinsic factor, you will likely be B12-deficient, which might lead to chronic nervous-system issues.

7 Leafy greens

Leafy greens such as spinach and kale are rich in magnesium, which may help you to feel calmer. Simply increasing our consumption of green leafy vegetables could offer a simple and affordable way of potentially protecting our brain from Alzheimer's disease and dementia.

To summarise

Your brain is the control centre for your body, and its function is closely linked to the health and well-being of other bodily systems. To optimise brain function and promote overall health, it is essential to prioritise good nutrition and make healthy dietary choices. This involves focusing on nutrient-dense foods like those listed above, while limiting or avoiding processed and high-sugar foods that can have negative effects on your body and brain.

By nourishing your body with a healthy and balanced diet, you can support your brain's ability to adapt and change in response to different situations and experiences.

Digestive health and detoxification: The power of fibre

Gut health is a hot topic at the moment. There is so much emerging research in this field, it's as if scientists have discovered a brand-new organ in the body. In a way, they have. We are learning more and more about how gut bacteria can positively impact not just our digestive health, but our overall health and well-being.

Let's talk about our gut microbiome

The name comes from *micro* (meaning 'small') and *biome* (meaning 'a habitat of living things').

While not particularly glamorous (let's face it, the gut is a dark and fairly dank place), our gut microbiome plays a significant role in nearly every function of the human body, and its importance should not be underestimated. It's home to trillions of bacteria, yeasts, viruses and microbes, all co-existing, but also competing with each other for both space and food.

During our lifetime, we can shape our microbiome – mainly through our dietary choices, but also in the following ways:
- **Medications:** our use of prescription drugs and antibiotics
- **Environment:** the diversity of bacteria we're exposed to daily
- **Stress:** the level of physical, emotional or psychological strain in our lives
- **Exercise:** a sedentary lifestyle has a negative effect
- **Sleep:** poor sleep quality can compromise our gut health

Poor gut health can contribute to many diverse health conditions, including dementia, heart disease, cancer and autoimmune diseases such as arthritis.

What's the goal?

As women, our health, our fertility and our longevity are all heavily reliant on the balance of microbes living within our gut. The goal is to have a broad and diverse microbiome, with as many different strains of beneficial bacteria as possible. Ideally, the beneficial bacteria should account for around 85 per cent of the bacteria in our microbiome.

There will always be harmful microorganisms hanging around – yeasts, parasites and viruses – but as long as they are a minority, we're doing okay.

Dysbiosis is the medical term for an imbalance of gut bacteria. Think of it as the bad guys outnumbering the good guys, and contributing to a variety of health issues. They can even influence our eating behaviour – for example, by causing cravings for sugar and junk food.

What's the solution?

The one factor that you can control to improve your gut health is the amount of fibre in your daily diet.

Fibre is *the* key food that will feed your beneficial gut bacteria and keep the balance tipped in your favour.

To maintain health, our recommended daily fibre intake is 30–35g per day. It is estimated that the average person consumes only 15–19g per day – well short of the optimum amount.

Prebiotic fibre

Onions, chia seeds and flaxseeds are great fibre choices, but what makes them special is that they also contain prebiotic fibre, a type of plant fibre that our bodies *can't* digest.

Think of this special prebiotic plant fibre as a fertiliser that encourages the growth of gut-friendly bacteria, which in turn contributes to maintaining a robust immune system.

When you don't eat enough fibre, your gut-friendly bacteria are literally starved; their levels start to decline, which allows the harmful bacteria to flourish and dominate.

What's so extra about hemp seeds?

A study published in the *American Journal of Gastroenterology* found that hemp seeds are particularly beneficial for digestive health. The high amounts of both soluble and insoluble fibre in hemp seeds can aid elimination and relieve constipation and abdominal discomfort.

In addition, the prebiotic fibre in hemp seeds enables your gut-friendly bacteria to produce short-chain fatty acids (SCFAs), including butyrate. Butyrate has very powerful anti-inflammatory effects on the body, helping to reduce our risk of heart disease, reducing elevated cholesterol levels (triglycerides) and maintaining optimum digestive health.

Hemp seeds have many other nutritional benefits. They are high in protein and essential fats, and they are also a rich source of key minerals – for example, iron, calcium and magnesium, all of which are central to women's health and hormone balancing.

I like to get my hemp seeds from Linwoods Health Foods, which sells convenient pouches of flaxseeds, hemp seeds and chia seeds. Their Multiboost Organic Milled Hemp Seeds have a mild nutty flavour similar to walnuts and can be added to lots of recipes – from smoothies and overnight oats, to energy balls, breads and even curries!

To summarise

Increasing your prebiotic fibre intake is a simple, daily habit you can action. It's time for fibre to receive the spotlight it deserves. Look after your gut bugs with prebiotic fibre and they will look after you!

Heart health: The elephant in the room

One of the key changes that occurs during menopause, as a result of a woman's low levels of oestrogen, is the significant impact on heart health. Studies have shown that the risk of heart attacks increases fivefold after menopause, making heart disease the leading cause of death for postmenopausal women. This is due to a range of factors, including changes in lipid metabolism, increases in blood pressure and alterations in the structure and function of blood vessels.

The connection between sugar and heart disease

Most people think that eating too much fat and high-cholesterol foods (eggs, cheese, shellfish) will block their arteries and cause a heart attack. This is not completely accurate – it is, in fact, the *type* of fat that plays a more deadly role.

In 2015 a systematic review[10] of a randomised controlled trial was published in the British medical journal *Open Heart*. The review showed that, in 1970, dietary recommendations to reduce fat to less than a third of total energy intake had been introduced to 220 million Americans – and to 56 million citizens in the UK by 1983 – *without* any supporting evidence from randomised controlled trials. No evidence whatsoever!

This is probably why we've all heard the advice to eat low-fat, low-calorie meals, the implication being they can reduce the risk of heart disease. However, this is simply not true, because once the fat is removed from a product, it is usually replaced with something else – usually sugar.

We know from countless research studies that the root cause of elevated cholesterol levels and abdominal obesity is not fats but **sugar and refined white carbohydrates**.

If, in addition to white bread, white pasta and white rice (all foods that can convert quickly into sugar), you are also consuming cakes, biscuits and fizzy drinks, you will find yourself on a blood-sugar rollercoaster, where insulin is being released far too frequently. This increases your triglyceride levels, leading to stored fat in your bloodstream. Insulin is known as the fat-storing hormone, which results in plaque sticking to your artery walls and lowering HDL cholesterol (the good cholesterol).

Inflammation and what we can do about it

The root cause of nearly every chronic illness is inflammation. High sugar consumption can increase inflammation (as well as oxidative stress – how well your body deals with life's exhaust fumes), which damages the lining of the arteries, making it easier for the plaque to stick.

You can determine your risk and pre-empt a serious event by measuring inflammation and having your CRP (c-reactive protein) levels checked in a routine blood test with your GP.

Homocysteine is another useful blood biomarker, as it is a predictor of clots and thickening of the artery walls (atherosclerosis). Homocysteine is an amino acid that we produce ourselves. It is designed to be detoxified and excreted, but if our detoxification processes are functioning sub-optimally, it can build up and increase inflammation. (Homocysteine levels are not checked as part of routine GP blood tests but require additional functional testing.) B vitamins, in particular, control the detoxification process and can prevent this build-up, which is why optimising our intake of all our B vitamins is recommended.

Blue zones: the world's five longevity hot spots

Blue zones are geographical regions that are packed with centenarians, or humans who live beyond the age of 100, with very low rates of Alzheimer's and heart disease. A decade of research into these areas attributes this longevity to a plant-based diet, lifestyle and community-driven culture.

There are five longevity hot spots around the world:
- Loma Linda, California
- Nicoya, Costa Rica
- Sardinia, Italy
- Ikaria, Greece
- Okinawa, Japan

The good health and low rate of chronic health issues, such as cardiovascular disease and dementia, is a testament to the plant-rich diet of the inhabitants of the blue zones. In addition, they are all community-driven cultures, which play a significant role in the inhabitants' good health and longevity, as researched by Professor George Slavich at the University of California, Los Angeles.

Professor Slavich points to evidence that shows that the quality and quantity of an individual's social relationships are a stronger predictor of chronic disease-related mortality than physical inactivity, alcohol use and smoking. Compared to people who are socially connected, those living in isolation are more likely to suffer from viral infections and inflammation.

The western diet and cholesterol

The typical western diet has a lot to answer for: obesity, diabetes, cardiovascular disease … We consume too much saturated fat, too many sugar-sweetened fizzy drinks, too much salt, too many animal-sourced foods, too much wheat – and simply not enough fruit and vegetables.

Non-hereditary high cholesterol (hypercholesterolaemia) is related to both a poor diet and lifestyle factors such as inactivity, smoking and stress. Upon diagnosis of elevated cholesterol, your GP will usually recommend three months of improved diet and lifestyle interventions, followed by a re-test of serum cholesterol levels. If, after three months, there has been no improvement, your doctor will most likely discuss treatment options with you, including the drug treatment statin therapy.

While statin therapy can be a beneficial treatment, most patients are unaware of the associated side effects. Typically, patients can experience intense muscle aches and pains, as well as fatigue. Many complain of zero energy, which further inhibits their ability to exercise.

If you have been diagnosed with non-hereditary hypercholesterolaemia, you should consider the drug-free approach to lowering your cholesterol, using diet and lifestyle interventions. That's not to say that diagnosed familial hypercholesterolaemia will not respond in kind to the same diet and lifestyle interventions, it's just a bit more difficult.

So, what can you do?

For every 1 per cent drop in cholesterol levels, there is a 2 per cent decrease in the risk of developing heart disease. So, let's look at a few evidence-based nutritional strategies to lower your cholesterol.

Cholesterol-lowering foods

Green leafy veg
Spinach, kale, Brussels sprouts

Avocado

Chia and flaxseeds
Ground or whole

Nuts
Almonds

Salmon
Fresh, organic if possible

Olive oil
Extra virgin, cold pressed

Gluten-free wholegrains
Oats, quinoa, brown rice

Beans and legumes
Lentils, chickpeas

Sweet potato
Mashed, roasted, steamed

Garlic
Added raw to food

Turmeric
Ground, dried, fresh root

Green tea
Matcha green tea

→ Aim to emulate a blue-zone diet. One of the most important features of the diets of blue-zone inhabitants is the combination of olive oil (a source of monounsaturated fats and antioxidants) and the intake of omega-3 fatty acids from oily fish (salmon, mackerel, sardines, kippers, herrings), as well as plant-based omega-3 sources (flaxseed and chia seeds).

→ Eat less saturated fat by reducing the consumption of animal products (processed meat, red meat and dairy products).

→ Increase consumption of fibre-rich plant foods, which help to control blood sugar – reducing cortisol release and enabling cholesterol to bind to the fibre and be effectively eliminated. To help lower cholesterol, aim for 30–35g of fibre-rich foods per day[II].

→ Foods such as oats and barley contain a type of fibre known as beta-glucan, which helps to reduce cholesterol. Daily consumption of a minimum of 3g of soluble oat fibre typically lowers cholesterol by 8–23 per cent.

→ Garlic can lower cholesterol levels and have positive effects on blood flow. Fresh, raw garlic is best for this, and can be grated or minced and added into soups, stews and casseroles *after* cooking to increase efficacy and therapeutic outcomes.

→ Increase heart-healthy monounsaturated fats – that is, olive oil, nuts and seeds.

→ Follow a low-glycemic diet – replace processed foods and refined white carbohydrates/sugars with whole foods.

→ Maintain ideal body weight with daily exercise.

The low-GL diet

GL (or glycaemic load) is the unit of measurement of both the quantity and quality of carbohydrates contained in certain foods, as well as the effect these foods have on our blood sugar. The goal is to maintain blood-sugar balance, and a low-GL diet enables this.

The low-GL diet is a hybrid of the Mediterranean diet and a low-carb diet, with an emphasis on plant-based sources of protein. This makes it naturally high in fibre, which reduces our risk for developing chronic health conditions such as heart disease, type 2 diabetes and Alzheimer's disease. By focusing on more plant-based protein, you are also mitigating the cancer risks associated with a high-meat and high-dairy diet, as well as reducing any stress on the kidneys and loss of bone mass.

The low-GL diet is the ideal way to support your heart health. You can read more about it in the last section of part two (p35).

To summarise

Blood-sugar peaks and troughs trigger the release of adrenal hormones (adrenaline, dopamine and cortisol) . This, in turn, increases inflammation, which can lead to heart disease. Keeping your blood sugars balanced is the best way to tackle this; it also helps you to lose weight and feel less stressed and gives you more energy. Those interested in trying the drug-free approach to lowering cholesterol should start including 50g of tofu and 25g of oats in their daily diet. The combination of protein- and fibre-rich foods that are also low in saturated fats is extremely effective in the fight against heart disease.

The truth about sugar

When we think of sugar, we think of the white granulated kind that you would find in the sugar bowl – but that is just one type of sugar (also known as sucrose). Sugar can be defined as any kind of soluble, sweet-tasting carbohydrate. It comes in many different forms: liquid (which is just sugar granules dissolved in water), syrup (syrups and treacles), sugar alcohols (xylitol, sorbitol) and artificial sweeteners.

Sugar labelling on food products can be confusing, evasive and even misleading, partly because sugar goes by many different names, several of which – such as dextran or molasses – don't sound anything like 'sugar'. As a rule of thumb, anything that ends with the letters 'ose' is sugar – for example, fructose, lactose, sucrose, glucose and maltose. Often, several of these are contained as hidden sugars in food products that are then marketed as health-promoting foods.

How to read a food label

The ingredients of a product are listed in the nutritional information in descending order by weight. If sugar is listed in the top five ingredients, that means that a good chunk of that food is made up of sugar – even if the final product doesn't taste sweet.

Food labelling is not straightforward, and many manufacturers misleadingly list the nutritional information in a way that doesn't reflect the amount we are actually consuming. I am referring to their 'serving size'. A good example of this is breakfast cereal; the recommended serving size is usually 30g. If you have never seen 30g of cereal in a bowl, weigh it out next time and see for yourself: it's a teeny-tiny amount! The average person eats four or five times as much. The nutritional information for 30g of cereal (which has a fairly low number of calories and a low amount of sugar) can therefore lead to a false perception of how much sugar we are really consuming.

Hidden sugars

During food processing, sugar is added to enhance flavour, texture, shelf life and other properties. Manufacturers are aware of sugar's addictive properties, which is why they use it.

So much of our supermarket food contains added sugar. Some of the worst offenders are the aforementioned breakfast cereals, yoghurt and bread, but sugar also lurks in places where we least expect it, such as in savoury foods like pasta sauces, mayonnaise and crisps.

Food and drink items that typically contain hidden sugars include:

→ **Cereal**, including hot cereals like flavoured quick oats (which are marketed as a healthy breakfast option).
→ **Packaged bread**, including sliced pans, par-baked bagels and baguettes. Brown bread (malted wheat and barley) often contains added sugar, too.
→ **Snacks** such as free-from (gluten-free) foods, vegan snacks and granola bars (also marketed as healthy options).
→ **Drinks** like flavoured coffees, energy drinks, blended juices and certain flavoured teas (such as the TikTok sensation bubble tea).
→ **Protein bars**, the majority of which are just confectionery with added protein.
→ **Sweetened yoghurts** and yoghurt drinks (including low-fat and fat-free yoghurt), and even cholesterol-lowering dairy drinks.
→ **Bottled sauces** such as dressings, condiments and marinades (tomato sauce, ketchup, mayonnaise, relish, chilli sauce, etc.).
→ **Restaurant food**, as sugar is used liberally in their sauces and dressings for extra flavour.

Highly processed sugars to be aware of

Highly processed sugars, also known as 'hyper-manipulated' sugars, have become increasingly common in modern diets. These types of sugars are refined and processed to a high degree, often resulting in a substance that is significantly different from natural sugar. The high level of processing can lead to a range of negative health effects, including weight gain, inflammation and increased risk of chronic diseases such as diabetes and heart disease. In fact, research suggests that highly processed sugars may be even worse for our health than natural sugar. This is due to factors like the high glycaemic index – which can cause a rapid spike in blood sugar levels – and the lack of nutrients and fibre that are present in natural sugar sources.

Maltodextrin
Derived from grains as starch and used in foods as a thickener, maltodextrin is rapidly absorbed into our bloodstream. Research studies[12] show correlations between the consumption of processed foods containing maltodextrin and the increasing prevalence of inflammatory bowel disease in the general population.

High-fructose corn syrup (HFCS)
Corn starch refined into corn syrup, HFCS, is 30 per cent less expensive than regular sugar, and many food manufacturers have begun using it as a cheaper alternative. It is made up of glucose and fructose (it can contain up to 90 per cent fructose), and it is rapidly absorbed into our bloodstream. There are serious health concerns with HFCS – namely, insulin

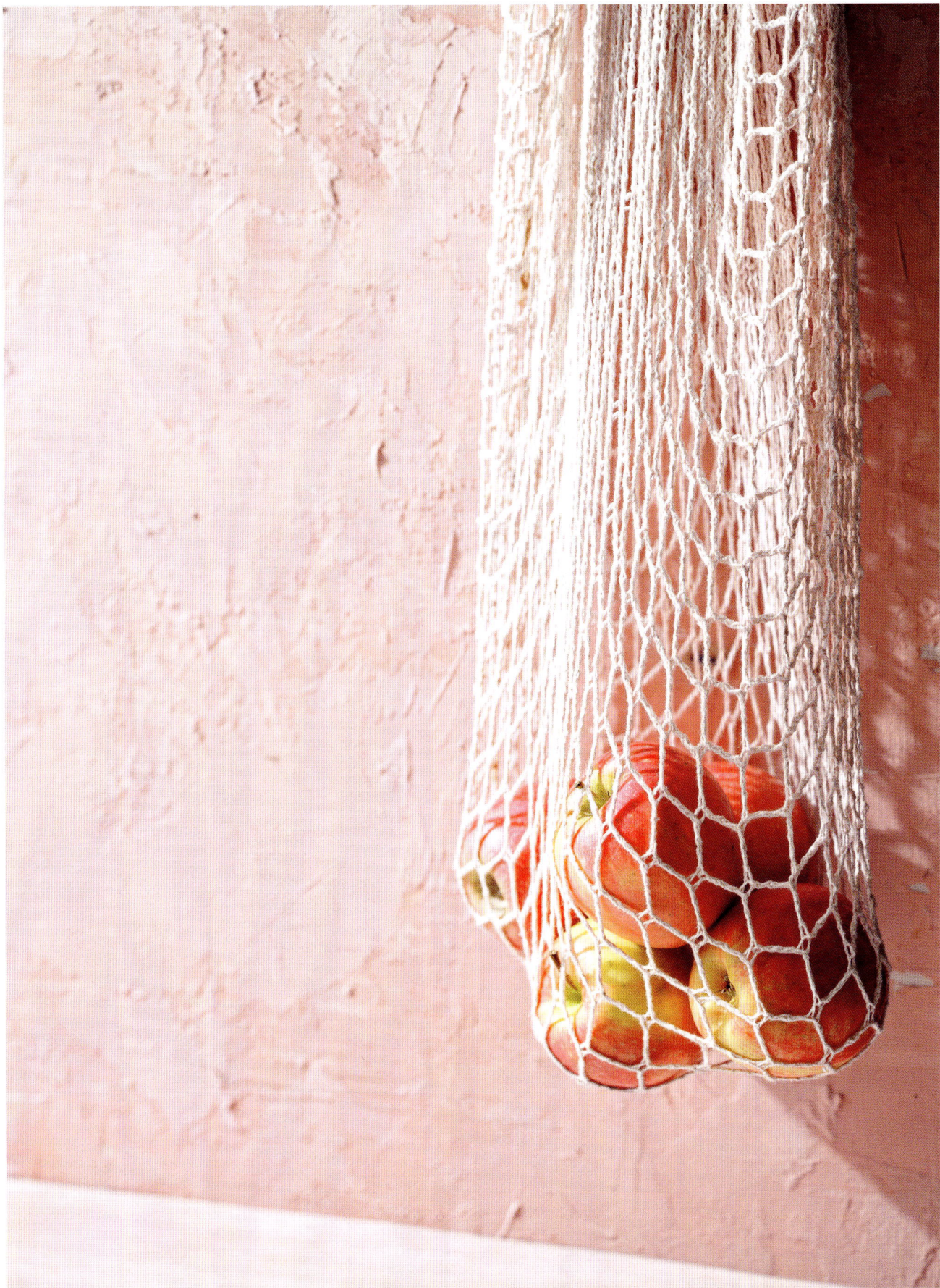

resistance and type 2 diabetes[13], non-alcoholic fatty liver disease (mostly in kids), metabolic syndrome and obesity. Avoid this stuff at all costs!

Artificial sweeteners

Many women use artificial sweeteners as substitutes for sugar to help them control their weight. However, artificial sweeteners can actually have the opposite effect. They contain zero calories, which can cause weight gain by increasing our appetite. To explain: our body is expecting calories in combination with a sweet taste. An absence of calories can often trigger food cravings, sending us off to get calories elsewhere and leading to weight gain.

Stevia

Derived from the leaves of the stevia plant, stevia is 200–300 times sweeter than sugar. It is considered a good choice for weight loss because it contains no calories. However, as with artificial sweeteners, this confuses our body, increasing our appetite and potentially leading to weight gain.

Xylitol

Xylitol is found naturally in the fibres of many plants, including birch trees. It looks like table sugar, but it is actually sugar alcohol. Low in calories and tooth-kind, xylitol is largely considered to be a good natural sugar alternative, with many diabetics using it, because it doesn't require insulin to be metabolised. However, it can cause bloating and diarrhoea, and it is not suitable for anyone with digestive issues (for example, IBS). It is also important to know that xylitol has been highly processed and there is limited research available for its safety.

How much sugar?

The WHO recommends a maximum of 6 teaspoons (approximately 12g) of sugar per day. This is their upper-limit recommendation, *not* the recommended daily amount (RDA).

Ideally, we don't want to be anywhere close to consuming this amount of sugar daily – and yet the average person consumes three times that amount. To put this into perspective, a single fizzy drink, or one of those so-called sports drinks, would put you over the limit. These contain some of the highest amounts of sugar in a single bottle.

The fact is, sugar adds zero nutritional value, and it causes measurable harm to our body over time. Health conditions such as hypertension, diabetes, obesity, non-alcoholic fatty liver disease, cardiovascular disease, dementia and premature ageing are all associated with excess sugar consumption.

How sugar affects the brain

Sugar is a high glycaemic food. High glycaemic foods cause a higher elevation in blood glucose, which produces a greater addictive drive.

Sugar lights up the brain, activating the regions of the brain associated with feelings of pleasure, happiness and reward response. It also gives us a dopamine hit – known as a 'sugar high'. This can cause us to consume increasing amounts of it to get that same high. Over time, this cultivates a progressively worsening addiction to sugar and other low-nutrient foods containing high amounts of sugar.

The bottom line: sugar is cheap and highly addictive

Food manufacturers know just how addictive sugar is. Many employ food scientists to hyper-manipulate the addictive properties of sugar to make it even *more* irresistible. If you have ever wondered why you can't stop after eating just one biscuit, and end up eating the whole lot, this is why. It's not your fault; you aren't weak-willed. It boils down to profit: the more sugar we eat, the more sugar we want, and the more sugar we buy.

Seasonal supermarket bulk buys don't help, either. Before Christmas or Halloween, you will often see large tins of biscuits, sweets and chocolates piled to head height in the shop aisles. The impossibly low price (usually just a couple of euros) encourages us to buy in multiples, further strengthening our addiction to highly processed, addictive, harmful sugars.

Weaning yourself off sugar

Follow the steps below to wean yourself off sugar. It will take a little time, and at first you may experience headaches similar to caffeine-withdrawal headaches. You may also feel very tired for a few days. This is to be expected, as your body is detoxifying and adjusting.

1. Get rid of all the savoury foods that contain added sugar (mayonnaise, ketchup, sauces, etc.) from your cupboard.
2. Think about how often you are having sweet foods and foods with added or hidden sugar – fruit yoghurt, healthy-seeming cereal bars, biscuits … Either reduce these in your diet or remove them entirely. Reducing sugar can prolong the process, and you might find that it's better to just rip the plaster off and deal with the withdrawals in the short term.
3. Stop adding sugar to your hot drinks and other foods. Start by reducing it over several days or even weeks. It may take some time to adjust to coffee or tea without sugar but stick with it; it will happen.
4. Cut down on coffee and tea if you associate them with biscuits or cake. Instead, opt for non-caffeinated herbal teas that have a mild sweetness to them, such as those containing fennel and cinnamon.
5. Try taking certain supplements (for example, chromium and cinnamon), which can help to curb sugar cravings. Other effective craving-killers include liquorice or peppermint tea, or a large glass of water with a little salt or a tablespoon of apple cider vinegar.
6. Brush your teeth. If you find yourself in the habit of eating something sweet after dinner, simply brushing your teeth can really help!

After five completely sugar-free days, you should notice a difference in your overall sense of well-being. You will no longer crave sugar as much – or maybe not at all. You will feel more energised and clear-headed, and therefore be able to make better dietary choices going forward. Sugar clouds your judgement, keeping you in a constant cycle of craving it and consuming it.

If you still find yourself bothered by sugar cravings, try to give these a 20-minute cooling-off window. Remind yourself that you have experienced this before, and it will pass. Often by the time the 20 minutes are up, the craving will have disappeared. You can also try exercise – even a short walk or a few trips up and down the stairs can have a beneficial effect. If you still want sugary food, however, save it until after you've eaten your lunch or dinner, so that the inevitable glucose uptake will have a lesser impact.

Changing tastebuds

Once you wean yourself off sugar, you'll start to notice the naturally occurring sweet taste of some whole foods (carrots, apples and beetroot, for example) or of spices like cinnamon and vanilla. Carrots, raisins, dates, figs and bananas are all great natural sugar alternatives; apart from being naturally sweet, they also contain beneficial fibre, which improves their nutritional density. You may want to use eating apples instead of cooking apples in recipes – you'll still get all the flavour (including the sweet taste) without the added sugar.

Better alternatives (though they're still sugar!)

There are also lots of sugar alternatives on the market. My advice is to use these sparingly, however, because even though they haven't been hyper-manipulated, they are still sugar and will cause a glucose spike. This glucose peak will trigger insulin into action, to get glucose out of our bloodstream and into our cells. The more often insulin is triggered, the more health issues this can potentially cause.

These sugar alternatives are available in good health-food shops:

Real organic maple syrup

Organic maple syrup contains 34 beneficial compounds that have antioxidant and anti-inflammatory benefits. It contains 15 times more calcium than honey, it is high in zinc and manganese and it is suitable for IBS sufferers, since it doesn't cause gastric symptoms.

Beware of fake maple syrup that may not contain any real maple syrup at all, but instead is made with golden syrup, maple flavouring, colouring and other highly processed ingredients.

Organic coconut sugar

This is rich in B vitamins and contains 17 amino acids, polyphenols and antioxidants. It also contains inulin, a type of beneficial fibre that feeds our gut bacteria.

Chicory root syrup

Relatively new to the market, chicory root syrup is one of the best available sugar alternatives because it scores low on the glycaemic index (so won't spike your blood sugars) and contains prebiotic fibre that feeds our beneficial gut bacteria to help them thrive. It looks and tastes like honey and is often marketed as a honey alternative. It's ideal for drizzling on porridge or using in things like salad dressings. I like to get mine from Homespun, an independent Irish company (see p280).

Fruit is not the enemy

Fruit is full of powerful antioxidants that offer multiple health benefits.

Some fruit – such as berries (blueberries, blackberries and raspberries, for example) – score lower than others on the glycaemic index. This means that they are among some of the best low-sugar fruit options you can choose from, along with apples and pears.

All fruit, when eaten whole, contains fibre, which slows the uptake of glucose into the bloodstream. This naturally controls your glucose curve. However, when you drink fruit juice such as orange juice, where the fibre has been removed, the opposite happens: a massive glucose spike occurs, triggering insulin release, which over time can do more harm than good.

My advice? Eat the whole orange and ditch the fruit juice.

To summarise

Reducing sugar intake has many overall health benefits, and using sugar alternatives – in moderation – can provide a lower-calorie and lower-glycaemic option to help us maintain a healthy weight. Breaking our dependence on sugary foods promotes healthier habits in the long run, enabling us to become less dependent on sweet-tasting flavours permeating all that we eat.

As we reduce our sugar intake over time, our tastebuds can adapt and become more sensitive to sweetness again. This means that we may start to notice and enjoy the natural sweetness in foods that we previously thought were bland or unappetising. It will likely be a gradual process, but, over time, our taste preferences can shift towards a more balanced and varied diet that emphasises whole, nutrient-dense foods.

The meno-middle: Why am I gaining weight?

Weight gain at this life stage can be very frustrating. Despite everything you may be doing, you just can't seem to shift those extra pounds – which all seem to have collected around your middle. What's going on? The meno-middle, as it is sometimes referred to, is unfortunately not only a source of frustration but an additional health risk that requires your attention.

Women with a concentration of fat around the middle (or central adiposity, to give its medical term) are at an increased risk of breast cancer, despite their oestrogen being in decline. This is because an enzyme known as aromatase – produced predominantly in fat cells – changes androgens (which are typically thought of as male hormones, but women produce them too) into oestrogen, causing a condition known as oestrogen dominance. This increases our risk of hormone-dependent cancers such as breast cancer. Meno-middle also increases inflammation, predisposing women to insulin resistance and Alzheimer's disease.

The good news is that you *can* lose fat around your middle – and reduce every known risk factor for breast cancer, cardiovascular disease, type 2 diabetes and dementia – without starving yourself or eating bland food. Let's look at how.

Okay, here's what's happening ...

In short, your metabolism has slowed down. This is largely triggered by the imbalance of hormones, but other factors may also be at play:

1   You are not building muscle
To rev up your metabolism and get it back up to speed, you need to build muscle. Cardio-based workouts are all very well, but you also need to include strength training with weights or body-weight exercises like yoga or Pilates.

2   You are not getting enough sleep
Sleep is crucial to your metabolic function. It affects your hunger hormones, stress hormones, mood and energy. Have you ever had a poor night's sleep and found yourself ravenous the next day? This is because your hunger and satiety hormones (leptin and ghrelin) are negatively affected by poor sleep.

3   You're stressed
Stress negatively affects your hormones, which slows your metabolism. In other words, stress can cause you to store fat! I'll return to this in a moment, because this can be a key factor for middle-aged women. Busy lives and new stressors – such as juggling childcare or ageing parents – often leave women feeling as though they have little time for themselves and can understandably lead to weight gain. Try to incorporate more stress-busting and self-care into your day to offset this.

4   You're undereating
Going too long without food or skipping meals trains your metabolism to slow down to preserve energy, resulting in a sluggish metabolism that doesn't burn food as fuel but instead stores it as fat.

5   An imbalance of macronutrients
Too many carbs, poor-quality fats, not enough quality protein ... I see this frequently in clinic. In your fight against the meno-middle, it is vital to get the correct macronutrient ratios.

6   Insulin resistance
If you store a higher proportion of fat around your middle, there is a good chance you are insulin resistant. If your cells have been bombarded with insulin for an extended period, its release no longer triggers the same affect and starts to fail to do its job (that is, to move glucose into cells). Glucose levels then remain high, causing high insulin levels that tell your body to store fat. Caffeine, high-GL foods, stress and sugar all mean that you will likely lose blood-sugar control, causing you to feel exhausted and steadily gain weight. Insulin resistance is the root cause of many chronic health issues. The solution? Treat the cause, not the symptoms, and reduce your risk.

Hormone hacks to make your body a pro fat burner

So, what can you do? Weight loss is 80 per cent diet and 20 per cent exercise, but the emphasis is often placed the other way around. You'll likely need to make some lifestyle changes, especially in terms of optimising your diet – not just for weight loss, but to future-proof your health.

1   Eat whole foods
Our hormones require the key nutrients found in whole foods to stabilise and thrive. Conversely, processed foods cause hormonal havoc, bringing fat loss to a halt. Opt for fibre-rich foods like cruciferous veg (such as cauliflower and broccoli), healthy fats that are crucial for the production of our hormones (think olive oil, nuts and seeds and avocados)

and complex carbs (such as quinoa, oats and sweet potatoes), which regulate our hunger hormones and our stress hormone, cortisol. Lean protein – organic chicken or soy, fish, eggs and tofu – can help to build and repair muscle.

2 **Reduce stress**
As I've already said, a stressed body is the perfect environment for fat storage and messed-up hormones. Stress raises cortisol, which causes us to store fat, especially around our waist. High cortisol also causes fatigue, depression and cravings, and it suppresses our immune system, making us more susceptible to frequent infections and illness. If you want to lose fat, you need to address your stress levels and incorporate stress-busting techniques into your daily routine.

3 **Intermittent fasting**
This is a big topic, but here are some of the basics. Intermittent fasting (IF) is not a diet: it is a timed eating schedule with a range of health benefits. The main benefit of IF is its ability to reduce inflammation in the body. Fasting for 12 hours overnight (for example, 7pm–7am) gives your digestion a break, which enables your body to rest and repair at a cellular level. I liken this to internal housekeeping. IF can also help with weight loss; when you fast, your insulin levels go down and fat cells release stored glucose, to be used by the body instead of being converted to fat.

Other health benefits include an improved hormone profile; the maintenance of skeletal muscle mass; decreased blood-glucose levels; and increased insulin sensitivity, lipolysis (breakdown of fats) and fat oxidation, and improved growth-hormone levels.

Getting started with IF

For those who are keen to try intermittent fasting, I recommend getting started with the 12:12 schedule – meaning that you have a 12-hour eating window followed by a 12-hour fasting window. Eventually you might be able to stretch the fasting window to 14 hours.

There are other methods of fasting – for example, the 5:2 diet, which encourages you to reduce your calories to approximately 600kcal two days per week and eat normally the other five days. In my opinion, this method encourages an unhealthy relationship with food: restriction, bingeing and purging. Going long periods without food and skipping meals forces your metabolism to slow down to conserve energy. In addition, 600kcal is an extremely low number of calories and not enough to maintain your metabolism or blood-sugar balance. The 5:2 method is more punishment than nourishment, and it will make it even more difficult to lose weight, especially if you are also stressed and consuming several cups of coffee to keep going.

Instead, try fasting for 12–14 hours overnight. The rest, repair and rejuvenation that your body carries out in a fasted state when asleep is far more beneficial to you at this life stage than skipping meals and starving yourself during the day.

Stress and fat around the middle

Our bodies deal with stress – whether that's the age-old stress of having to flee danger or modern-day equivalents such as money worries, relationship woes and work deadlines – by raising the stress hormone cortisol, along with adrenaline and blood sugars. Signs of excess cortisol include feeling both 'tired and wired', poor sleep or insomnia, sugar cravings and excess body fat.

During times of stress, we are hard-wired to crave sugar and other stimulants. This is because, in anticipation of an increased energy requirement to flee the danger (the so-called 'fight or flight' response), the body feels that it needs to increase levels of fat (lipids) and sugar (glucose) in the bloodstream.

However, more often than not, we're not in danger – we're just sitting at a desk, or sitting in traffic, feeling stressed. Unless there is a surge of physical activity, all that extra energy generated to flee the danger will be re-deposited as fat around the middle.

Fat targets our mid-section to be close to the liver, where it can quickly be converted back into energy if needed (to flee that danger). The more stress, the more fat is deposited!

A stressed body is a perfect environment for fat storage. As women, we are often professional plate spinners and many of us suffer from chronic ongoing stress without any natural release. Work, family, kids, housekeeping … Many of us are always multitasking and doing things for others. Unless you have reserves, you will inevitably drop and smash some of those plates, so put yourself and your well-being on your to-do list!

Open a well-being account for yourself. Think of it as a bank account with no overdraft facility and no credit card. Make regular deposits in the form of rest, relaxation, meditation, exercise, sleep and a healthy diet. Withdrawals will happen from time to time – late nights, poor diet, no exercise or too much stress – but if you keep making regular daily deposits, you will have the reserves to deal with the withdrawals.

It's called balance!

To summarise

When we are chronically stressed – that is, *all the time* – our body thinks we are under attack, so it keeps making more cortisol to cope with our (non-existent) life-or-death situation.

The net result of chronic stress is that our body is permanently in survival mode and will therefore forfeit all other 'unnecessary' functions to stay alive. Weight loss is considered an unnecessary function. The last thing our body will do in response to stress is relinquish any excess stored fat, because it thinks it may need it.

Designing a healthy diet and how to use this book

I don't mention calories in any of the recipes in this book. Although they have a role to play, calories are not the priority – nourishment is. This book is laid out to emphasise the eight different categories you need to optimise now in order to future-proof your health and feel good.

When you start to eat this way, two things will happen:

1. You will feel satisfied and experience fewer cravings. You will also eat less and less of the high-sugar, calorie-dense foods you used to rely on for energy. In effect, the calories will take care of themselves.
2. You will have more energy and naturally feel inclined to be more active, which will help to keep you at a healthy weight.

The optimal-health food pyramid

I wanted to give you a visual of what constitutes a healthy menopause diet to help you get the correct ratios and optimise your daily intake of these foods.

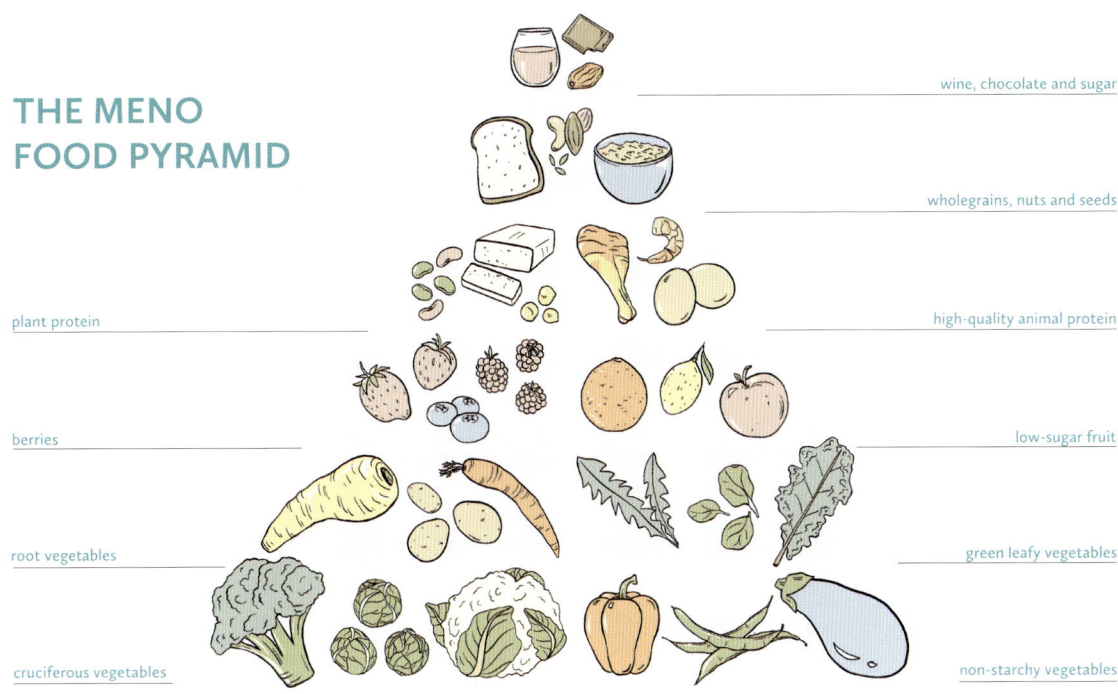

PART TWO: FUTURE-PROOFING YOUR HEALTH

This 'meno' food pyramid represents the low-glycaemic (low GL) way of eating, which is a slightly modified version of the Mediterranean diet, one of the most health-promoting diets ever studied. As you can see from the pyramid, a meno diet is predominantly plant-based; that's because plants deliver a multitude of health benefits that support so many of our bodily systems.

Let's talk through the levels.

1–4 Cruciferous, non-starchy, green leafy and root vegetables

At the bottom of the pyramid, and recommended in large quantities, are cruciferous vegetables (brassicas), non-starchy vegetables (Mediterranean vegetables), green leafy vegetables and root vegetables. Including a diverse and varied selection of all of these is how you will reap the most health benefits.

5–6 Berries and low-sugar fruit

In the middle are low-sugar fruits (apples and pears, for example) and a wide selection of brightly coloured, antioxidant-rich berries.

7–8 Plant protein and quality animal protein

Next up are quality animal proteins (organic, if possible) and plant-based proteins such as beans, lentils and tofu. This hybrid of plant and animal sources works well – for example, a variety of oily fish (salmon or mackerel) and quality sources of organic chicken, eggs and shellfish, in combination with plant proteins.

9 Wholegrains, nuts and seeds

Wholegrains – that is, brown rice and pasta, rye bread, porridge oats, nuts and seeds – are considered a staple of our diet and can be increased in quantity according to our activity levels. The more active we are, the more complex carbohydrates like these we can include. Nuts and seeds are a great source of fibre, protein and healthy fats, and they should be included across most meals.

10 Wine, chocolate and sugar

At the very top of the pyramid are wine, chocolate and other foods containing lots of sugar, such as dried fruit and honey. These are intended to be enjoyed occasionally (not every day) and in small amounts.

Your 16 nutrients for tracking

My goal with this book was to provide you with delicious-tasting food that also contains all the key nutrients you need to optimise now, **in their effective doses**.

The recipes have been analysed using professional Nutritics software, and each recipe displays the key nutrients in my Meno 8 categories, plus eight more. These 16 nutrients are displayed as a bar chart at the bottom of each recipe, providing at-a-glance information, so you can be aware of your gram or microgram intake and your percentage of the recommended daily amount (RDA).

The RDA of each nutrient is covered in each of the Meno 8 chapters, so you know what to aim for. The nutritional information has been calculated per portion or recommended serving size, so that you can easily keep track of your nutrient intake. Using fibre as an example: the optimal daily intake is approximately 30–35g. You'll no longer need to wonder if you are achieving this goal, since you will be able to quickly see the fibre content of every recipe you make.

16 Key Nutrients

Fibre	Magnesium	Vitamin A	Vitamin B3
Omega-3	Iron	Vitamin C	Vitamin B6
Protein	Zinc	Vitamin D	Vitamin B9
Calcium	Potassium	Vitamin E	Vitamin B12

Multi-use recipes

Several of the recipes in this book can be used in multiple ways. This was an important factor for a recipe to make the cut. It can be time-consuming to cook everything from scratch with multiple ingredients, so I wanted to make it worth your while, resulting in several uses for your hard work.

You will notice that many of the condiments, sauces and dressings can be shared and used in multiple recipes, which are listed with a cross-reference. Lots of the recipes also freeze well, so that you can batch-cook, further simplifying the process of prioritising your nutrition.

The low-GL diet

Eating low GL is not a restrictive diet, but rather a way of eating for life that is easy, delicious and sustainable. It will stop you from feeling tired and hungry and craving sweet foods. Simply put, it's about keeping your blood sugars balanced.

Foods have a GL value, which measures the effect they have on our blood-sugar levels. Starchy carbohydrates (that is, bread, rice, pasta and potatoes) are all high-GL foods that raise our blood sugar and cholesterol levels. High-glycaemic foods also cause more of the fat-storing hormone, insulin, to be released, as well as boosting the production of the stress hormone, cortisol. All the extra glucose in our bloodstream gets stored as fat, increasing our triglycerides (blood fats). Over time, we become sensitive to insulin, so we keep making more, pushing our cholesterol levels even higher!

The low-GL approach for weight loss

If you are reading this and have been trying to lose weight the conventional way – low fat, low calories – at this point you are likely an expert in what *doesn't* work. Many weight-loss diets are extremely restrictive, causing us to rely on willpower, which (we all know …) doesn't last.

The low-GL approach is very straightforward: for weight loss, you need to eat a maximum of 40–45 GLs per day (10 GLs for main meals and 5 GLs for snacks), spread evenly throughout the day and always with protein. If you are taller or exercise a lot, you can increase this by approximately 20 per cent.

When you eat 45 GLs of carbohydrates, you will have automatically eaten both a smaller quantity and a better quality of carbs, as far as your blood sugar is concerned. Once you reach your target weight, you can continue eating this way indefinitely and simply increase your good carbs for maintenance.

Why a low-GL diet is better than a low-fat, low-calorie diet

If you eat a lot of shop-bought, low-fat foods, you will inevitably be eating more carbohydrates, not to mention sugar. A low-fat diet is usually a high-carbohydrate diet and eating more carbohydrates – especially refined white carbohydrates – causes a vicious cycle of see-sawing blood-sugar levels that leads to weight gain and that can damage your health.

Several animal studies have provided evidence of how low-GL diets cause more fat loss than conventional low-fat diets. The major driver of appetite is your blood-sugar level. Instead of focusing on calories, focus on the GL value of the food. It's not that calories don't count – they do – but the easiest way to eat less is to feel full, and that's how low-GL foods make you feel. Low-GL diets are much easier to stick to because you feel satisfied and fuller for longer. This helps you achieve your goal of long-term weight loss.

Five-day planner – healthy meals for a healthy week

I've put together a suggested Monday–Friday meal plan using recipes from later in this book. I've always found that a five-day plan feels less restrictive than trying to map out the full week; at the weekend, you should still make healthy choices, but this allows for a little more flexibility.

Portion sizes

Your hand is all you need! It's proportionate to your body, its size never changes and it's always with you. Simply put, your hand is the perfect tool for measuring food and nutrients.

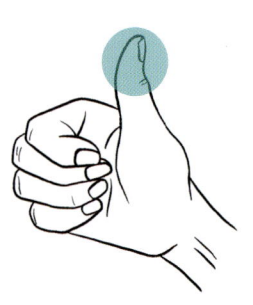

1 thumb =
a serving of
fats

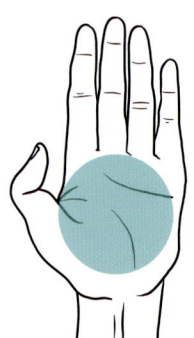

1 palm =
a serving of
protein

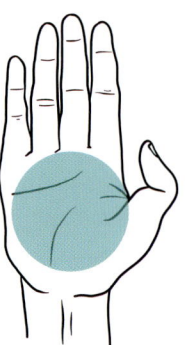

1 palm =
a serving of
carbohydrates

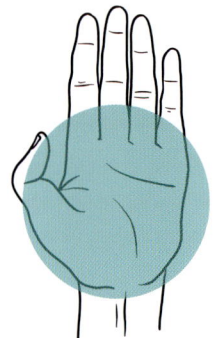

1 full hand =
a serving of
vegetables

Hybrid: meat and plants

	MONDAY	TUESDAY	WEDNESDAY	THURSDAY	FRIDAY
Breakfast	**Life-giving green juice** and **Tofu scramble*** *make double and reheat on Tuesday	**Life-giving green juice** and **Tofu scramble**	**Oat and flaxseed porridge** with **blueberry compote**	**The glow bowl** with berries and **Pecan cinnamon granola*** *make enough glow bowl mix for two days	**The glow bowl** with berries and **Pecan cinnamon granola**
Lunch	**Tomato, chilli and fennel soup** and **Porridge bread** with mashed avocado, smoked salmon and red onion* *make several portions and repeat for lunch on Wednesday	**The lit-from-within chicken salad** with wholemeal noodles	**Tomato, chilli and fennel soup** and **Porridge bread** with mashed avocado, smoked salmon and red onion	**Mackerel niçoise salad** with **Balsamic dressing** and **Flaxseed crackers**	**Roasted carrot and yellow pepper hummus**, **Flaxseed crackers** and **Rocket, pine nut and Parmesan salad**
Dinner	**Daily dahl*** *make enough for several portions and repeat on Wednesday	**Lentil Bolognese** with spiralised courgetti* *make double and reheat on Thursday	**Daily dahl**	**Lentil Bolognese** with spiralised courgetti	Grilled salmon with **Cauliflower pea mash** and steamed broccoli

Plants only

	MONDAY	TUESDAY	WEDNESDAY	THURSDAY	FRIDAY
Breakfast	**Lime chia pudding**, topped with **Pecan cinnamon granola*** *make double to have again on Wednesday	**Probiotic lime green smoothie** and **Sweet potato and apple breakfast cookies*** *make a batch of cookies and freeze	**Lime chia pudding**, topped with **Pecan cinnamon granola**	**Spirulina, lime and mint overnight oats**, plus **Beetroot, ginger and fennel juice*** *make enough juice for two days	**Tofu scramble** with avocado and tomatoes, plus **Beetroot, ginger and fennel juice**
Lunch	**Minestrone bean stew** with **Parsley gremolata*** *make several portions and repeat for lunch on Wednesday	**Falafel wrap*** *make double falafel and repeat on Thursday	**Minestrone bean stew** with **Parsley gremolata**	**Falafel wrap**	**Roasted carrot and yellow pepper hummus**, **Flaxseed crackers** and **Rocket, pine nut and Parmesan salad**
Dinner	**Mushroom and lentil shepherd's pie** with **Flash-cooked tender stem broccoli*** *make double and repeat on Wednesday	**Roasted aubergine involtini**, served with **Rocket, pine nut and Parmesan salad** in **Balsamic dressing**	**Mushroom and lentil shepherd's pie** with **Flash-cooked tender stem broccoli**	**Crispy tofu Thai red curry** with wholegrain brown basmati rice* *make enough curry paste for two batches and repeat on Friday	**Crispy tofu Thai red curry** with wholegrain brown basmati rice

Part three:
The Meno 8

1. Phytoestrogens

What are they, and how do they work?

Phytoestrogens (also known as isoflavones) are plant-derived oestrogens that mimic the effects of your oestrogen, as if your body was naturally producing more. They **do not** increase your body's oestrogen levels, which will remain low in menopause and will continue to decline with age.

The main benefit of phytoestrogens for menopausal women is their mild oestrogenic binding effect on the body's oestrogen receptors. This can be likened to an anti-oestrogenic effect, because this binding action means those sites become blocked, preventing your oestrogen from binding to the receptors. This blocking action weakens the cancer-causing potential of old circulating oestrogen.

What are the other benefits?

The benefits of including phytoestrogens in your diet range from helping to normalise oestrogen levels to boosting antioxidant and anti-inflammatory activity in the body. We know from a number of both human and animal studies that consuming phytoestrogens from dietary sources can be a very effective means of preventing and managing menopause symptoms. More importantly, it also reduces our risk factors for some of the Big Four – namely, osteoporosis and heart disease.

Phytoestrogens are safe

Many of my clients, initially, question the safety of isoflavones, particularly soybeans. In light of this, I want to offer some reliable, evidence-based information, so that you can make an informed choice for your peace of mind. A 1996 study[14] reviewed 861 articles (human cell-line studies, human epidemiologic studies, randomised trials and review articles) containing information regarding menopause, cancer and cardiovascular disease. The findings revealed that:

All studies concurred, that phytoestrogens are biologically active in humans or animals. These compounds inhibit the growth of different cancer cell lines in cell-culture and animal models.

Human epidemiologic evidence supports the hypothesis that phytoestrogens inhibit cancer formation and growth in humans. Foods containing phytoestrogens reduce cholesterol levels in humans. Animal and human data show benefits in treating osteoporosis through consuming foods containing these compounds.

This review suggests that phytoestrogens are among the dietary factors affording protection against cancer and heart disease in vegetarians. With this epidemiologic and cell-line evidence, intervention studies are now an appropriate consideration, to assess the clinical effects of phytoestrogens because of the potentially important health benefits associated with them.

Where can I get my phytoestrogens?

Foods high in phytoestrogens include soybeans, soy-containing foods, flaxseeds, nuts, wholegrains, apples, fennel, celery, parsley and alfalfa seeds. In cultures where menopausal women eat a predominantly plant-based diet, rich in phytoestrogens, fewer menopausal symptoms (from hot flushes to reduced bone loss) are experienced. Let's take a closer look at some of these phytoestrogen-friendly foods.

Alfalfa seeds

These are a member of the pea family and classed as a legume. They contain multiple beneficial compounds, particularly phytoestrogens and lignans. They are also a rich source of vitamin C, as well as vitamins B2 and B3, folic acid and minerals like zinc, magnesium, copper and more.

Alfalfa seeds are also rich in other phytochemicals called saponins. Animal trials have shown that saponins can exert a beneficial effect on cardiovascular disease, lowering LDL cholesterol (the bad type) in the liver, without affecting levels of HDL (good) cholesterol. The saponins in alfalfa sprouts can also boost immune function, increasing the activity of our natural killer cells.

The antioxidant superpowers of alfalfa sprouts surpass those of several main players in the antioxidant family – for example, kale and Brussels sprouts. They can also disarm some of the most powerful free radicals (hydroxyl and peroxyl), turning them into stable, non-harmful compounds.

Sourcing and storing tips
Alfalfa sprouts come in small plastic containers in which they have been hydroponically grown. They are available in supermarkets or from your local greengrocer, but I recommend buying them from dedicated growers. The quality is excellent, and they are always fresh, resulting in optimum nutrition benefits.

Only buy refrigerated sprouts, rinse them well before use and always keep them in the fridge to avoid any risk of salmonella contamination. Fresh sprouts have a clean, fresh aroma, with white or cream-coloured stems. Avoid anything that is off-colour or that has a musty aroma or any slimy spots.

Growing your own
You can also grow alfalfa sprouts yourself in a couple of days. Once sprouted, they will keep well in the fridge for up to five days. Use them daily (and liberally) as part of sandwich fillings, salads, omelettes or smoothies for maximum health benefits.

Soybeans

Soybeans have many known anti-cancer properties. Soy isoflavones are a good example of these, and they are especially protective against breast and prostate cancers. The comparatively low rates of breast and colon cancers in China are attributed to high soybean consumption.

The two isoflavones found in soybeans are daidzein and genistein. These are the primary isoflavones for reducing menopause symptoms; they act as phytoestrogens and can bind to oestrogen receptors such as in breast tissue, essentially blocking these sites and reducing the effects of oestrogen. This weakens its cancer-causing potential.

Soy isoflavones have also shown beneficial effects as regards preventing bone loss and osteoporosis. The amount of isoflavones present in different soy-based products can vary widely; tofu and tempeh, for example, generally contain higher levels of isoflavones than soy milk.

Further soybean benefits
In addition to isoflavones, soybeans contain high levels of protein (which is considered equal to animal proteins in terms of quality) and essential fats. This essential fat content

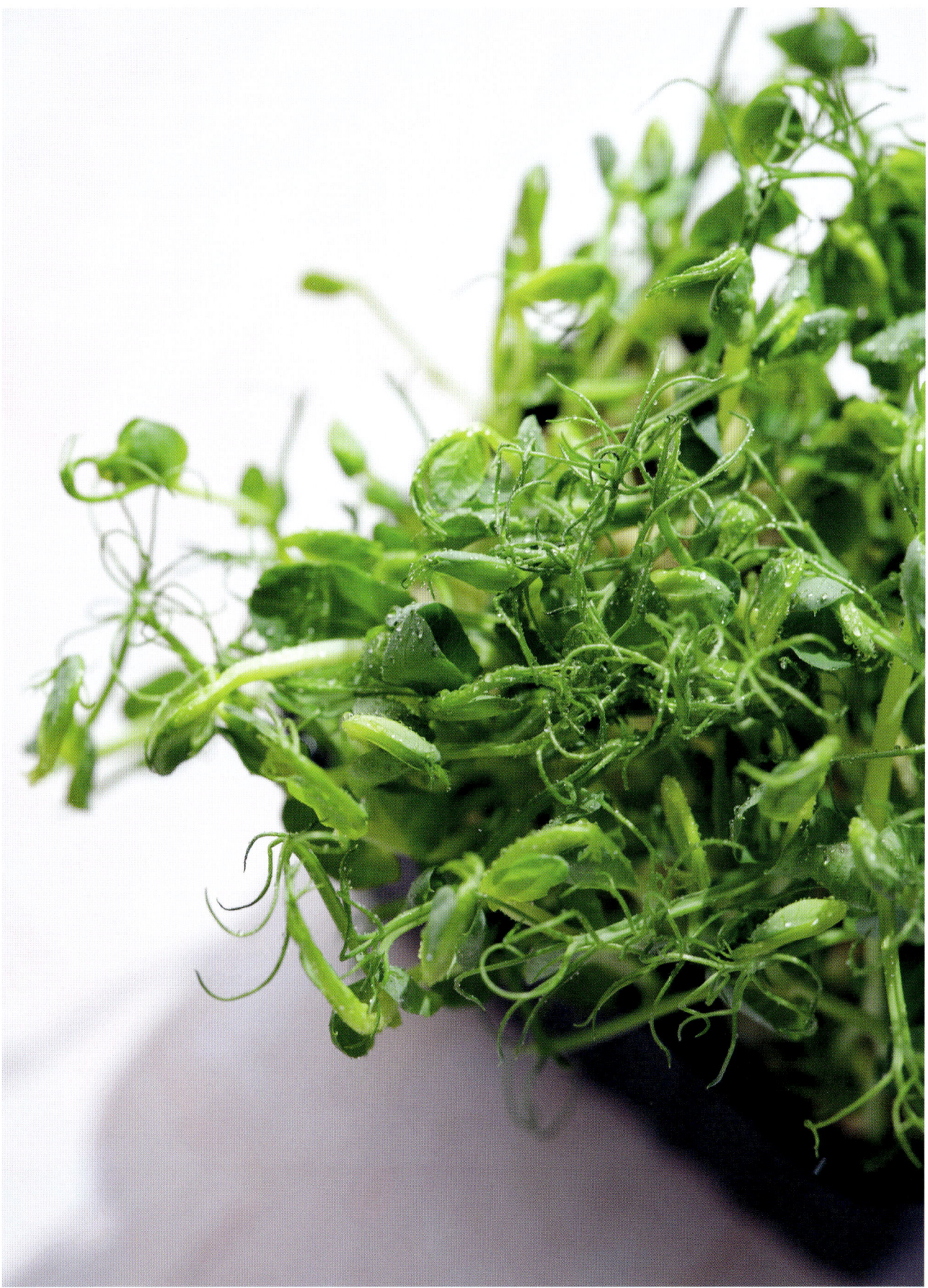

supports the cholesterol-lowering abilities of soybeans. The total fat content of soy is approximately 18 per cent, of which 85 per cent is unsaturated, comprising linoleic and oleic acid.

Soybeans are also particularly high in phytosterols, which enhance immune function, and lecithin, which is the major component of cell membranes. Also known as phosphatidylcholine, lecithin is an excellent emulsifier, which helps oils and water to mix. Lecithin contributes to nervous-system health, as it helps to maintain the myelin sheath (the protective layer around nerve cells). It is also a building block for the neurotransmitter acetylcholine.

Soybeans also contain fibre, 94 per cent of which is insoluble and 6 per cent is soluble. Much of the soybean fibre's effectiveness is due to its ability to bulk our stools. It is also heart-protective – reducing blood cholesterol and triglyceride levels – improves glucose tolerance and increases insulin sensitivity. This makes soybean fibre very beneficial for treating constipation, diarrhoea, high cholesterol and diabetes.

Flaxseed (linseed)

Flaxseed is the most abundant source of a type of phytoestrogen known as lignans. Flaxseeds have many other nutritional highlights too – for example, they are a good source of fibre, magnesium, potassium and manganese, as well as iron and copper.

The benefits of lignans contained in flaxseed include:
- Improving blood lipid profiles by reducing total cholesterol[15].
- Significant anti-cancer benefits, as demonstrated in a 2002 study[16] by Dr Paul Goss, the director of the breast cancer prevention program at Toronto Hospital. Other studies have concluded (through tracking reduction in oestrogen levels) that reducing oestrogen reduces the risk of breast cancer.

Phytoestrogens and cancer

The activity of oestrogen is involved in most breast cancers, and research shows that it may well be implicated in thyroid cancer, too. In 2002, a population-based, multi-ethnic study[17] from the American Association of Cancer Research looked at phytoestrogen consumption and thyroid-cancer risk, concluding that:

> We observed that thyroid cancer risk was reduced among women who consumed larger amounts of traditional and non-traditional soy-based foods (i.e. tofu) along with soybean and alfalfa sprouts.
>
> Soy-based foods and soybeans are rich sources of the isoflavones genistein and daidzein, and alfalfa sprouts contain large amounts of a particular isoflavone (formononetin).
>
> These isoflavones as well as certain lignans were associated with reduced risk.
>
> Furthermore, these associations were observed among both white and Asian women, as well as among pre-and postmenopausal women.

Soy isoflavones offer breast-cancer protection to postmenopausal women, too. You don't need to eat huge amounts – approximately 100mg per day of isoflavones (about 1.25g) is shown to be protective against breast cancer. Soy isoflavones may also help to improve vaginal dryness and irritation.

Phytoestrogens and bone health

We know that HRT (hormone replacement therapy) oestrogen is bone protective and widely prescribed for women to support bone health, but a diet rich in isoflavones could be a good alternative, especially for women who are unable to use HRT or simply don't want to. Consuming approximately 300mg of isoflavones is equivalent to 0.45mg of conjugated oestrogens, or an average dose of common HRT preparations.

Ultimately, increasing the amount of plant foods that you eat – especially those high in phytoestrogens – while reducing the number of animal foods in your diet can have benefits across many of the areas in which menopausal women are at risk. See p79 for my phytoestrogen-rich recipe section.

2. Fibre

What is it, and how does it work?

Fibre comes from plants – mostly the cell walls of plants, to be precise. There are different types of fibre, all of which can improve every aspect of our digestive health, heart health and blood-sugar regulation, not to mention help us to maintain a healthy weight.

There are two main types of fibre:
→ **Soluble fibre**, which dissolves in water, retains water and forms a gel-like substance in the colon. It slows down digestion and nutrient absorption from the stomach and intestine.
→ **Insoluble fibre**, which does not dissolve in water and passes through our digestive tract relatively intact and undigested. Insoluble fibre can help to speed up the passage of food (transit time). It also adds bulk to the stool and can help relieve constipation.

If you include both types of fibre in your diet on a daily basis, you will reap the most health benefits – this table will give you some ideas of where to find which type.

Sources of fibre

SOLUBLE FIBRE		INSOLUBLE FIBRE		
Oat bran	Slippery elm	Wheat bran	Spinach	Avocado
Guar gum	Apples (skin)	Oat bran	Peas	Sunflower seeds
Psyllium husks	Onion (skin)	Beans, lentils and legumes	Flaxseeds	Wholegrain pasta
Glucomannan (konjac root)	Seaweeds	Barley, quinoa, rye and oats	Almonds, walnuts	Wholegrain bread

What is fibre made of?

The exact composition differs from plant to plant, but most plant cell walls contain:
- 35 per cent insoluble fibre
- 45 per cent soluble fibre
- 15 per cent lignans
- 3 per cent protein

Dietary fibre is a combination of these components, so supplementation of a single type of fibre cannot replace or replicate the benefits of a diet rich in a variety of high-fibre foods. It is the variety of high-fibre foods that yields the most benefit, not the nutrient in isolation.

How much fibre do we need?

Research shows that 90 per cent of the population doesn't consume enough fibre daily. On average, as a nation, we are only getting approximately half of what we should be getting. This is because of our growing dependency on refined grains, processed foods and ready meals.

We need 25–30g of fibre a day to maintain health, and approximately 35g or more per day to optimise health. Fibre can come from vegetables like Brussels sprouts, peas, artichokes, avocados, berries, nuts and seeds, especially chia seeds and flaxseeds. You can use the table below to check exactly how much fibre a serving of some of these foods contains. Remember, you're aiming for a daily target of 35g.

Fibre-rich food sources

FIBRE-RICH FOOD	PORTION SIZE	TOTAL FIBRE CONTENT (G PER SERVING)
Chia seeds	100g	34.4
Popcorn	100g	13.4
Almonds	100g	13.3
Oats	100g	10.1
Raspberries	125g	8
Chickpeas	100g	7.6
Lentils	100g	7.3
Avocado	100g	6.7
Pear	1 medium-size	5.5
Artichoke	100g	5.4
Apple	1 medium-size	4.4
Kale	100g	3.6
Brussels sprouts	100g	3.6
Banana	1 medium-size	3.1
Carrots	100g	2.8
Beetroot	100g	2.8
Quinoa	100g	2.8
Broccoli	100g	2.6
Strawberries	125g	2

Why fibre is important

Fibre is an essential component of a healthy diet and has numerous benefits for our overall well-being. Here are some of the ways in which fibre contributes to our health:

→ High-fibre foods contain vitamins and minerals, specifically B vitamins, folic acid, essential fatty acids (omega-3), antioxidants including vitamin E and selenium, and many other micronutrients.
→ Fibre provides the primary food source (prebiotics) for our beneficial gut bacteria.
→ High-fibre foods help to slow down glucose absorption, regulate our blood-sugar levels and support detoxification.

Transit time, faecal weight and elimination

Transit time is the time it takes for food to travel from the point of entry in the mouth to elimination in a bowel movement. People who consume a high-fibre diet (30–35g per day) have a transit time of approximately 30 hours and an average faecal weight of 500g. In contrast, people who eat a typical western diet (low in fibre) have a slower transit time – usually 48 hours or more – and an average faecal weight of only 100g.

A prolonged transit time extends your exposure to various toxins, waste and cancer-causing compounds in the intestines. The longer you hold on to faecal matter, the greater your exposure to these toxins, hence the importance of a daily bowel movement.

How fibre can help with common menopausal health issues

At this life stage, our digestion often becomes sluggish, and we can find ourselves quickly and easily **constipated**. When I'm working with clients, this is often the first place I start: supporting their digestive health and improving the frequency of bowel movements to get their metabolism going again.

You should have a bowel movement daily; ideally, twice a day. It should be well formed and easy to pass. The way to achieve healthy motility is by including both soluble and insoluble fibre in your diet, as well as foods high in prebiotic fibre, such as chicory, artichokes, plantain, onions, leeks and asparagus.

The best type of insoluble fibre to increase bowel-movement frequency is wheat bran or oat bran, which are both rich in cellulose, a principal part of the plant wall. Cellulose arrives in our large intestine in its undigested form and acts as the primary food source for our beneficial bacteria. Wheat bran can also bind water, which enables it to increase faecal weight and size. I recommend adding wheat bran or oat bran to porridge or overnight oats (see pp104, 238) or the porridge bread recipe (see p102). Magnesium supplementation may also ease constipation by helping to calm the nervous system.

If, at the other end of the scale, you suffer from **diarrhoea**, the best type of fibre to help bulk your stool is psyllium husks – a soluble gel-forming fibre (classed as a mucilage). Another helpful gel-forming fibre is glucomannan (from the konjac root), which also happens to be one of the most potent cholesterol-lowering compounds. Gel-forming fibres are also very effective at reducing after-meal glucose spikes, as well as reducing insulin levels in diabetics. Foods such as prunes can similarly have a gentle laxative effect.

Fibre: the key to lowering cholesterol

The health benefits of water-soluble, gel-forming fibres like glucomannan and oat bran have been widely researched. We know, for example, that oat beta-glucan is capable of lowering serum cholesterol and triglyceride levels. The mechanism is simple: old cholesterol can bind to the gel-forming fibre and be safely and effectively excreted in faecal matter. In addition, gel-forming oat- or wheat-bran fibres can reduce cholesterol production in the liver.

Many nutrients act synergistically with each other, bringing additional health benefits when combined. A research study[18] published in the *British Journal of Nutrition* in 2007 shows how combining soluble fibre with plant sterols (phytochemicals found in tofu, legumes, almonds, seeds and porridge oats) is more effective in lowering cholesterol than statins. Studies have also shown that regular consumption of 1–3g of plant sterols per day lowers LDL cholesterol by approximately 15 per cent. For example, the combination of oat bran and plant sterols, which have been widely researched for their cholesterol-lowering abilities, is a very effective method of reducing cholesterol.

Plant sterol sources

FOOD TYPE	SOURCE	TOTAL PLANT STEROL CONTENT (MG/100G WEIGHT)
WHOLEGRAINS	Oat flakes	45
	Wheat germ	345
	Wheat bran	200
	Brown rice	87
LEGUMES	Peas	135
	Beans	127
NUTS AND SEEDS	Peanuts	117
	Almonds	138
	Walnuts	108
	Pecan nuts	108
	Pistachio nuts	108
VEGETABLES	Beetroot	25
	Broccoli	37
	Cauliflower	31
	Brussels sprouts	37
	Leek	19
	Dill	32
	Parsley	28
	Peas	30
	Red pepper	22
	Sweetcorn	28
	Alfalfa sprouts	20

Try to include a mix of raw and cooked plant sterols in your diet every day; you can use the table opposite to check the total plant-sterol content of some of your favourite foods.

Supporting weight loss

Fibre supplementation can be an effective method to support weight loss. For starters, fibre keeps you full for longer, but it also does much more than this. Fibre enhances blood-sugar control – in other words, it keeps your blood sugars balanced, decreasing glucose spikes and insulin release, which leads to weight loss.

The best type of fibre for weight loss is the soluble gel-forming fibre mentioned previously – that is, glucomannan and psyllium husks, but pectin (found in apples and citrus fruits) and seaweed fibres such as carrageenan are also excellent. Simply add the gel-forming fibre to water and drink before meals. The gel-forming mucilage fibre binds to water in the stomach and small intestines, forming a gelatinous mass that slows the absorption of glucose, keeping you feeling full for longer and reducing the absorption of energy by 30–180kcal per day.

It's worth noting that these water-soluble fibres are also fermented by our gut bacteria, which can potentially produce a good bit of wind and lead to increased flatulence or even abdominal discomfort. Start with a small amount of soluble fibre (1g in water) and slowly increase to 2g and so on, until you reach the recommended daily dose of 15g, split into three doses.

The maintenance of intestinal flora

Our gut flora are very delicate, and can be easily damaged by medications (antibiotics, anti-inflammatories, antacids, corticosteroids), as well as by processed foods, alcohol and the poor absorption of key nutrients.

As much as 75 per cent of our immunity resides in the gut. Many experts believe that the starting point in improving systemic immune health and reducing chronic inflammation is by optimising our microflora balance and the health of our mucous membranes (think gut lining).

So, what has all this got to do with fibre?

Our friendly gut bugs, which are the foundation of our overall health and well-being, rely heavily on dietary fibre as their primary food source. Can you guess what happens when they don't get fed? Yep, they die off.

A low-fibre diet (our typical western diet) is associated with an increase in endotoxin-producing bacteria (the bad guys) and a much lower number of *Lactobacillus* varieties (the good guys), which we want in abundance in our gut.

Eating a diet rich in a variety of fibres from multiple sources creates the ideal environment for more beneficial bacteria to grow and thrive. It also promotes the action of short-chain fatty acids (SCFAs), which are responsible for lowering inflammation.

Short-chain fatty acids (SCFAs)

When our friendly bacteria get their feed of fibre (especially the fibre found in apples, citrus and legumes), they produce what is known as short-chain fatty acids (SCFAs). These are very effective at lowering systemic inflammation. There are several different types of SCFAs, but the ones with the most beneficial outcomes for our health are:

- **Propionate**, which helps to lower cholesterol because it inhibits a key enzyme (HMG-CoA reductase) responsible for cholesterol synthesis in the liver.
- **Butyrate**, which is associated with impressive anti-cancer activity and is used in the treatment of ulcerative colitis.

Legumes

Legumes are among the oldest cultivated plants: fossil records demonstrate their use in the diets of prehistoric people. Although they are sometimes referred to as poor people's meat, I like to think of them as healthy people's fuel! Legumes provide similar numbers of calories to grains, but nearly two to four times the amount of protein, as well as 7–8g of fibre per 100g serving.

Research shows that legumes – in particular, soybeans – contribute considerable health benefits: from lowering cholesterol to blood-glucose management to reducing cancer risk. Brightly coloured beans (for example, red kidney beans) also provide high amounts of antioxidants – even more than blueberries.

The problem with legumes is that they can increase flatulence and digestive discomfort (bloating and trapped wind). The flatulence-causing compounds in legumes are primarily oligosaccharides, which the body cannot digest. They pass through our system until they reach the large intestine, where our gut bacteria break them down, producing gas in the process.

Correct cooking can reduce the number of oligosaccharides and therefore the excess wind. Sprouting is also a good way to make legumes more digestible, as well as increasing their nutritional value.

To summarise

Fibre is an extremely effective tool in your arsenal for lowering cholesterol and supporting weight loss, so make sure that you get enough of it in your diet – aim for 35g of fibre daily for optimum health benefits. At the same time as increasing your fibre intake, make sure that you drink enough water: a minimum of 2 litres daily to avoid constipation.

Certain types of (insoluble) fibre found in legumes, apples and citrus fruits feed our friendly bacteria, enabling them to convert the fibre to powerful inflammation-lowering compounds that can inhibit cholesterol production in the liver, as well as increase powerful anti-cancer activity. Look after your gut bugs with a fibre-rich diet, and they will look after you!

3. Omega-3

What are they, and how do they work?

Omega-3 essential fatty acids (to give them their full title) are good fats that we need to get from dietary sources – hence the word 'essential'. We cannot produce these ourselves but they are crucial for our health, so they need to be present in our diet.

The type of fat we consume has a significant influence on our health and well-being. Good fats like omega-3-rich fats play many important roles in the body – structurally, for example, to optimise our cell membranes, or as building blocks for hormone production. This is particularly relevant for women – not only in this life stage, but throughout our lives.

Fat has a bad rep

Misleading dietary recommendations from the 1970s and 80s have demonised fat for decades. Even now, many women completely avoid this food group, opting instead for fat-free or zero-fat foods. In addition, we often consume too much of the wrong type of fat – that is, saturated fats found in animal products, as well as trans fats found in ultra-processed foods. This combination of zero-fat foods and the wrong type of fat is very damaging, and it denies our body the basic raw materials to produce certain key hormones and neurotransmitters.

But remember, it is the *type* of fat that is important. Once the fat is removed from a product, it is generally replaced with something else – mostly sugar, and therein lies the problem. Furthermore, the combination of saturated fat or ultra-processed trans fats (or both) with refined carbohydrates is in fact the deadly combination we should be avoiding.

We now know that a diet high in sugar and refined white carbohydrates is the root cause of elevated cholesterol levels and one of the main drivers of abdominal obesity – not fats!

Why are omega-3 fats classed as good fats?

This is to do with how they influence our cell membranes. Every human cell has a protective fatty membrane known as the phospholipid bilayer. Eating lots of heart-healthy, omega-3-rich fats ensures that the phospholipid bilayer remains fluid, enabling the cell to hold on to water and other vital nutrients, and therefore to function properly.

In contrast, by consuming poor-quality fats (such as hydrogenated oils), the cell membranes are much less fluid and therefore much less communicative with other cells. As a result, they lose their ability to signal hormones such as insulin. Over time, this can lead to insulin resistance, pre-diabetes, diabetes and obesity.

The sources of omega-3 essential fats

Alpha-linolenic acid (ALA) is a type of omega-3 fatty acid that is abundant in plant-based sources such as flaxseed and chia seeds. It is also present in oily fish, but to a lesser extent. Oily fish are a rich source of other types of omega-3 fatty acid called EPA and DHA, which are not commonly found in plant-based sources.

It is therefore recommended to consume a combination of oily fish and plant-based omega-3, as well as to supplement with 1g of fish oils per day*. Oily, or cold-water, fish include salmon, mackerel, herring, halibut, kippers and sardines. Research suggests eating good-quality oily fish twice a week (approximately 350g per week) protects against heart disease. This translates to approximately 400mg of omega-3 fats per day.

*Please note that you should inform your doctor before taking fish-oil supplements, especially if you are taking blood-pressure-lowering medication: fish oils can lower your blood pressure further.

A closer look at flaxseed

Flaxseed (or linseed) is an extremely rich source of ALA, a true omega-3 essential fatty acid. In fact, ALA has twice the amount of omega-3 fatty acids as fish oil!

So, why do we recommend consuming mostly oily fish as an omega-3 source?

The problem is that flaxseed has more of a diluted effect on the body than omega-3 fish oils. This is because ALA has to be converted to become bioavailable – usable by the body. In addition, the conversion process is dependent on the presence of a specific enzyme (delta-6 desaturase). Due to several factors – from nutrient deficiencies to the regular consumption of saturated fats or alcohol – some people have less of this enzyme. As a result, they may be poor converters of ALA and not get the full value of omega-3 in flaxseeds.

Flaxseed is also an abundant source of plant lignans. These are fibre compounds that can bind to oestrogen receptors and interfere with the cancer-promoting effects of oestrogen on breast tissue.

Flaxseed is a true superfood, and you should aim to include two tablespoons of ground flaxseeds in your daily diet. You can add it to smoothies, sprinkle it into live probiotic yoghurt and add it to bread or energy ball recipes. Try coating tofu in ground flaxseeds before baking.

How to select and store

Flaxseeds can be purchased whole or ground. Ground flaxseeds are prone to oxidation, so always purchase in a resealable vacuum-sealed pouch. Once open, reseal and store in the fridge (they will keep for up to six months). Whole flaxseeds have a longer shelf life. I like to get mine from Linwoods Health Foods, which sells convenient, resealable pouches of cold-milled flaxseed in many variations, as well as a range specifically for menopause called Menoligna; see the Resources section for more information (p280).

Flaxseed oil should always be purchased in a dark, resealable bottle. Once open, store in the fridge. Never use flaxseed oil in cooking – it has a low smoke point, so once it comes into contact with a direct heat source, it will begin to smoke and denature, becoming damaging to our health.

How omega-3 essential fats benefit our health

As we now know, one of the chronic health conditions that menopausal women find themselves at an increased risk of is Alzheimer's disease. So, what can we do to reduce that risk? Can diet play a role? Absolutely! Indeed, preventative measures are the only cards we hold in the fight against Alzheimer's and dementia.

The review[19] below confirms that nutrition plays a key role in preventing a decline in intellectual function:

> There is strong evidence that the incidence and prevalence of Alzheimer's Disease are affected by diet, with high-risk factors found to include alcohol, fat, refined carbohydrates, salt, and total caloric consumption.
>
> Preventative factors are found to include antioxidants, essential trace minerals,

estrogen for post-menopausal women, fish and fish oil, and anti-inflammatory therapeutic agents.

Thus, healthy diets should be considered the first line of defence against both the development and progression of Alzheimer's Disease, as well as all other chronic degenerative diseases.

The finding that the highest correlation between diet and Alzheimer's Disease incidence and prevalence is found 3–5 years before the study period, suggests that diet modifications late in life can still influence the risk of developing Alzheimer's Disease.

Overall, this review highlights the importance of adopting healthy eating habits from an early age. It also emphasises, however, that modifying our diets to improve their quality later in life can still have a positive impact on our risk of developing Alzheimer's disease. This finding is encouraging and motivating, as it suggests that even small dietary changes can make a difference in this area.

Further benefits of omega-3s

A 2022 study[20] highlights the extensive health benefits of omega-3 fatty acids in fish.

This systematic review combined data from 17 studies (11 human studies and 6 animal studies) to see what effect omega-3s had on emotion – specifically anxiety and depression – and cognition during the menopausal transition. The review found that for menopausal women, fish-oil supplementation was shown to have an anti-anxiety effect, helped to maintain inflammatory balance along with antidepressant and neuroprotective activities, and had neuroimmune-modulating actions. It also found less psychological distress, decreased depressive symptoms and significant improvements in depression scores in those who took omega-3s.

Eating natural, unprocessed fats can also protect your heart

It is a common misconception that eating too much fat- and cholesterol-containing foods (such as eggs, cheese and shellfish) will block our arteries and cause a heart attack. This is not completely accurate. We now know that cholesterol-containing foods like these do not contribute to elevated cholesterol – it is the *type* of fats in our diet that plays more of a role.

Poor-quality fats consist mainly of processed vegetable oils, including soy, canola, margarine and hydrogenated fryer oils. These should be avoided in all forms.

This list also includes industrially produced baked goods – that is, par-baked goods and those from supermarket bakeries, including cakes, buns and biscuits. You know the ones I am referring to – they are generally cheap, sold in multipacks and have a long list of unpronounceable ingredients.

The problem with poor-quality fats is that they have generally been treated with high heat, high pressure or both, and therefore cause damage to our cell-membrane function. Without a healthy, flexible membrane, cells can't function properly and over time this impacts our health.

Omega-3 fats are good fats, and they're heart-healthy: they can reduce our cholesterol, as well as the level of harmful triglycerides in the blood. This, in turn, reduces inflammation, which is linked to the root cause of heart disease.

Olive oil – nature's golden elixir

In addition to omega-3 essential fats from oily fish and flaxseed (ALA), I also recommend that you increase your intake of monounsaturated fats in the form of olive oil, as your daily fat of choice.

The health benefits of extra virgin olive oil (EVOO) are vast. It is high in monounsaturated fatty acids (MUFAs), the most important of which is called oleic acid. Oleic acid is known to be extremely heart-healthy, with positive effects on cholesterol and inflammation. It is also capable of fighting free-radical damage (or oxidative stress), which causes ageing. Olive oil is especially healthy for your brain; it improves focus and memory, and also helps to regulate mood. A study found that individuals who added a litre of high-quality EVOO to their diets every week experienced more than a 40 per cent reduction in risk for dementia, as well as a more than 60 per cent reduction in the risk of breast cancer in women.

Shopping for olive oil

When buying olive oil, always buy extra virgin. It's the only grade that retains the natural health-promoting phenols, as it's cold-pressed, meaning that it's minimally processed. All other olive-oil grades – 'virgin', 'pure' and 'light' – have been chemically refined to mask defects, and this process destroys the healthful phenols.

However, even if a supermarket olive oil label *claims* 'extra virgin', you've still got to be careful. Many supermarket oils are past their best (rancid), not pure (chemically processed) or even counterfeit! Thanks to the health benefits of EVOO, demand has increased exponentially worldwide, and to capitalise on this, lower-quality olive oil is often labelled and marketed as EVOO. To get the most health-promoting benefits possible, it's important to be sure of the source of what you are buying.

Wherever you shop for your olive oil, freshness is the most important factor in terms of nutritional benefit. Olives are fruit and maintain their window of peak freshness for about six months after they have been harvested – but harvest-fresh oil is almost impossible to find in supermarkets. When shopping for olive oil, forget the 'best before' or 'use by' date; you need to find EVOO with a **harvest pressing** date on the label of no more than six months earlier than your date of purchase. As well as the nutritional benefits of such fresh olive oil, the flavour will be much nicer! I recommend buying online or directly from the producers; they sell EVOO fresh from the harvest that is bursting with flavour and goodness.

Storing olive oil

There are three things to avoid in the storage of your EVOO: **light**, **heat** and **air**. Let's look at why, and what can be done about each one.

1. In short, sunlight is damaging to the delicate, antioxidant-containing polyphenols in EVOO. The oil also contains chlorophyll, the naturally occurring chemical that plants use for photosynthesis (the greener the EVOO, the more chlorophyll it contains). When EVOO is exposed to sunlight, a chemical process called photo-oxidation occurs that denatures and destabilises the oil, reducing its overall quality. You may have noticed that some olive oil is packaged in dark bottles – this is to reduce its exposure to light. You can further reduce the potential for photo-oxidation by storing your EVOO in a dark cupboard or pantry.
2. The ideal temperature for storing EVOO is 13.5 degrees Celsius (although up to 21 degrees is acceptable). Avoid hotspots such as next to your cooker, next to the radiator,

on top of the fridge or in direct sunlight; the oil will degrade and turn rancid sooner than it should. To safeguard the flavour of your EVOO, not to mention its health benefits, aim to store it in a cool, dry location.

3. The most challenging threat to your EVOO is oxygen, as it's the hardest to avoid. As soon as you open the bottle, your oil is exposed to the air, which causes oxidation. A sealed container will keep as much oxygen as possible from coming into contact with your oil and damaging it. Large boxes or litre tins work well because you dispense only what you need, or you can decant into smaller bottles and refill as necessary.

To summarise

Consuming too many saturated fats and trans fats (found in meat, processed foods and hydrogenated vegetable oils) poses a risk to your health. Furthermore, these poor-quality fats in conjunction with refined grains and/or sugar are an even more dangerous combination.

In addition, not eating enough monounsaturated fats (from nuts, seeds and olive oil, as well as omega-3 fats found in oily fish, flaxseeds and chia seeds) is associated with an increased risk of cancer and about 60 other conditions, including heart disease, stroke, high blood pressure and diabetes.

4. Calcium and magnesium

What are they, and how do they work?

Both calcium and magnesium are classified as major minerals in the body. The other major minerals are chloride, sodium, sulphur, potassium and phosphorus.

Enzymes require minerals to function, and if a mineral is missing, the enzyme cannot do its job. For example: to activate vitamin A, our enzymes require zinc; its absence can result in a type of visual impairment known as night blindness.

Tips for better mineral absorption

Juicing provides better mineral absorption in comparison to consuming whole fruits or vegetables. This is because the fibre contained in fruits and vegetables can sometimes interfere with our absorption of minerals. By separating the minerals from the fibre in the juicing process, you get a concentrated form of nutrients in a more bioavailable form, which your body can utilise straight away. Green leafy veg is the best source of many of the major minerals, especially calcium, and by juicing your greens, your body will benefit more.

Calcium, and where to find it

Calcium is the most abundant mineral in the body. Our bodies depend on calcium for the contraction of our muscles, to regulate our heartbeat and to assist in the clotting of our blood. A calcium deficiency is a major contributing factor to both osteoporosis and high blood pressure.

Though likely the most well-known, cow's milk dairy is not the only source of calcium. Many plant-based calcium sources are just as good, and they are the sources that I recommend to my clients. There's more detail on this in the bone health section in part two (see p11), but essentially the most health-beneficial calcium sources are seaweed, green leafy vegetables and legumes. These contain antioxidants, complex carbohydrates, fibre and iron, while adding very little fat and no cholesterol to your diet.

The recommended daily intake of calcium to maintain bone mineral density is 1,200mg. You can check your calcium intake using the online tool from the International Osteoporosis Foundation (www.osteoporosis.foundation/educational-hub/topic/calcium-calculator). If necessary, the following table shows several good sources of dietary calcium to optimise your daily intake:

Magnesium, and why we need it

Magnesium is one of the most important minerals; indeed, it plays a part in over 300 different enzyme reactions and is considered life essential. As much as 60 per cent of our magnesium is found in our bones; 30 per cent is found in our muscles and only 1–2 per cent is found in the blood (so blood tests don't give an accurate picture of our body's magnesium levels).

Magnesium is mostly needed by the heart (to control blood pressure, cholesterol, palpitations) and the brain (to combat mood disorders such as anxiety and depression, and for sleep). Other benefits of magnesium include links to bone health, as it can increase bone density and lower the risk of osteoporosis; asthma relief (as an anti-inflammatory); diabetes management; and the improvement of joint health and immune function.

Calcium-rich food sources

FOOD TYPE	SOURCE	TOTAL CALCIUM CONTENT (MG PER 100G SERVING)
SEAWEED	Kelp	1,093
	Dulse	296
LEAFY GREENS	Kale	249
	Turnip greens	246
LEGUMES	Peas	135
	Soybean	73
	Tofu	128
NUTS AND SEEDS	Sesame seeds	120
	Almonds	138
	Walnuts	99
	Pecan nuts	73
	Brazil nuts	186
VEGETABLES	Parsley	203
	Broccoli	103

Magnesium deficiency

Most symptoms of magnesium deficiency are very similar to menopause symptoms. These include restless leg and muscle twitches (especially in bed at nighttime), constipation, anxiety and brain fog – as magnesium is needed for neurotransmitter function – heart palpitations, teeth problems, headaches and poor sleep.

Sound familiar? A magnesium deficiency may be due to one or more of the following factors:

- The diuretic effect of caffeine and alcohol means that we pee more, losing key minerals in the process
- Soil depletion of key minerals (from modern farming methods such as crop spraying) means that the foods we eat simply contain less magnesium
- People who suffer from coeliac disease and those with low stomach acid have compromised absorption of minerals, which can lead to a magnesium deficiency
- Chronic stress leads to poor gut health, which depletes magnesium stores

How much we need, and where to find it

The RDA of magnesium to maintain optimal health is approximately 300mg. Many nutritional experts agree that magnesium intake should be based on body weight: 6 milligrams per kilogram of body weight.

Supplementary sources of magnesium and their carriers

All minerals need a carrier molecule to be transported around the body. The different carriers will determine levels of absorption. This is because some of the carriers will detach the magnesium only reluctantly, resulting in low absorption.

Think of carriers as plugs.

- **Magnesium oxide**
  The oxide plug is hard to detach, which results in low absorption. This is best avoided, unless you are constipated (it has a mild laxative effect and supports bowel transit time).

Magnesium-rich food sources

FOOD TYPE	SOURCE	TOTAL MAGNESIUM CONTENT (MG PER 100G SERVING)
DRIED SEAWEED	Nori	770
DRIED HERBS	Dried basil	492
	Dried coriander	694
NUTS AND SEEDS	Pumpkin seeds	535
	Flaxseed	392
	Cumin seeds	366
	Brazil nuts	376
	Cashews	273
	Almond butter	303
GRAINS	Wheat bran	490
	Wheat germ	336
	Buckwheat	229

- **Magnesium citrate**
  The citrate plug is the easiest to detach, which results in good absorption. This works best in an acidic environment – that is, with good levels of stomach acid, so that our body can convert and use it. Take your magnesium citrate first thing in the morning before food, away from other supplements, to ensure optimum absorption.
- **Magnesium glycinate**
  The glycinate plug offers excellent absorption. The coupling with an amino acid (glycinate) is ideal for pain, anxiety and insomnia. It is also great for immune function, muscle function, tiredness and fatigue.

The process of absorption

Just like calcium, magnesium is absorbed in the gut; 40 per cent is absorbed in the small intestine and 5 per cent is absorbed in the large intestine. The rest – 55 per cent – exits the body as waste.

Consider the following tips for optimal magnesium absorption:
- Take magnesium just before bed (on an empty stomach) or first thing in the morning before food.
- Transdermal magnesium absorption is also very effective, especially at night to aid restful sleep. Try a magnesium spray: 5–6 sprays directly on to your arm or leg will give you an approximate dose of 150mg. The absorption through the skin is very effective and you will quickly feel the benefits. This is ideal for anyone with compromised digestive function (that is, who may have low stomach acid) as it avoids the stomach.

A final word on magnesium

Magnesium is one of my core menopause nutrients. Magnesium deficiency is extremely common, especially among women at this life stage, so I strongly recommend increasing your dietary intake of this important mineral, as well as including a good practitioner-grade magnesium supplement to optimise your levels.

Magnesium works very closely with calcium to support our bones; it is also very heart protective, reducing blood pressure and improving heart muscle contraction. Lastly, magnesium's role in preventing the recurrence of kidney stones is widely accepted, with the combination of dietary sources and supplementary sources yielding the best outcomes.

5. Antioxidants

What are they, and how do they work?

Antioxidants deal with the 'exhaust fumes of life': pollution, toxins, chemicals, nutritional deficiencies and even stress. They are heart-healthy, and can also slow ageing.

Antioxidants are contained in all brightly coloured fruits and vegetables. I've already mentioned 'eating the rainbow'; by this I mean choosing a wide variety of fruits and vegetables for your diet, in as many colours as possible – the main ones being red, dark green, yellow, orange and purple. You can find some good examples of these colourful sources in the table below.

The different-coloured pigments contain powerful antioxidants to protect us against disease. The substances found in brightly coloured fruits and vegetables are known as phytochemicals. They are powerful agents in the fight against cancer and often work in harmony with key antioxidant vitamins – that is, vitamin A, vitamin C and vitamin E.

The benefits of the different colours in plant foods

Here's a crash course on the different plant colours and how their phytochemical content impacts our health:

→ **Blue or purple** signals the presence of anthocyanins, which have been found to prevent blood clots and delay cellular ageing. They may even slow the onset of Alzheimer's disease. You find it in foods like aubergines, beetroot, blueberries, red cabbage and purple potatoes.
→ **Green** indicates the presence of phytochemicals like sulforaphane, isocyanates

Antioxidant phytochemical colours and food sources

RED (LYCOPENE)	DARK GREEN (ISOTHIOCYANATES, SULPHUROPHANE)	YELLOW OR PALE GREEN (CAROTENOIDS)	ORANGE (BETA-CAROTENE)	BLUE OR PURPLE (ANTHOCYANINS)
Apples	Asparagus	Avocados	Apricots	Aubergine
Peppers	Artichokes	Bananas	Peppers	Beetroot
Cherries	Peppers	Bell peppers	Squash	Blackberries
Cranberries	Broccoli	Bok choy	Carrots	Blueberries
Pink grapefruit	Brussels sprouts	White cabbage	Sweet potatoes	Red cabbage
Radishes	Cucumbers	Cauliflower	Oranges	Cherries
Raspberries	Beans	Celery	Papaya	Plums
Plums	Kale	Courgettes	Pumpkin	Grapes
Strawberries	Peas	Fennel	Mangos	Currants
Tomatoes	Spinach	Limes	Yams	
Watermelon	Swiss chard	Lemons		
		Onions		
		Pineapple		
		Squash		

and indoles, which are anti-carcinogenic and detoxifying. Many green veggies are part of the brassica family, which includes broccoli, Brussels sprouts, bok choy, rocket, kale and cauliflower.

Orange means the compounds alpha-carotene and beta-carotene are present. The former protects against cancer, as well as benefiting skin and eye health, while beta-carotene is a precursor to vitamin A and a powerful antioxidant within the body. Look for foods like carrots, pumpkin, acorn squash and sweet potatoes.

Pale green or white is caused by compounds called allicins, which have powerful anti-cancer, anti-tumour, immune-boosting and anti-microbial properties. These are present in garlic, onions, leeks and other vegetables. Many of these same foods also contain antioxidant flavonoids like quercetin and kaempferol.

Red indicates a carotenoid called lycopene, which is protective against heart disease and cancer thanks to its powerful antioxidant activity. It is found in tomatoes, bell peppers and carrots. Asparagus also contains a good amount of lycopene – proof that you can't always judge a book by its cover…

Yellow or green means a food contains the carotenoids lutein and zeaxanthin, which are especially beneficial for the eyes and help protect the heart against atherosclerosis. Vegetables in this group may not always appear yellowish. In addition to yellow summer squash and orange bell peppers, spinach, collard greens, mustard greens, turnip greens, peas and even avocados all contain these powerful nutrients.

Hit your daily targets

Antioxidants are measured in ORAC (oxygen radical absorbency capacity) units, which translate to how good a particular food is at dealing with the exhaust fumes of life. Your goal is 6,000 ORAC units per day. Below is a table of 25 different foods. Each food delivers approximately 2,000 ORAC units, so choose at least three of these foods to hit your daily target.

Anti-cancer phytochemicals

Anti-cancer phytochemicals are natural compounds found in many plant-based foods that have been shown to have powerful

Foods high in ORAC units

60g of blackcurrants	125g of pistachios	200g of cooked lentils	180g of kidney beans	1 medium artichoke
60g of blueberries	7 walnuts	90g of broccoli florets	⅓ medium avocado	1 apple
60g of strawberries	8 pecans	1 orange	60g of cherries	1 medium beetroot
60g of raspberries	⅓ tsp cinnamon	½ tsp turmeric	400g squash	70g of kale
8 asparagus spears	150ml of red wine	4 pieces of dark chocolate (85%)	½ tsp oregano	30g of raw spinach

antioxidant and anti-inflammatory effects. These compounds may help to protect against cancer and other chronic diseases by neutralising free radicals and reducing oxidative stress in the body. Carotenes and flavonoids are two phytochemicals that have been studied extensively for their potential anti-cancer properties.

Carotenes enhance our immunity. They are mostly found in yellow and orange fruits and vegetables: carrots, squash, apricots, citrus and yams, but also in spinach and kale.

Flavonoids act as antioxidants with immune-enhancing properties. They have a direct anti-tumour effect. They are found in most dark berries (blueberries, blackberries and cherries), but also in tomatoes and greens.

It's important to ensure that your body has an adequate supply of phytochemicals and other nutrients by incorporating food rich in these compounds into your diet. Fortunately, there are many delicious foods that are high in antioxidants, including carrots, blueberries and green tea. Let's take a closer look at some of these.

Carrots

Carrots are rich in beta-carotene, the precursor to vitamin A. Two carrots provide roughly four times the RDA of vitamin A, as well as high levels of vitamin C, vitamin K and fibre. In 100g of carrots, there are 41 calories, 9.6g of carbohydrate (4.5g of which sugars) and 3g of fibre.

The antioxidant compounds in carrots, specifically beta-carotene and carotenoids, can protect against cardiovascular disease and cancer[21]. Carrots are also well known for promoting good vision, especially night vision, and for reducing the incidence of cataracts, the leading cause of blindness in the elderly.

Remove the leafy tops before storing carrots. If you don't, these will draw moisture from the roots and cause the carrots to spoil faster. Store the carrots away from apples, pears and potatoes (which will cause them to become bitter) in the coolest part of the fridge.

Cooking carrots breaks down the fibres that enhance the bioavailability of beta-carotene for the body to utilise. Simply lightly steam for optimum benefits. For inspiration, check out recipes like my roasted carrot and yellow pepper hummus (see p117) or carrot, ginger and celery soup (see p199).

Açai

Açai berries are small, purple berries that are rich in anthocyanins. They have a very high ORAC score and are therefore a potent antioxidant. They are also high in fibre, B vitamins, trace minerals and monounsaturates (MUFAs) and oleic acid (also in olive oil). The fountain-of-youth smoothie bowl recipe (see p202) uses açai berry powder.

Pomegranate

The pomegranate has a long history of medicinal uses that goes back to ancient Greece and Egypt. It is rich in polyphenols and high in fibre; its vibrant red colour is due to its anthocyanins, which deliver potent amounts of antioxidants.

It is especially beneficial for heart health, since it can increase nitric oxide (NO), a molecule that plays a critical role in regulating blood-pressure levels. When NO levels are low, blood vessels can become constricted, which can in turn increase blood pressure and thus the risk of heart disease. In addition to increasing NO production, polyphenols in pomegranate may also help reduce inflammation and oxidative stress, which are both risk factors for heart disease.

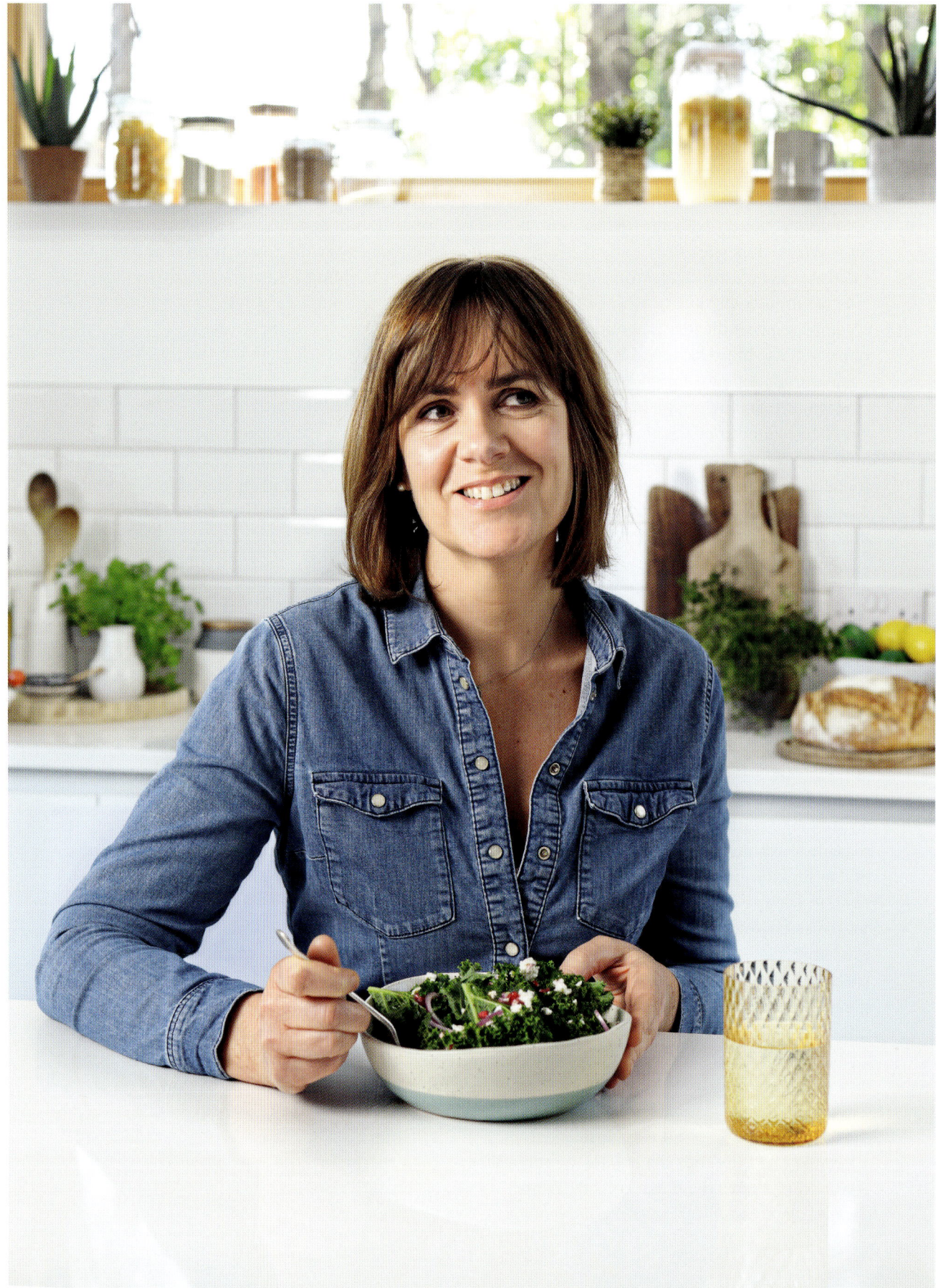

Blueberries

A good source of vitamin C and fibre (pectin), blueberries are also an excellent source of flavonoids – specifically, anthocyanins, which are responsible for the blue, purple and red colour pigments in fruits and vegetables. The antioxidant capabilities of blueberries are rated the highest among nearly all fruits.

A research study[22] published in *The Journal of Neuroscience* indicates that blueberries help to protect the brain from age-related cognitive decline, such as Alzheimer's disease. The research states that 'in addition to their known beneficial effects on cancer and heart disease, phytochemicals present in antioxidant-rich foods may be beneficial in reversing the course of neuronal and behavioural ageing'.

The current medicinal use for blueberries is for the prevention of age-related macular decline and improving night-time vision. Additional research indicates a protective element in the prevention of cataracts and glaucoma. There is also evidence of the medicinal benefits of blueberries in the treatment of urinary tract infections (UTIs). Blueberries contain the same protective compounds as cranberries, which can help to prevent frequent UTIs.

Store your blueberries by washing them in a little apple cider vinegar and water to remove any pesticides. Dry them off in a salad spinner and pat dry with a kitchen towel, then place in a glass food-storage container lined with kitchen paper – the drier the better, to prevent the spread of mould. Frozen blueberries are a great alternative to fresh blueberries in winter, and they're ideal for use in cooking.

Chocolate

Chocolate is rich in beneficial plant sterols and flavonoids. What's the flavonoid content per 100g of chocolate? Well, that depends on the percentage of cocoa solids:

- 100g of milk chocolate contains approximately 13mg of flavonoids
- 100g of chocolate with circa 50 per cent cocoa solids contains approximately 53mg of flavonoids
- 100g of chocolate with circa 85 per cent cocoa solids contains approximately 135mg of flavonoids

For the biggest flavonoid bang for your buck (and to gain the most medicinal benefits), choose chocolate with a minimum 70 per cent cocoa solids – ideally 85 per cent or above.

One of the key areas of research around chocolate focuses on its cardiovascular benefits. A surprising finding confirms that the saturated fat contained in chocolate does not elevate cholesterol levels. The flavonoids in chocolate are also protective against damage to the lining of the arteries[23]. In short, chocolate is good for your heart!

It is not just the high levels of flavonoids contained in chocolate but also other key compounds that can increase the bioavailability of the flavonoids in the body. The flavonoids are called pro-anthocyanins, which are also found in grape seeds, apples, berries and pine-bark extract. Additionally, chocolate provides arginine, an amino acid that makes nitric oxide. Nitric oxide causes blood vessels to dilate, improving blood flow and reducing blood pressure.

Dark chocolate is so high in antioxidant-rich polyphenols (which protect it from oxidation) that it will keep for a long time if stored correctly. It can pick up odours from other items, however, so never store them near onions and garlic, for example (unlikely, but it has to be said!). It is best to store your chocolate in an airtight container, or the fridge or freezer. Warm temperatures can cause surface white streaks called 'blooms' – this is the result of the cocoa butter rising to the surface. Chocolate with blooms is still safe to eat, though its flavour may be affected.

Green tea

The major polyphenols of green tea are flavonoids, which are responsible for its health benefits. The type of flavonoid contained in green tea is known as EGCG (epigallocatechin gallate), which is responsible for its antioxidant activity in the body.

Several animal studies[24] confirm that green-tea polyphenols can inhibit cancer by blocking the formation of cancer-causing compounds. Green tea is especially important in preventing breast cancer and prostate cancer. A 1998 study[25] specifically confirms that 'results indicate that increased consumption of green tea before clinical cancer onset is significantly associated with improved prognosis of stage I and II breast cancer'.

Drinking high-grade green tea is a good way to get your daily dose of caffeine. A 170ml cup of green tea contains approximately 10–15mg of caffeine, while a small espresso coffee (60ml) contains approximately 90mg of caffeine. The caffeine in green tea provides more relaxed awareness in comparison to the sledgehammer effect of regular coffee. In addition, green tea can increase your body's antioxidant activity, while also providing anti-cancer benefits.

Heat, moisture and light degrade the delicate medicinal properties of green tea. Store your green tea bags in an airtight container or glass jar. Once open, use them up quickly. Matcha-grade loose tea or powder should be stored in a cool dry place, away from direct light or heat. Matcha is one of the highest-grade green teas used in traditional Japanese ceremonies. It works well in desserts and chia puddings, too.

Key antioxidant vitamins

As we've seen, antioxidants can be found in many foods, and some of the most potent include vitamins A, C and E. These vitamins can help to protect us against cellular damage, can reduce inflammation and can support overall well-being for healthy ageing.

Vitamin A

A major player in our immune status, vitamin A is more widely recognised for the role it plays in our vision: a vitamin A deficiency can result in night blindness. Vitamin A is also beneficial for the structure of our skin, with many skin conditions responding well to the addition of vitamin A.

It is found in the highest concentrations in liver, cow's milk and fortified foods. However, it can also be formed from beta-carotenes (yellow and orange veg) and dark-green leafy veg like spinach and kale. Since vitamin A is a fat-soluble vitamin, it is prone to toxicity in high doses from animal sources. However, vitamin A from beta-carotenes found in plants exerts no toxicity.

Vitamin E

Another fat-soluble vitamin, vitamin E is sometimes referred to as ∂-tocopherol (from the Greek for 'to bear children') as a result of a study carried out in 1922 to restore fertility in rats. The main function of vitamin E is to protect against damage to cell membranes (especially nerve cells) and to promote skin healing.

Vitamin E is a key antioxidant required by the body, as it has a protective effect against heart disease, cancer and strokes. It is one of the top three antioxidants that round up the free radicals that can accelerate ageing.

The RDA is set at approximately 10mg or 15 IU (international units) per day, but a more accurate way of determining your requirement is based on the number of polyunsaturated fats you consume. The higher the amount, the greater your requirement for vitamin E.

Sources of vitamin E per 100g:
- **Wheat-germ oil:** 64 IU of vitamin E
- **Sunflower seeds:** 27 IU of vitamin E
- **Sunflower oil:** 18 IU of vitamin E
- **Almonds:** 13 IU of vitamin E
- **Wheat germ:** 6 IU of vitamin E
- **Avocados:** 2 IU of vitamin E

Vitamin C

Vitamin C is a water-soluble vitamin. This means that you pee it out all the time, which highlights the importance of eating vitamin C-rich foods every day, with every meal.

The primary function of vitamin C is the manufacture of collagen, the main protein substance of the body. Collagen supports the structures that hold our body together – that is, ligaments and tendons. Vitamin C is also critical to immune function and plays an important role in wound healing.

During increased times of physical, psychological or emotional stress, we can find ourselves peeing more, indicating a greater need for vitamin C during these times. Ensure you include extra vitamin C-rich foods in your diet, plus a high-quality supplement to keep your immune system strong.

Classic symptoms of vitamin C deficiency include bleeding gums, slow wound healing and excessive bruising. If you find yourself more susceptible to infections, or experiencing more frequent colds and flu, it is wise to increase your vitamin C intake. If you smoke, you naturally have a far greater requirement for vitamin C in comparison to a non-smoker.

The RDA for vitamin C is 60mg per day. When we think of vitamin C-rich foods, many of us immediately think of citrus fruits; however, red peppers, green leafy veg, broccoli and kiwis contain at least twice the amount of vitamin C in citrus fruits – so bear this in mind when trying to optimise your intake.

It's also important to note that vitamin C is destroyed by exposure to air. A slice of melon left in the fridge will lose up to 49 per cent of its vitamin C content in less than 24 hours, so it is best to consume freshly prepared fruits and vegetables to preserve their vitamin C content.

To summarise

In today's world, we are exposed to a variety of environmental stressors and toxins that can cause damage to our cells and tissues over time. This damage, known as oxidative stress, is thought to contribute to the development of chronic diseases such as cancer, heart disease and diabetes. One of the most effective ways to counteract this damage is to consume a diet rich in brightly coloured fruits and vegetables, which are packed with antioxidants that can help neutralise harmful free radicals and reduce oxidative stress in the body.

Other antioxidant-rich foods, such as nuts, seeds, wholegrains and oily fish, can also provide important nutrients that support overall health and well-being. By making an effort to incorporate these foods into our daily diets, we can help protect our bodies from the damaging effects of modern-day living and support optimal health and longevity.

6. Protein

What is it, and how does it work?

After water, protein is the most plentiful nutrient in our body. Protein is necessary for the structure of nearly every molecule in the body – in particular, hormones, neurotransmitters and enzymes.

Our recommended daily amount (RDA) of protein is usually calculated by body weight using this formula:

BODY WEIGHT IN KG X 0.80G = YOUR RDA OF PROTEIN

One of my key dietary recommendations for menopausal women is to increase the number of plant proteins they are eating and to reduce the number of animal proteins.

Why? A high intake of animal protein is linked to heart disease, many cancers, high blood pressure and kidney stones, as well as osteoporosis. Studies show that increased intake of animal protein from dairy products can lead to the excretion of calcium in the urine. A vegetarian diet rich in plant protein is associated with a reduced risk of developing these conditions.

Protein quality

Complete proteins contain all nine essential amino acids. Animal sources – that is, meat, fish and dairy – are examples of complete proteins.

Plant sources of proteins (grains and legumes) often lack one or more of these essential amino acids. However, they can become complete proteins when they are combined with each other. Combining two plant protein sources (for example, rice and beans) results in a complete amino-acid profile.

Good sources of plant proteins

- **Organic-certified soy products**, such as tofu. A 125g portion of tofu contains approximately 10g of protein, while 235ml soy milk provides around 6.5g of protein. In terms of protein quality, soy is considered equal to animal foods. Organic soy protein can also help to lower cholesterol in contrast to animal protein (casein in milk), which tends to raise cholesterol.
- **Quinoa** is one of only two grains that contains all nine essential amino acids (buckwheat being the other one). Quinoa is rich in magnesium, iron, zinc and B vitamins too. It is a great protein source for vegans.
- **Legumes** like adzuki beans, black beans, kidney beans, lentils and soybeans are good and inexpensive plant protein sources. They are low in calories, low in fat and high in fibre, all of which support heart health and help to lower cholesterol.

While beans and lentils are good sources of plant protein, they do not contain all nine essential amino acids like animal protein. They are typically low in two amino acids: tryptophan and methionine. I therefore recommend combining legumes with wholegrains, which are commonly higher in these missing amino acids. When eaten together, this results in a complete package of all nine essential amino acids, similar to that found in meat.

Legumes can also pose some digestive problems. They can cause increased intestinal gas, bloating, burping, flatulence or even discomfort. These common effects are caused by the oligosaccharides (starch-like molecules in the outer shell of the bean), which ferment in the gut. Soaking the beans or lentils in water overnight reduces gas production.

- **Hemp protein** is an exceptionally high-quality plant protein in terms of amino acid composition, containing all nine essential amino acids (similar to meat, milk and eggs). 100g of hemp seed contains approximately 29g of protein.

Hemp protein is easily digested and contributes to good levels of antioxidant activity. You can easily and effectively increase the nutritional value of your breakfast porridge, smoothies or bread recipes by adding either milled or shelled hemp seed.

The health benefits of hemp seed extend far beyond just protein. It is rich in the essential omega-3 fat linolenic acid, as well as being an excellent source of iron and B vitamins, plus trace minerals. Read more about the additional benefits of hemp in the digestive health section of part two.

Good sources of animal proteins

- **Eggs** contain the second-highest-quality food protein after whey protein (from cow's milk). They are considered a near-perfect food, with almost equal parts quality protein and fat (one large egg contains 6.3g of protein and 5.3g of fat, 1.3g saturated). Eggs are rich in vitamin K, and a good source of B vitamins, selenium and vitamin D. They are also rich in choline, a key component of our cell-membrane structures that is very important for brain function and health.

In the past, people with high cholesterol were told to avoid eggs. However, new research[26] confirms that instead of contributing to heart disease, eggs can actually lower the risk.

Where possible, always choose organic eggs. Free-roaming, organically raised hens are given a high-quality feed (usually omega-3 rich), which we then benefit from in turn. By contrast, industrially raised hens are given processed grains, often sprayed with pesticides and antibiotics. Industrially produced eggs contain no omega-3 fatty acids.

- **Chicken** is a good source of protein and vitamin B6, with free-range, organic chicken the best option in terms of quality. At the bottom of the page is a breakdown of the protein and fat numbers based on the cut of meat.
- **Salmon** is an oily, cold-water fish. Oily fish is extremely beneficial for heart and brain health, and salmon is an excellent source of protein (approximately 25g per 100g of salmon), potassium, selenium and vitamin B12, as well as niacin (vitamin B3).

Wild salmon usually contains higher amounts of omega-3s and protein than farmed salmon, which has higher omega-6 fatty acids (which drive inflammation). Wild

Protein and fat content of chicken

CUT	PROTEIN (G/100G)	TOTAL FAT (G/100G)	SATURATED FAT (G/100G)
Breast (skinless)	31	3.6	1.0
Leg (skinless)	28	5.7	1.5
Thigh (skinless)	27	8.4	2.3

Alaskan salmon tends to be the cleanest source of fish, as it typically contains the lowest levels of heavy metals and pesticides.

A research study[27] spanning more than 25 years examined the association between the consumption of omega-3-rich fish and the incidence of coronary heart disease (CHD), and concluded that 'Among women, higher consumption of fish and omega-3 fatty acids is associated with a lower risk of CHD, particularly CHD deaths'.

→ **Prawns** are an excellent source of protein, iron, selenium and vitamin B12, with 100g of prawns containing approximately 21g of protein and 195g of cholesterol. Scientific evidence[28] shows that despite their high levels of cholesterol, prawns do not raise serum levels of bad cholesterol (LDL-C); in fact, they can raise HDL-C.

Store your prawns by buying them fresh from your fishmonger and putting them in the fridge as soon as possible, on a bed of ice on the bottom shelf. If using frozen prawns, defrost in a bowl of cold water or allow them to thaw slowly overnight in the fridge.

Protein and mental health

Protein plays a key role in supporting our mental health. On a daily basis, we need an abundance of very specific raw materials that are contained in amino acids (the building blocks of proteins). We then need certain co-factor nutrients to convert these raw materials into neurotransmitters (the brain cells that support our brain chemistry).

Below is a summary of the different foods, amino acids and nutrients that play key roles in our mental health:

→ To make **dopamine** and **adrenaline** (the neurotransmitters that conduct signals), you need the amino acid tyrosine, which is found in high-protein foods such as eggs, soy foods, spirulina, poultry, dairy, fish and seeds (pumpkin and sesame).

→ To make serotonin (the happy hormone), which is the precursor to **melatonin** (the sleep hormone), you need the amino acid tryptophan, also found in high-protein foods.

You will get all you need if you eat some form of *complete* protein every day – that is, protein that contains all nine essential amino acids. For vegetarians, I recommend eggs, organic soy (tempeh, tofu), quinoa or a combination of beans and grains.

The co-factor nutrients that are required to convert these raw materials are:

→ **All the B vitamins** and **folate** are crucial for methylation. This is the complex biochemical process that the body uses to produce the brain chemicals and the myelin sheath that supports the nerve cells. Green leafy veg are the best source of folate. Research has shown that deficiency in either vitamin B12 or folate contributes to depression.

→ **Vitamin C** is a water-soluble vitamin that we need to consume every day, ideally with every meal. It is also a powerful antioxidant. It is contained in foods like yellow peppers, citrus, kiwi, strawberries, broccoli, sprouts and salad greens.

→ **Zinc** is one of the most important and abundant trace minerals in the brain. Zinc deficiency has been linked with depression and attention deficit hyperactivity disorder (ADHD). The best sources of zinc are green leafy veg, pumpkin seeds, sesame seeds, almonds and tofu.

→ **Copper** is an essential mineral that plays a key role in a number of bodily functions, including the production of red blood cells, the maintenance of nerve cells and support of the immune system. Good sources include soy, oysters, shitake mushrooms, sesame and sunflower seeds, as well as Brazil nuts, cashews and hazelnuts.

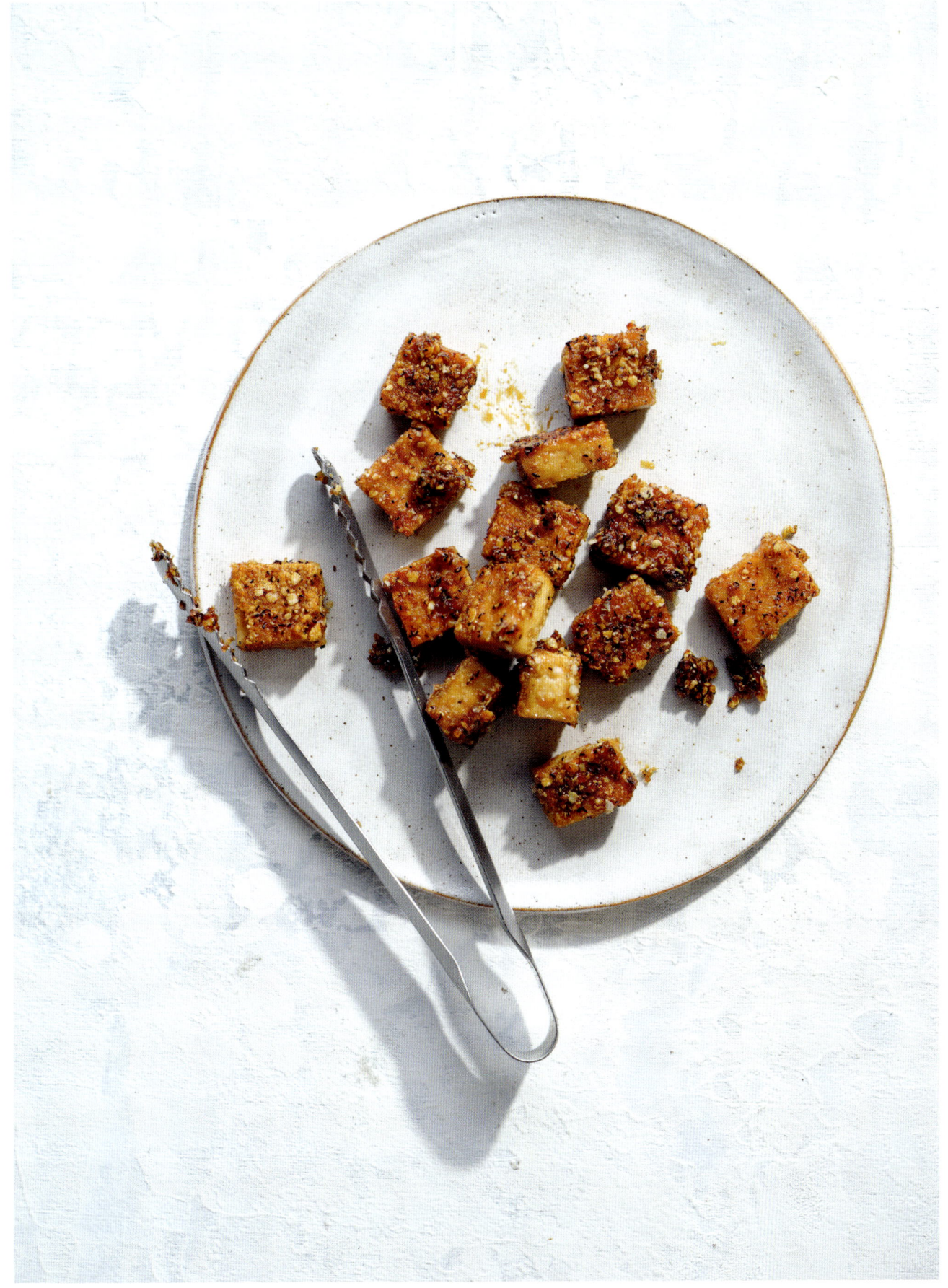

Protein and detoxification: optimising sulphur-containing foods

Sulphur is a component of four amino acids, and it is found in protein-rich foods like eggs, legumes and grains. Sulphur-containing proteins support phase II liver detoxification, which is when toxins are converted to water-soluble metabolites, enabling us to eliminate them via urine or a bowel movement. This is of particular benefit to women's health: the safe and effective elimination of old oestrogen prevents oestrogen dominance, which can lead to hormone-dependent cancers.

To summarise

Protein is an essential nutrient that is needed by the body to build and repair tissues, produce enzymes and hormones, and support a healthy immune system. Our bodies do not have a storage system for protein, unlike for carbohydrates and fats, so this means we need to consume it regularly to meet our bodies' needs. It can be found in a variety of foods – while many people think of meat and eggs as the primary sources of protein, there are also excellent plant-based sources such as legumes, nuts and seeds.

As we age, our bodies become less efficient at processing and using protein, so we may need to consume a greater volume of it to maintain muscle mass and support overall health. By including a variety of protein-rich foods in our diets, we can ensure that we are getting the nutrients we need to support optimal health and well-being as we get older.

7. Probiotics

What are they, and how do they work?

Probiotics are friendly bacteria that we want in abundance in our gut. The key strains are *Bifidobacterium* and *Lactobacillus.*

Prebiotics work in conjunction with probiotics; they are the nutrients that friendly bacteria need to survive and thrive – essentially, the food for probiotics. The key nutrients of prebiotics are fructooligosaccharides (FOS), short-chain fatty acids (SCFAs) and inulin (a type of insoluble fibre).

Introducing fermented foods

Fermented foods have played an important role in the diets of almost every society throughout the world. Examples of fermented foods include yoghurt, sourdough bread, apple cider vinegar, sauerkraut, kombucha and kimchi. Fermented foods are considered to be live, and are associated with wide-ranging health benefits, including that:

- Fermenting not only preserves food but also enhances the nutrient content of that food by increasing vitamin and enzyme levels
- Fermentation improves the digestibility of food, because the carbohydrates and sugars are broken down in the fermentation process, making it easier to absorb the nutrients contained
- The minerals in cultured foods are more readily available to the body

To grasp the principles of fermentation, it is a good idea to understand some of the basic science regarding the process, and that of lacto-fermentation in particular.

Lacto-fermentation

During fermentation, microorganisms such as yeast and bacteria convert sugars and other nutrients into alcohol, organic acids or gases. In the case of beer or wine, yeast is used to convert the sugar in grapes or grains into alcohol, resulting in the final product.

Fruit and vegetables, meanwhile, are converted into a fermented state by bacteria that turn their sugar into lactic acid. This process is what gives fermented foods their distinctive sour taste and helps to preserve them. This is known as lacto-fermentation.

The 'lacto' portion of the term refers to a specific species of bacterium, namely *Lactobacillus*. You may be familiar with *Lactobacillus acidophilus*, the acid-loving bacterium commonly used to make yoghurt. Beyond preservation advantages, *Lactobacillus* organisms produce antibiotic and anti-carcinogenic substances that contribute to good health – yet another reason to have an abundance of *Lactobacilli* residing in our intestinal tracts. The diets of every traditional society have included some kind of lacto-fermented food.

Let's take a closer look at some of the fermented foods that are popular today.

Yoghurt

Natural probiotic yoghurt contains live strains of bacteria (usually *Lactobacillus acidophilus*) that are very beneficial for our digestion. Depending on the yoghurt, there will be varying numbers of viable bacteria strains: home-made yoghurt usually contains higher numbers due to longer fermentation times in comparison to shop-bought yoghurt. Yoghurt can be helpful to alleviate stomach upset or excess intestinal gas.

There are anecdotal claims that yoghurt containing *Lactobacillus acidophilus* produces its own antibiotic effect, improves immunity, helps with allergies, improves skin health and more; however, these claims are still unproven, and research studies are under way.

Sourdough bread

Sourdough is a fermented food containing natural probiotics. It is easier to digest than regular bread because the flour is soaked for longer, and these natural probiotics feed your gut flora with good bacteria.

Unfortunately, real sourdough bread is not readily available. A lot of so-called sourdough breads on sale in supermarkets don't contain a naturally occurring yeast culture. I call them 'sour-faux'. They mostly have added yeast and a whole lot of additives that you simply don't need. This is not real sourdough bread and does not come with any health benefits.

If you want real sourdough bread, you can either make it yourself or buy from a reputable sourdough baker (check out realbreadireland.org). Making sourdough bread requires know-how, but this can be easily learned. I teach classes both in person and online, or you can try my four-seed rye sourdough bread recipe (see p256), a health-promoting, fibre-rich bread that requires little or no skill to make. All you need is a starter culture; please see the Resources section (p280) for more information.

Apple cider vinegar (ACV)

Apple cider vinegar is made by fermenting the sugar from apples and turning it into acetic acid – the active ingredient. Raw ACV contains the 'mother' and strands of proteins, enzymes and friendly bacteria that give it a murky appearance but also all the health benefits. A common dosage ranges from one teaspoon to two tablespoons per day. The best way to incorporate apple cider vinegar into your diet is to dilute it in a glass of water or to add it to salad dressings. Check out the recipe on p255 to make your own ACV.

ACV also has various other non-health-related uses, including hair conditioning, skin care and dental care.

The benefits of ACV

- **Kills harmful bacteria:** The active ingredient acetic acid can kill harmful bacteria or prevent them from multiplying. Studies show that it inhibits bacteria (like *E. coli*) from growing in food and spoiling it. It has a history of use as a disinfectant, cleaning agent and natural preservative.
- **Regulates blood sugars:** The most successful use of ACV to date is in patients with type 2 diabetes. ACV can help regulate high blood sugars and insulin sensitivity, especially after meals rich in refined carbs and sugars: it can reduce blood sugar by 34 per cent following the consumption of 50g of white bread. Two tablespoons of ACV before bedtime can reduce fasting blood sugar in the morning by 4 per cent. For these reasons, vinegar can be useful for people with diabetes, pre-diabetes and those who want to keep their blood-sugar levels low to manage their appetite.
- **Promotes weight loss:** Studies suggest that ACV can increase feelings of fullness and help you eat fewer calories, which leads to weight loss.
- **Improves cardiovascular health:** ACV lowers cholesterol and improves cardiovascular health by reducing triglyceride levels. It can also help to improve insulin sensitivity, which can lower the risk of diabetes (in turn a risk factor for heart disease); and it has been found to lower blood pressure, which is another important factor in reducing the risk of heart disease.
- **Anti-cancer benefits:** There is a lot of hype online about the anti-cancer effects of ACV. This needs to be researched more before any recommendations can be made.

Sauerkraut

Sauerkraut has been through the lacto-fermentation process, so it can help us maintain a healthy gut microbiome. It has a mildly acidic tanginess and can add a real flavour punch to salads or sandwiches.

Be aware that some shop-bought sauerkraut has been heated to prolong shelf life; this means the beneficial bacteria are no longer active. Always check the label or – better still – make your own. It couldn't be simpler (see my recipe on p250).

Kombucha

Originally from China, although it is also widely consumed in Eastern Europe, kombucha is the result of a fermentation process combining a kombucha mushroom with tea and sugar.

The kombucha mushroom is not actually a fungus, but a symbiotic culture of bacteria and yeast (SCOBY). Over the course of one or two weeks, the SCOBY – which looks somewhat like a pancake – converts the sugary tea solution into a kombucha drink.

This is a health-promoting beverage that contains many organic acids, active enzymes, amino acids, beneficial bacteria, probiotic microorganisms and polyphenols, as well as many B vitamins and vitamin C. It is used as a treatment for a huge range of health issues – from cancers and metabolic problems to arthritis, candida and kidney, stomach and bowel disorders.

Kombucha is a fun drink to make, and it tastes really good too. Given the right culturing time, the right conditions and a 'second ferment' to carbonate it or make it fizzy, it becomes a delicious drink, full of health benefits for people of all ages to enjoy.

To summarise

Probiotics have been found to provide a range of health benefits, from improving gut health and digestion to supporting immune function and mental health. Surprisingly, our gut microbiome, which is made up of trillions of bacteria and other microorganisms, is now considered to be a complex and dynamic organ system in its own right. Recent research has shed light on the important role that the gut microbiome plays in a wide range of bodily functions, including nutrient absorption, hormone production and immune-system function. By consuming probiotics in the form of fermented foods, we can help to support a healthy and diverse gut microbiome. This exciting area of research is still in its early stages, and there is much more to learn about the many ways in which the gut microbiome and probiotics can impact our health and well-being.

8. Brassicas

What are they, and how do they work?

Brassicas are vegetables that belong to the cruciferous family. This family contains more phytochemicals with researched anti-cancer properties than any other vegetable family[29].

A high daily intake of cruciferous vegetables can increase the action of enzymes that disable carcinogens. It has consistently been confirmed in population studies that the higher the intake of cruciferous vegetables, the lower the rates of cancer (particularly colon, prostate, lung and breast cancer).

The beneficial compounds in cruciferous vegetables are known as glucosinolates, and they are comprised of the following:
→ Indole-3-carbinole (I3C)
→ Sulphurophane
→ Diindolylmethane (DIM)

These glucosinolates work their magic by increasing antioxidant defence mechanisms. In addition, they improve our ability to detoxify effectively; for example, we know that I3C is particularly beneficial for the breakdown of old oestrogen for safe and effective elimination[30].

Let's take a look at some of the brassicas most commonly eaten today.

Cauliflower

Perhaps the most commonly eaten brassica, cauliflower is not as nutrient-dense as the other cruciferous vegetables but it still packs a good nutritional punch. It is rich in vitamin K, vitamin C, fibre, potassium and B vitamins. It has less chlorophyll and carotenes than kale and broccoli; this is due to its thick stalky leaves, which cover the florets and protect them from sunlight.

Cauliflower is also so versatile; it can be cooked and prepared in multiple ways, from cauliflower rice (see p264) or cauliflower mash to cauliflower steaks and lots more. I recommend storing your cauliflower stem-side down in the fridge to prevent moisture from developing in the florets, which could lead to mould.

Broccoli

Rich in vitamin C, broccoli is one of the most nutrient-dense foods, despite being low in calories. It contains similar amounts of protein to a cup of rice, but with less than one-third of the calories. It is also a high-fibre food containing plenty of the major minerals: magnesium, potassium and phosphorus.

Like cauliflower, broccoli contains glucosinolates (anti-cancer phytochemicals) – particularly I3C and sulphurophane, both of which enable the effective elimination of a form of harmful oestrogen (2-hydroxy-estrone) that has been linked to breast cancer. Sulphurophane is also very effective in treating digestive conditions like gastritis and acid indigestion. It has even been proven to help eradicate the notorious antibiotic-resistant *Helicobacter pylori*, which is responsible for ulcers and more.

Preliminary studies indicate that approximately 1kg of broccoli per week is adequate to benefit from these cancer-fighting compounds and cut your risk of cancer in half. Use broccoli in as many ways as possible, both raw and cooked. Raw broccoli is great in juices and smoothies, as well as part of a crudité selection. You can roast or lightly steam it ahead of time as part of your weekly meal prep and then add it to salads or omelettes.

Keep fresh green broccoli in the fridge in open packaging. Don't wash it before storing it. Avoid any moisture coming into contact with the broccoli to avoid bacteria forming on the florets, and use within four days.

Broccoli sprouts

Broccoli sprouts (or microgreens, as they are sometimes called) are miniature herb versions of their grown-up broccoli counterpart. They are rich in sulphurophane – in fact, they contain anywhere from 30 to 50 times the concentration of sulphurophane in comparison to full-sized broccoli.

Human trials[31] have demonstrated how the concentration of sulphurophane in broccoli sprouts can increase our detoxification enzymes, which increases our antioxidant activity, thus reducing our cancer risk. I3C is another important cancer-fighting compound contained in broccoli sprouts. The same concentration of sulphurophane and I3C found in 1kg of broccoli is contained within a mere 30g of broccoli sprouts, and I recommend including a mixture of both in your diet. Microgreens can be used in multiple ways: try adding them to smoothies or using them to top your salads, or as part of a filling for an omelette or sandwich. You can buy broccoli sprouts from microgreen growers or try your hand at growing them yourself.

Broccoli sprouts should be stored in the fridge, in the packaging in which they are purchased. If you grow them yourself, you can keep them in an airtight jar in the fridge. They should smell fresh and retain their colour. They will last for up to four days.

Kale

A true superfood, kale has many nutritional highlights. Firstly, it is a great source of calcium, and is therefore an excellent food source to include in your diet to reduce your risk of osteoporosis. Cooked kale delivers three times the concentration of calcium found in raw kale.

Kale is also rich in vitamin C: approximately

70g of kale gives you 70 per cent of your RDA of vitamin C. Considering that vitamin C is a water-soluble vitamin that we need to consume daily, in every meal, eating kale is a great way of optimising our intake of this important antioxidant.

Kale is also a great source of fibre and minerals. It contains copper, iron and calcium, all three of which are important for women's health and hormone balancing. In addition, kale has vitamins B1, B2 and E.

I recommend buying your kale leaves from either your greengrocer or local growers. De-stem the leaves and discard the stalk (which is very fibrous and difficult to digest). Wash the leaves well and spin-dry in a salad spinner before storing in a sealable, food-grade storage bag in the fridge. Your kale leaves will keep well like this for five to six days.

Kale is a versatile brassica; if using in a salad, mix or massage your dressing into the leaves ahead of serving. Kale is very fibrous, so it takes a while to break down. It is ideal to use in a make-ahead salad to take with you on the go. You can also finely slice it and add it to soups and stews, just before serving, for maximum nutrient impact, or add it raw to smoothies or juices. I also like to lightly steam kale and add to omelettes, pasta sauces or my tofu scramble recipe (see p80).

Cabbage

Cabbage is the head of the cruciferous vegetable family, which includes broccoli, cauliflower, Brussels sprouts, kale, radishes and turnips. There are three types of cabbage: red, green and savoy. All varieties contain a wealth of powerful nutrients, including:
→ Vitamin C
→ Vitamin B6
→ Vitamin B1 (biotin)
→ Folic acid
→ Calcium
→ Magnesium
→ Manganese

The anti-cancer properties of cabbage are the glucosinolates, also contained in all the other cruciferous vegetables mentioned above. These anti-cancer compounds are well documented[32], and it is recommended to regularly consume a wide variety of cruciferous vegetables to reduce your risk of cancer.

As well as these powerful anti-cancer benefits, cabbage is also very effective for the treatment of ulcers. Cabbage juice demonstrates rapid healing properties for peptic ulcers, and patients can often see results in seven days or less[33], as demonstrated in a study carried out by Dr Garnett Cheney at Stanford University in 1947:

> *Thirteen patients with peptic ulcers were treated with fresh cabbage juice, which, experiments have indicated, contains an anti-peptic ulcer factor. The average crater healing time for seven of these patients who had a duodenal ulcer was only 10.4 days, while the average time as reported in the literature, in 62 patients treated by standard therapy, was 37 days.*
>
> *The average crater healing time for the other six patients with gastric ulcers treated with cabbage juice was only 7.3 days, compared with 42 days, as reported in the literature, for six patients treated by standard therapy.*

The lack of public awareness about the benefits of cabbage juice for treating peptic ulcers could be due to a variety of reasons, including a lack of mainstream media coverage and limited research funding. Increased awareness via social media platforms, health forums and health blogs would encourage more people to consider natural remedies as a viable alternative to conventional medication for the treatment of peptic ulcers.

Cabbage is a very affordable superfood to start including more of in your diet. Buy cabbage whole and fresh – avoid pre-cut or shredded cabbage as the beneficial nutrients will have already been depleted. Store it in the fridge to retain maximum nutrient concentration. Once you cut open the cabbage, the vitamin C content will deplete quickly, so wrap it tightly in cling film or place it in an airtight container in the fridge.

Raw cabbage can also be shredded in a food processor and used for salads or coleslaw (see p92). It is also the base ingredient for sauerkraut (see p250), which amplifies and increases the cabbage's nutrient content even further through the fermentation process. Sauerkraut is a great addition to salads, sandwiches and wraps. For a tasty alternative to boiled cabbage, try my roasted cabbage steaks recipe (see p273).

To summarise

Brassicas are versatile and easy to incorporate into your diet. They can help to reduce the severity of menopausal symptoms, such as hot flushes and night sweats, and have several other health benefits, including supporting heart health by lowering levels of LDL cholesterol and improving bone health (as they are a good source of calcium). Brassicas also contain high levels of antioxidants – they are rich in compounds like vitamin C, carotenoids and flavonoids – and can help to protect against oxidative stress and chronic diseases.

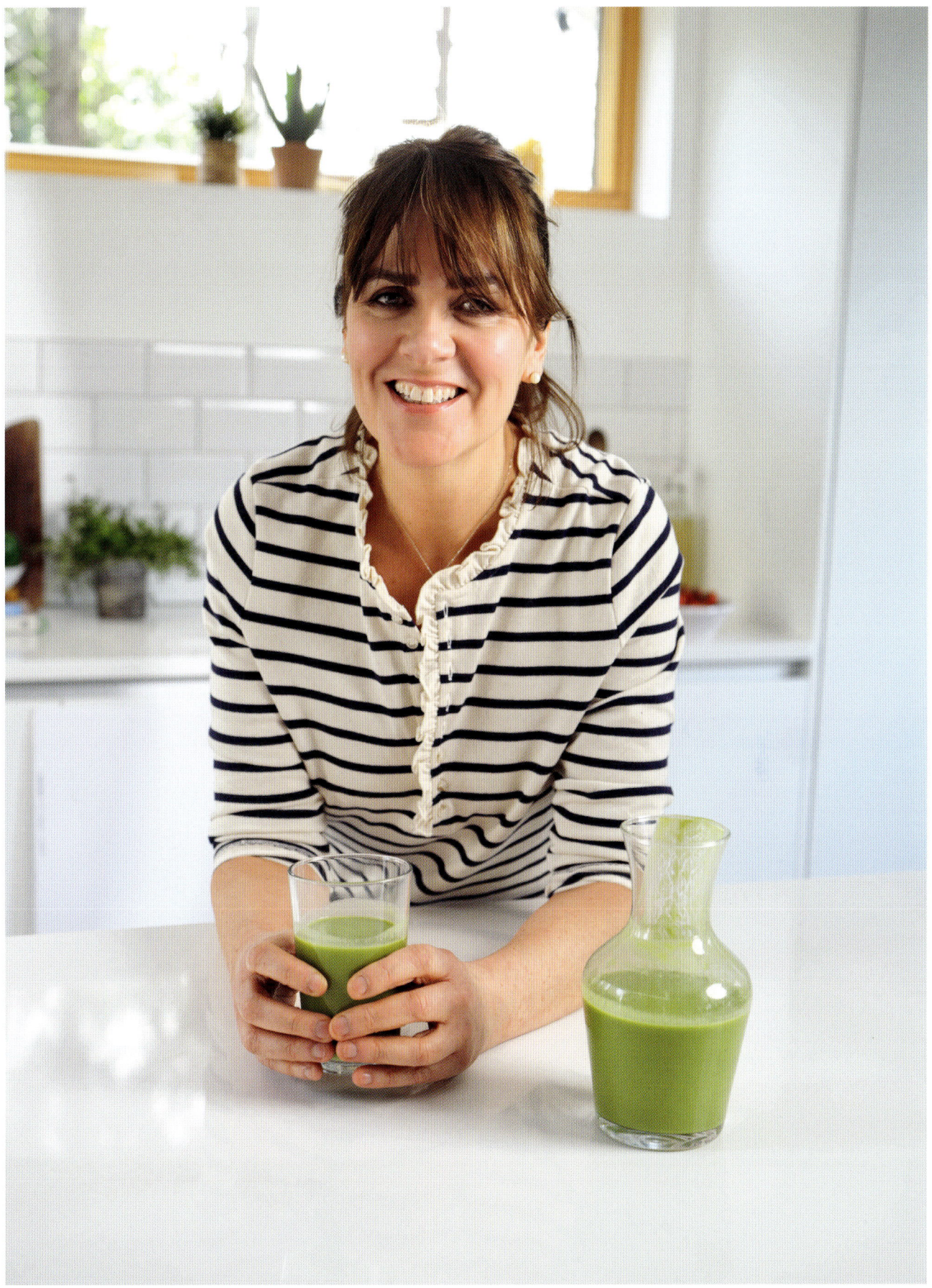

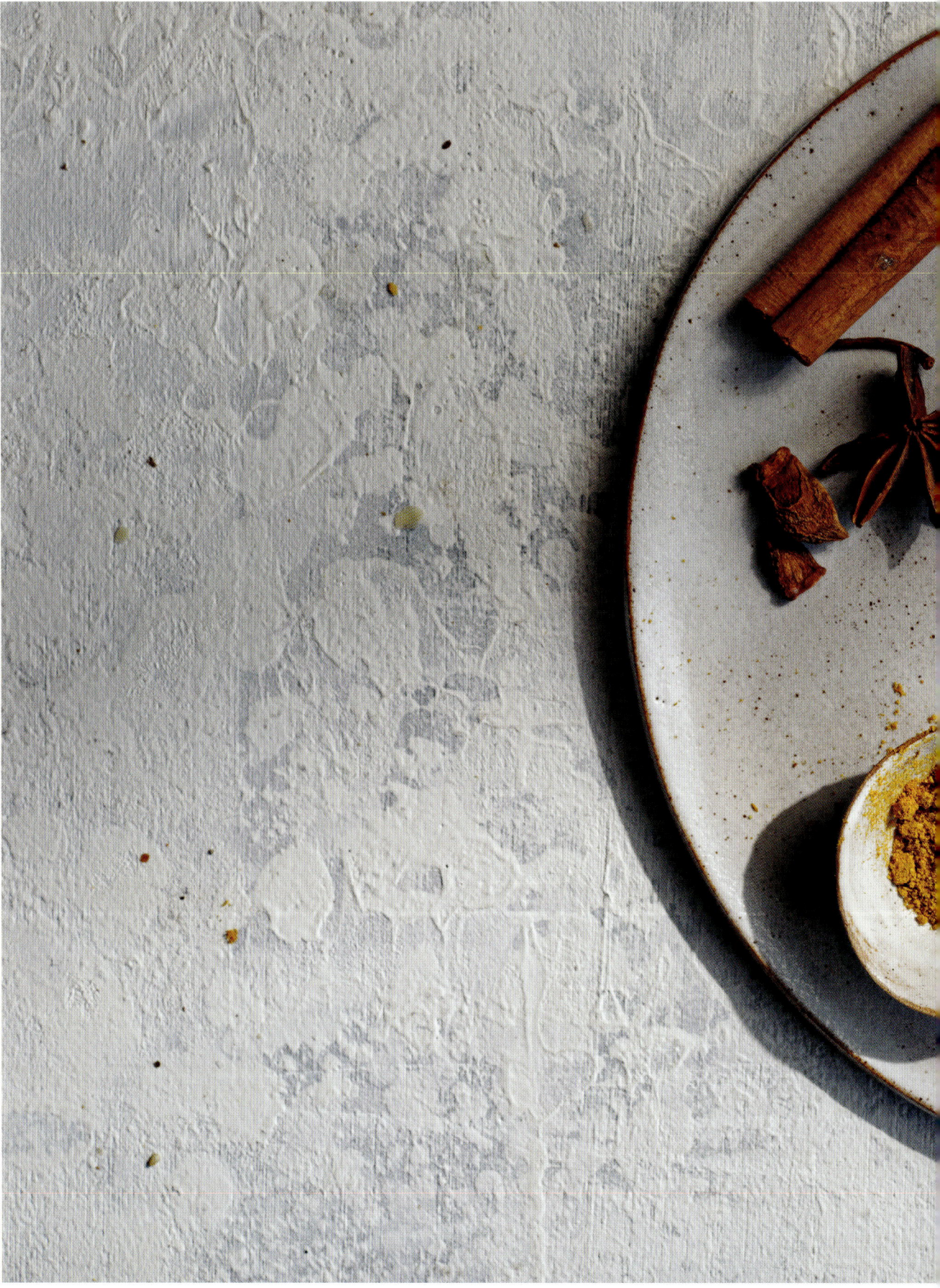

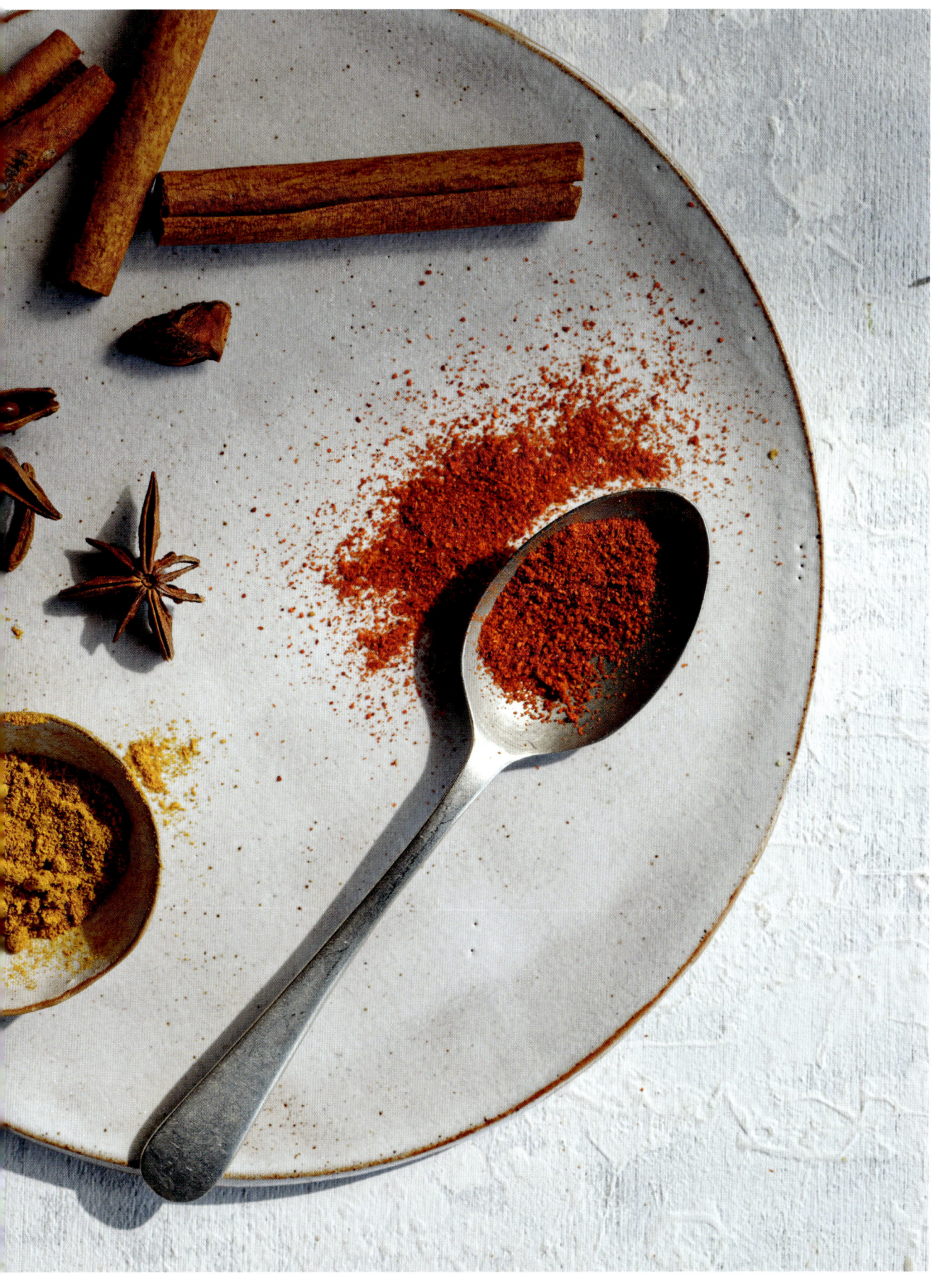

Part four: Recipes

1. Phytoestrogens

Phytoestrogens are naturally occurring plant compounds found in soy, flaxseed, nuts, wholegrains and more. They do not increase our levels of oestrogen but simply mimic the effect of the hormone, as if our body was naturally producing more. Including phytoestrogen-containing foods in your diet can help regulate your body temperature – reducing the frequency and intensity of night sweats – and improve your bone health, and have been associated with lowering the risk of heart disease and cancer. Phytoestrogens also have anti-inflammatory properties, which can improve overall bodily health.

All the recipes in this section are really tasty and will hopefully change your mind for the better about tofu! I particularly love the crispy tofu Thai red curry – it's a winner for a warming midweek meal.

Tofu Scramble

with spinach, garlic and mushrooms

Ingredients
1–2 tsp olive oil
1 clove of garlic, finely chopped
1 small white onion, finely chopped
100g mushrooms, sliced
200g firm organic tofu, broken into small pieces
1 tbsp nutritional yeast flakes, mixed into a paste with 1 tbsp water
handful of spinach leaves
1 tsp turmeric
1 tsp cumin
1 tsp lemon juice
1 tsp soy sauce
1 tsp chilli flakes (optional)

SERVES: 2

Not only does this filling veggie dish taste delicious, it also reheats well. If you haven't eaten tofu before, this is a good place to start, as this recipe requires no marination.

1. Heat the oil in a deep-sided frying pan and sauté the garlic for around 10 seconds.
2. Just as the garlic begins to brown, add the onion and mushrooms. Continue to sauté for 3–4 minutes until the onion begins to become translucent.
3. Add the tofu to the pan and cook for around 5 minutes, stirring to break the tofu up further until it resembles scrambled eggs in texture.
4. Add the yeast paste, the spinach leaves and all of the other ingredients to the pan.
5. Continue to cook, stirring continuously until everything is thoroughly mixed and warmed through. Serve on a slice of porridge bread or a grilled portobello mushroom, or with some avocado and cherry vine tomatoes.

PER 200G PORTION

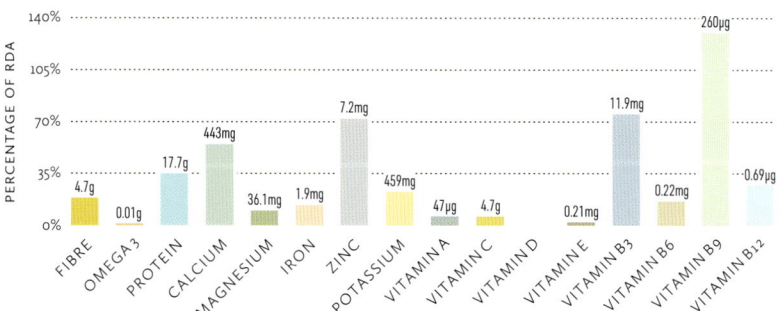

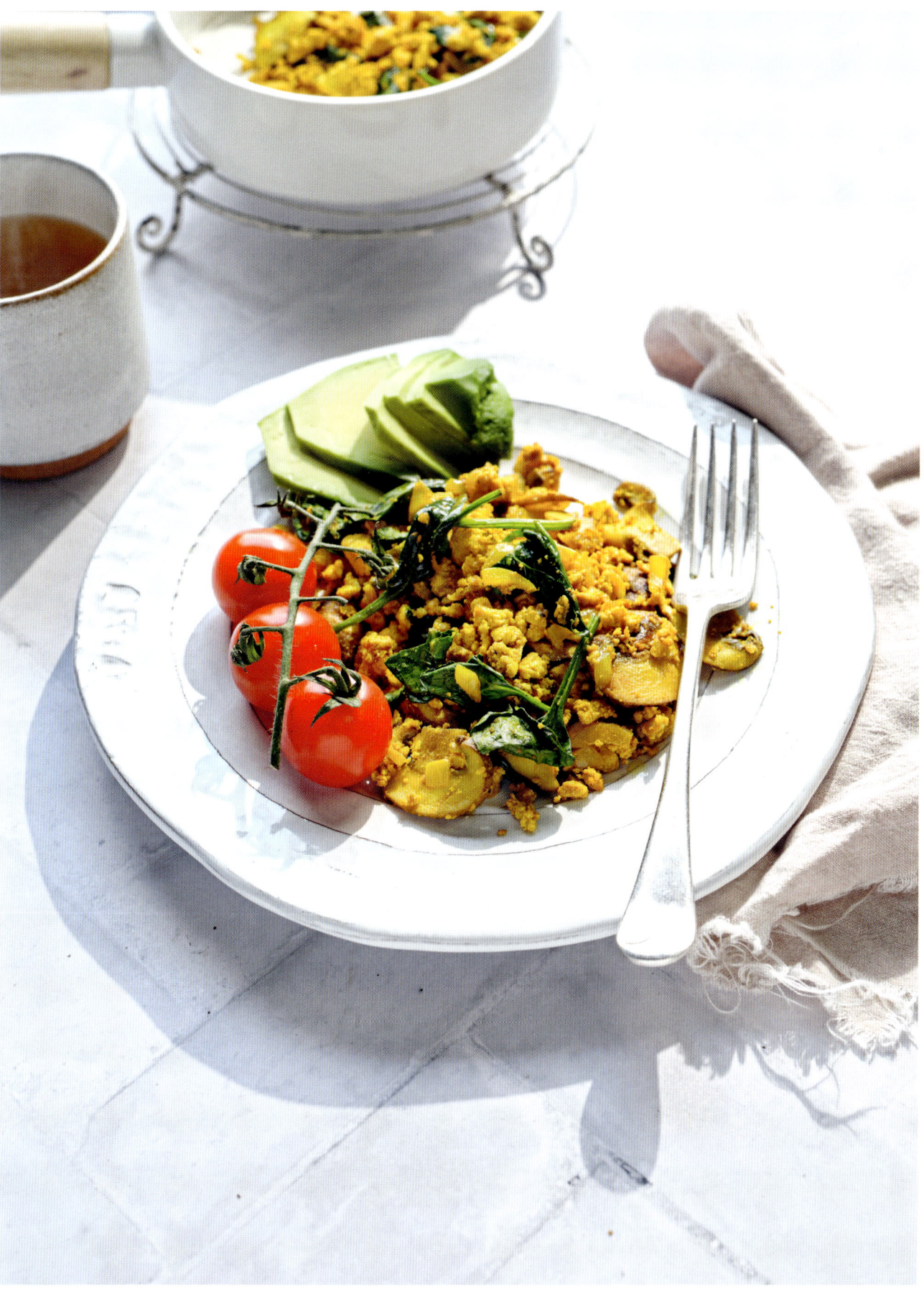

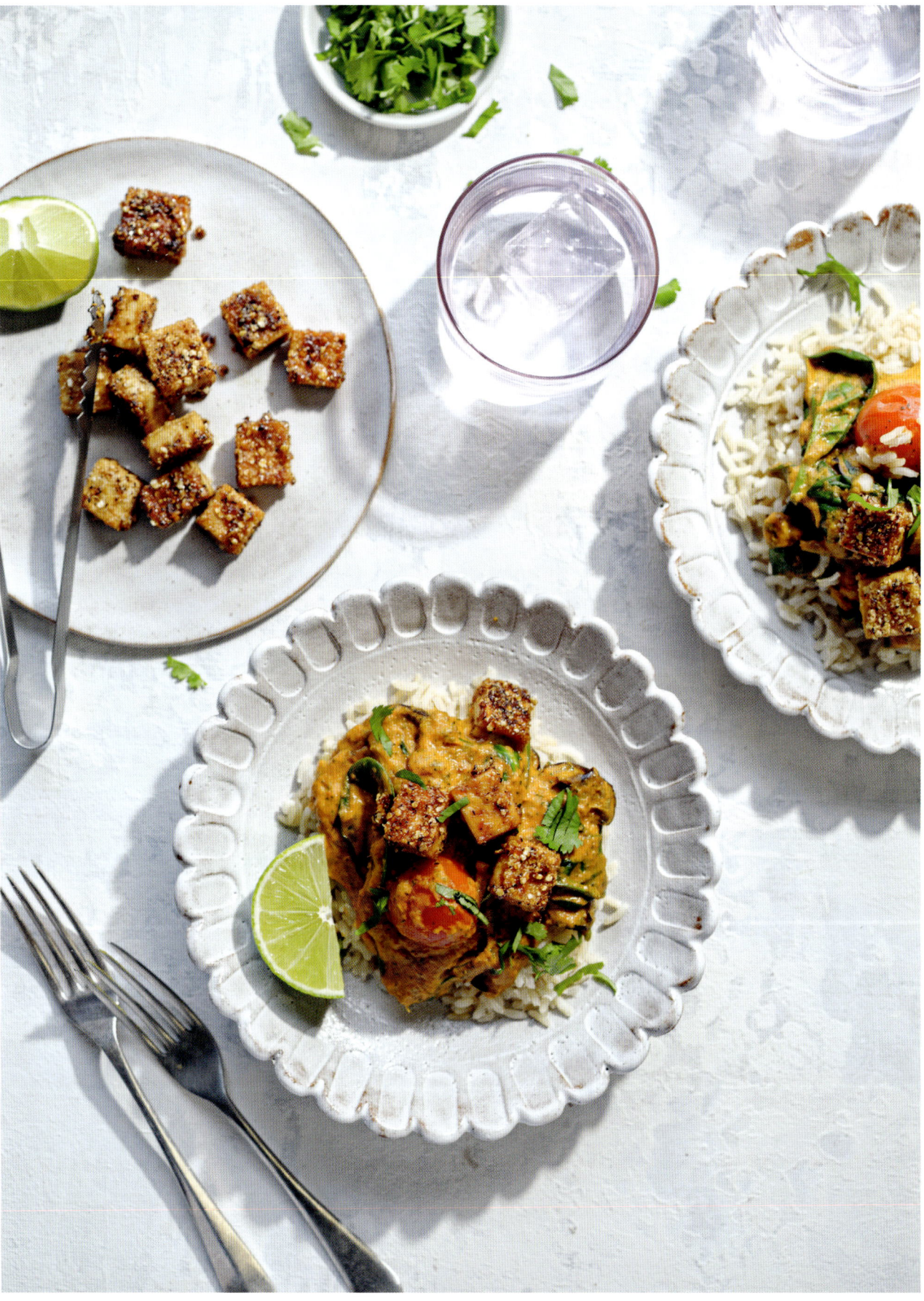

Crispy Tofu Thai Red Curry

with wholegrain rice

CURRY PASTE

- 2 sticks of lemongrass, peeled and chopped
- 1 tbsp tomato purée
- 4 roasted red peppers, skins and seeds removed
- 40g fresh coriander
- green tops of 1 bunch of spring onions
- ½ chilli or ¼ tsp dried chillies
- 4 fat cloves of garlic
- 30g freshly grated ginger
- 8–10 frozen lime leaves
- 2 tbsp soy sauce
- 1 tsp fish sauce (optional)
- 1 tsp sesame oil

SAUCE

- ½ aubergine, sliced into rounds
- 1 tbsp olive oil
- pinch of salt
- 140g light coconut milk
- 4 cherry tomatoes
- ¼ bag of baby spinach leaves

TOFU

- 200g tofu, cubed
- 30g quinoa flakes
- 1½ cloves of garlic
- 1½ tbsp soy sauce
- 1 tsp sesame oil
- 1 tbsp maple syrup
- 1 tbsp walnut oil

TO SERVE

- 200g wholegrain rice
- 2 tbsp flaked almonds, toasted
- 2 tbsp coriander, chopped
- pinch of red pepper flakes (optional)

SERVES: 2

Packed full of goodness, this versatile and tasty recipe can be adapted to include chicken or prawns. Some of its elements – for example, the Thai red curry paste – can be prepped in advance.

1. Preheat the oven to 180°C.
2. Make the Thai red curry paste by combining all the ingredients in a food processor or blender and blitzing to a smooth paste.
3. Lay the aubergine slices flat on a baking sheet. Brush with olive oil and sprinkle with a little salt, then roast in the oven for about 10 minutes, or until lightly brown. Remove from the oven and allow to cool. (This can also be prepped in advance.)
4. Start cooking the rice.
5. Put the tofu in a bowl with the quinoa flakes. Cover and shake, or simply mix until the tofu is well coated in the quinoa.
6. Combine the garlic, soy sauce, sesame oil and maple syrup for the tofu marinade in a small bowl, and set aside until ready to use.
7. Make the sauce. In a large wok, add 200g of Thai red curry paste, the coconut milk and cherry tomatoes. Gently heat through, mixing until everything is well combined, then add the baby spinach leaves and roasted aubergine slices.
8. Next, cook the tofu. In a separate frying pan, heat the walnut oil for a minute or so (it should get really hot). Add the cubed tofu pieces – they should sizzle when they hit the hot pan. Fry for a few minutes before using tongs to turn over. The goal is to get them really crispy on all sides. Once you have achieved this, quickly add your tofu marinade and mix well to coat all the pieces. Remove from the heat and set aside. >

9   To serve, plate up a good portion of rice (you can also use cauliflower rice, see p264), add 2 ladles of sauce beside it, top with 2 tablespoons of crispy marinated tofu, toasted flaked almonds and chopped coriander, and finish with red pepper flakes (if available).

Tip: The Thai red curry paste yields enough for at least four portions. You can freeze this, if needed, though it also keeps in the fridge for several days.

PER 630G PORTION (INCL. 100G RICE)

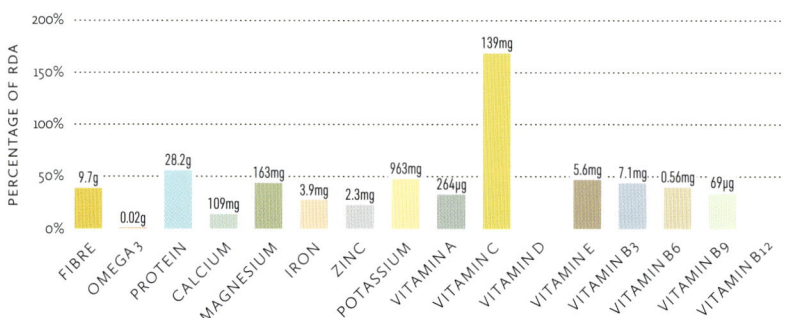

Roasted Aubergine Involtini

with Med veg tofu, tomato and sweet potato sauce

AUBERGINE LAYER

2 whole aubergines, finely sliced lengthways (about 0.5cm thick)

olive oil, for brushing

pink Himalayan salt, to taste

TOFU FILLING

200g roasted Mediterranean vegetables (see p197)

25g fresh basil leaves, de-stemmed

2 tbsp sun-dried tomatoes in oil

2 tbsp nutritional yeast

400g organic firm tofu

pink Himalayan salt and black pepper, to taste

TOMATO SAUCE

1 tbsp olive oil

2 red onions, finely chopped

4 cloves of garlic

800g tinned organic chopped tomatoes

1 small sweet potato, peeled and diced

salt and pepper, to taste

1 tbsp maple syrup

VEGAN PARMESAN

½ cup flaked almonds

1 tbsp nutritional yeast

1 tsp garlic powder

salt and pepper, to taste

SERVES: 6

A healthy plant-based twist on an Italian classic, this is great as either a starter or a main course. It can be served directly to the table and shared family-style.

1. Preheat the oven to 200°C and line two baking sheets with parchment paper (or use silicone baking sheets).
2. Lay the aubergine slices on the sheets and brush with olive oil on both sides. Season with Himalayan salt.
3. Roast until light golden brown (about 12–15 minutes).
4. Next, make the tofu filling. Put the roasted Med veg in a large mixing bowl and set aside.
5. Blend the basil leaves, sun-dried tomatoes and nutritional yeast in a food processor.
6. Break up the tofu in a mixing bowl with a fork. Add the basil and sun-dried tomato mixture and mash through. The texture should be slightly rough, not smooth like baby food.
7. Add the tofu mix to the roasted Med veg and combine well. Taste and season with salt and pepper if needed.
8. For the tomato sauce, heat the olive oil in a medium-sized saucepan.
9. Add the onions and 3 finely chopped cloves of garlic; place the lid on and allow to sweat for 6–8 minutes.
10. Add the tinned tomatoes and diced sweet potato to the pot. Season with salt and pepper, and cook for 15 minutes with the lid on.
11. Meanwhile, make your vegan Parmesan by blitzing together the almonds, yeast, garlic powder and seasoning.
12. Remove your pot from the heat. Grate in the last clove of garlic and add the maple syrup to taste. Blend until smooth.
13. To assemble the involtini, add 1 tbsp of tofu mix to each aubergine slice, spreading it out evenly end to end. Roll up and repeat for each aubergine slice.
14. Spoon some of the tomato sauce into the bottom of a casserole dish, and start adding the aubergine rolls, packing them in tight side by side until the casserole dish is full. >

15 Spoon some more of the tomato sauce over each aubergine roll.
16 Sprinkle with vegan Parmesan.
17 Bake at 200°C for 25 minutes. Sprinkle with more vegan Parmesan and serve piping hot.

PER 420G PORTION

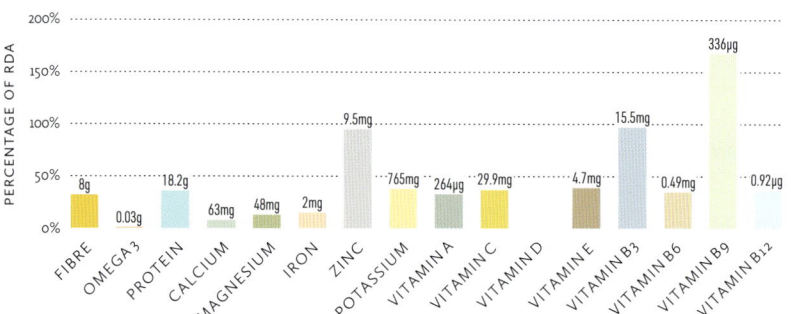

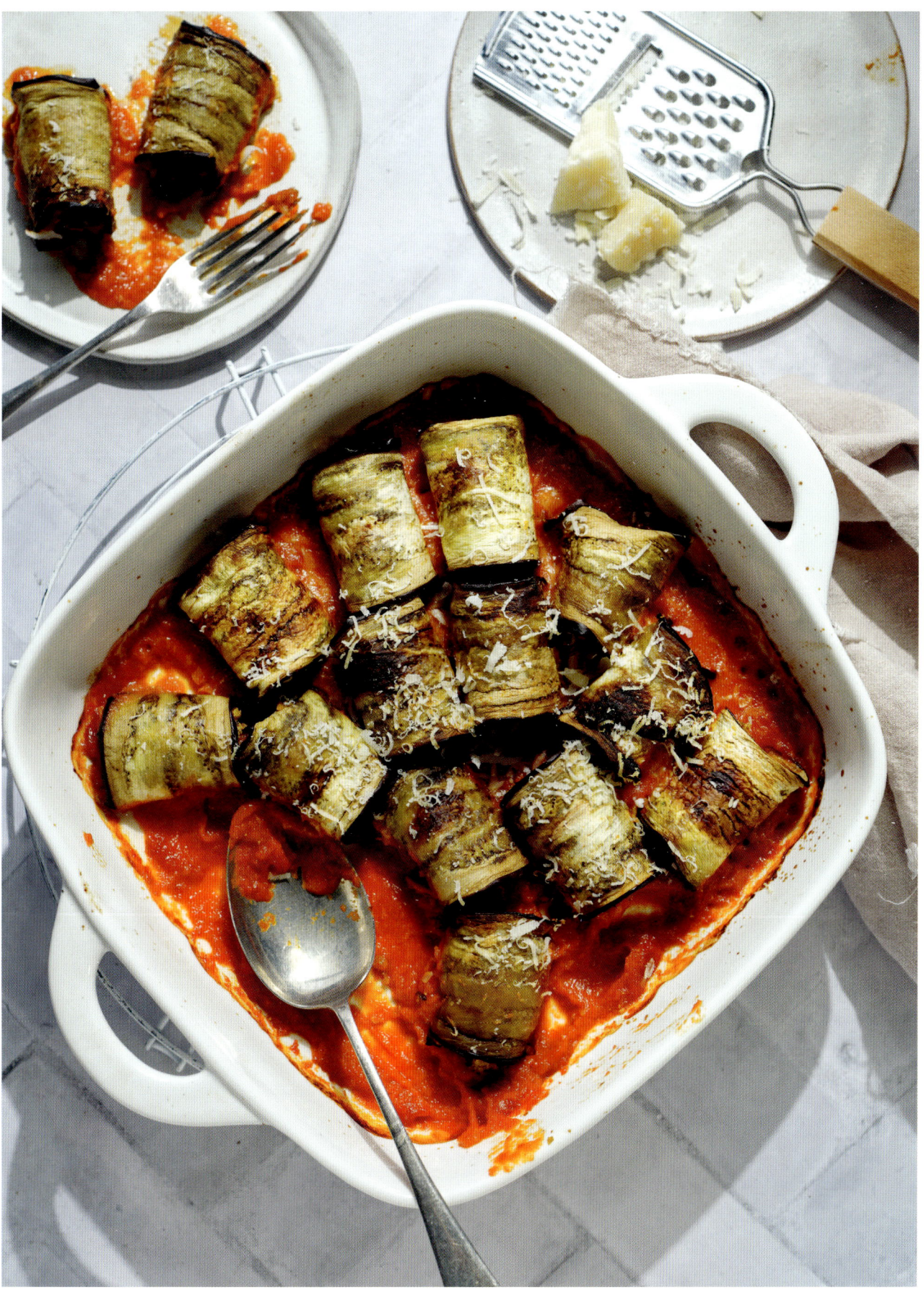

Ramen Bowl

with crispy tofu and miso

TOFU

200g tofu, cubed

30g quinoa flakes

1½ cloves of garlic

1½ tbsp soy sauce

1 tsp sesame oil

1 tbsp maple syrup

1 tbsp walnut oil

BROTH

200ml vegetable broth

200g soba noodles

thumb-sized piece of ginger, peeled and grated

75g sweetcorn

2 handfuls of baby spinach leaves

1 level tsp white miso paste

½ tsp pink Himalayan salt

1 nori seaweed sheet, cut into squares

¼ spiralised courgette

1 spring onion, finely sliced

TO SERVE

handful of coriander, chopped

½ avocado, sliced

handful of broccoli sprouts

SERVES: 2

This warming bowl of goodness is packed with phytoestrogens and plant protein.

1. Put the tofu in a bowl with the quinoa flakes. Cover and shake or mix until the tofu is well coated in the quinoa.
2. Mix the garlic, soy sauce, sesame oil and maple syrup for the tofu marinade in a small bowl; set aside until ready to use.
3. Heat some walnut oil in a saucepan. When the pan is hot, fry the coated tofu pieces, turning them until they are crispy and golden on all sides. Add the marinade to the hot pan and mix well for a minute on the heat. Remove the pan from the heat and keep warm.
4. Bring your veggie broth (I like to make this using Marigold bouillon powder) to the boil and cook the soba noodles in it for 5 minutes, until just tender. Using tongs, lift the noodles out of the broth and divide them between two serving bowls.
5. Add the ginger, sweetcorn and spinach leaves to the broth, and warm through for a minute over a low heat. Remove from the heat, add the miso paste, season with salt and and mix well before dividing the broth between the two bowls.
6. Add the remaining ingredients to the bowl: nori seaweed pieces, spiralised courgette and spring onions. Top each bowl with crispy tofu, chopped coriander, avocado and broccoli sprouts.

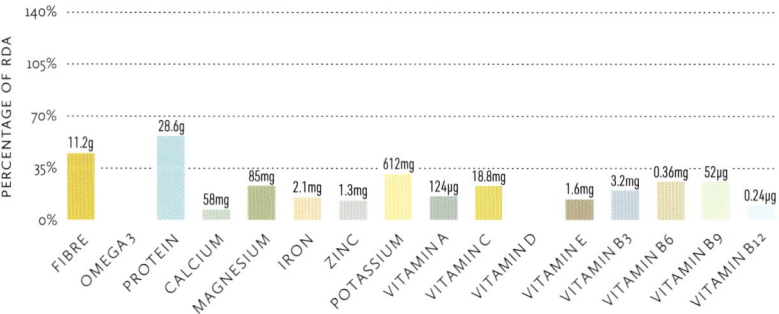

PER 650G PORTION

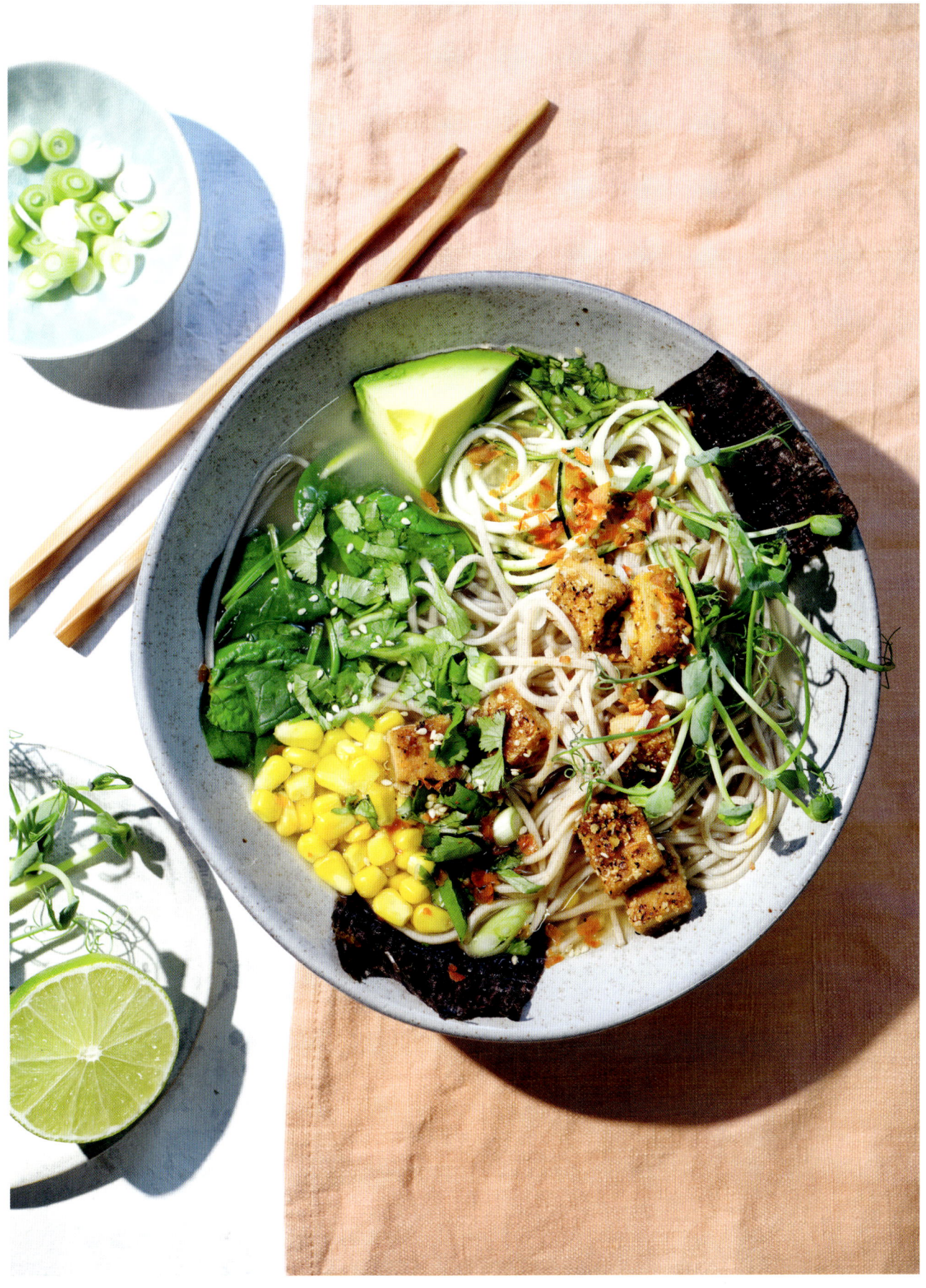

Sweet Potato, Lentil, Shitake, Tofu and Lemongrass Curry

with green banana sambal

CURRY

1 tbsp sesame oil

1 red onion, diced

1 leek, finely sliced

2 large cloves of garlic, minced

1 small red chilli, finely chopped

2.5cm piece of ginger, peeled and grated

1 tsp organic curry powder

1 tsp turmeric

1 tsp cumin

1 large sweet potato, peeled and chopped into bite-sized chunks

2 red peppers, cut into chunks

150g fresh shitake (or regular) mushrooms

230g organic lentils

400ml half-fat coconut milk

50–70ml veg stock

6–8 frozen lime leaves

crushed seeds of 3–4 cardamom pods

3 lemongrass stalks

pink Himalayan salt, to taste

crispy tofu (optional, see p83)

SAMBAL

1 small green banana, sliced into small chunks

1 tsp lemon juice

6g desiccated coconut

SERVES: 6

The tofu is optional in this fragrant curry, as there is adequate plant protein in the lentils and immune-boosting mushrooms.

1. Put the sesame oil, onion and leek in a large stockpot, and allow to soften.
2. Add the garlic, chilli and ginger and stir to combine.
3. Add the curry powder, turmeric and cumin, followed by the sweet potatoes, red peppers and shitake mushrooms. Mix everything, then add the lentils.
4. Add just over half the coconut milk and all the stock mixture, lime leaves and crushed cardamom seeds.
5. Bash the ends of the lemongrass stalks with a meat tenderiser to open up the flavours. Place these straight into the curry and cover with the liquid.
6. Season with Himalayan salt, bring up to simmer and allow to cook gently for 30–40 minutes until the sweet potato is soft.
7. Meanwhile, make your green banana sambal by adding all the ingredients into a bowl and mashing gently to mix well.
8. Once your curry is cooked, add the remaining coconut milk and the crispy tofu (if using).
9. Serve in a bowl alongside your banana sambal. My go-to accompaniments are brown basmati rice, toasted cashews and chopped coriander.

PER 365G PORTION

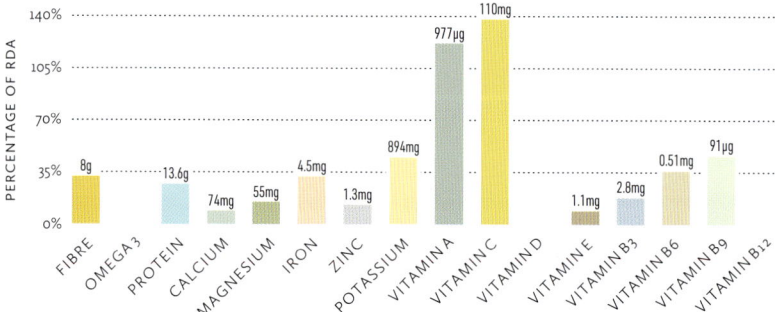

Edamame Bean Hummus

500g frozen edamame beans, shelled

60g tahini

1 tsp lemon zest

juice of 1 lemon

1 tbsp olive oil

60ml plant milk, such as organic soy milk

2 cloves of garlic

½ tsp cumin

½ tsp coriander

1 tsp pink Himalayan salt

ground black pepper, to taste

SERVES: 8

A new take on hummus – no chickpeas! Edamame beans are a type of soybean, packed full of fibre and isoflavones. This can be enjoyed as a snack with veg sticks or my tasty home-made savoury granola (see p122).

1. Boil a pot of water and add the frozen edamame beans. Bring back to the boil and cook for about 5 minutes. Remove from the heat, drain and allow to cool.
2. Combine all the other ingredients in a food processor.
3. When cool, add the edamame beans to the food processor and blitz until smooth.
4. If your hummus is too thick, add a drop of water and/or some more plant milk, and then serve. I like to finish it off with a drizzle of olive oil, fresh chopped herbs and a sprinkling of cumin.

Tip: Edamame beans can usually be found in the freezer section of the Asia Market or your local equivalent.

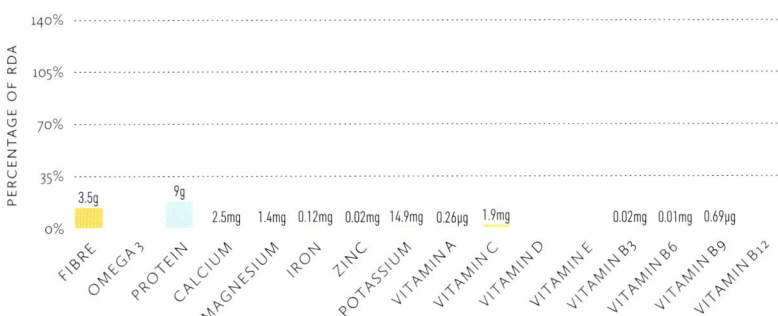

PER 85G PORTION

Edamame and Sesame Rainbow Slaw

¼ red cabbage

2 carrots

1 small fennel bulb

100g frozen edamame beans, shelled

2 spring onions, finely sliced

4 radishes, finely sliced

1 bunch of fresh coriander, chopped

6 tbsp ginger miso dressing (see p96)

sea salt and black pepper, to taste

handful of broccoli sprouts

20g white sesame seeds, toasted

1–2 tbsp savoury granola (see p122)

SERVES: 10

Edamame beans and sesame seeds are rich in isoflavones – plant compounds that mimic the oestrogen we produce ourselves. This salad is the ideal accompaniment to a falafel wrap (see p223) or a lentil and mushroom burger (see p228), or you can serve it as a side for a summer barbecue.

1 Shred the red cabbage, carrots and fennel in a food processor, one at a time, and put in a large bowl.
2 Flash cook the edamame beans in boiling water, drain and allow to cool.
3 Add the spring onions and radishes to the bowl with the rest of the vegetables.
4 Add the cooled edamame beans and coriander, drizzle over the dressing and toss together until well coated. Season with sea salt and black pepper.
5 Top with broccoli sprouts, toasted sesame seeds and savoury granola, and serve.

PER 90G PORTION

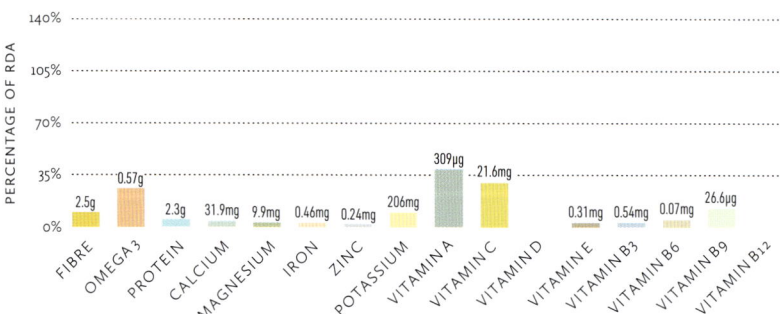

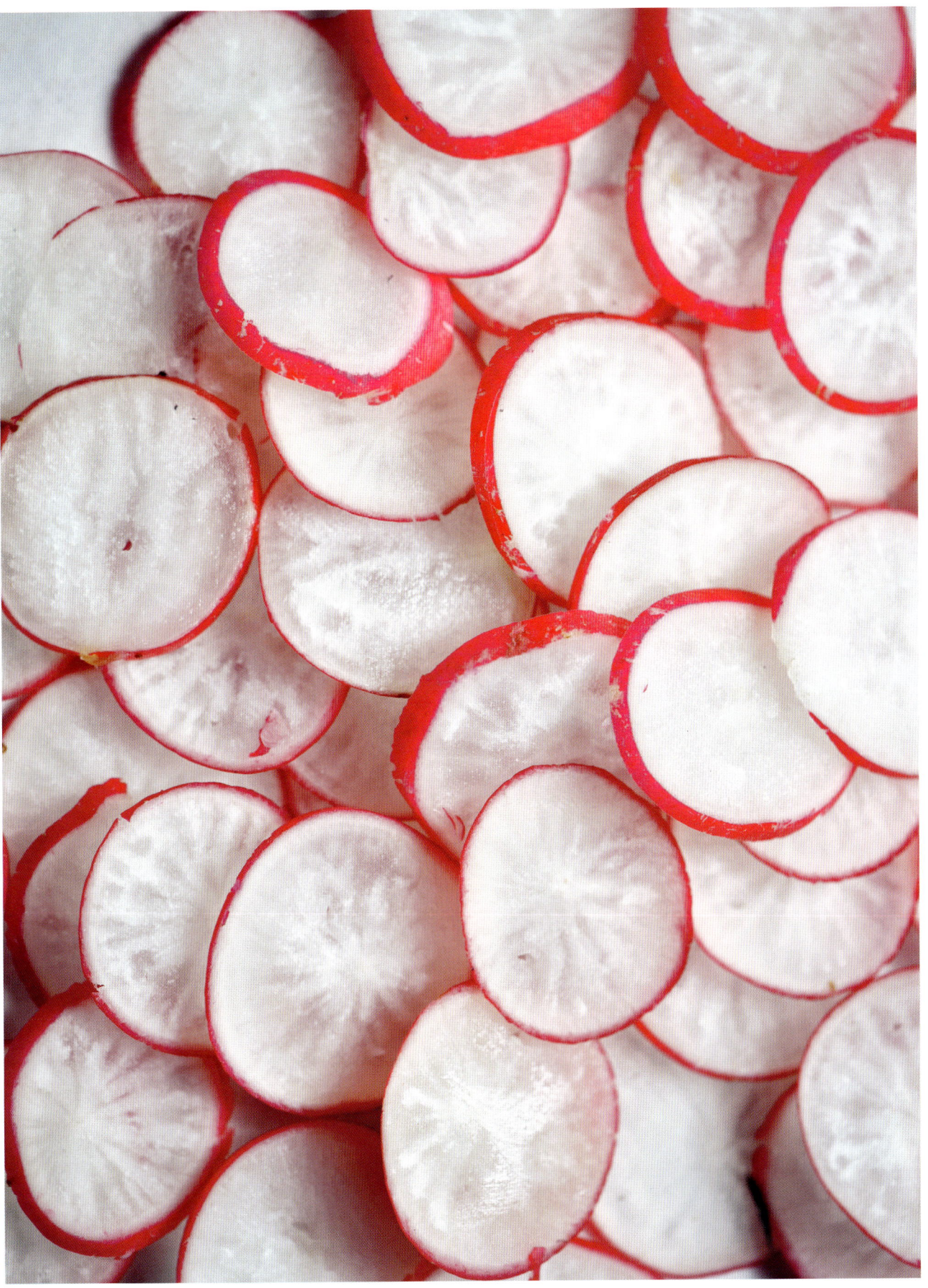

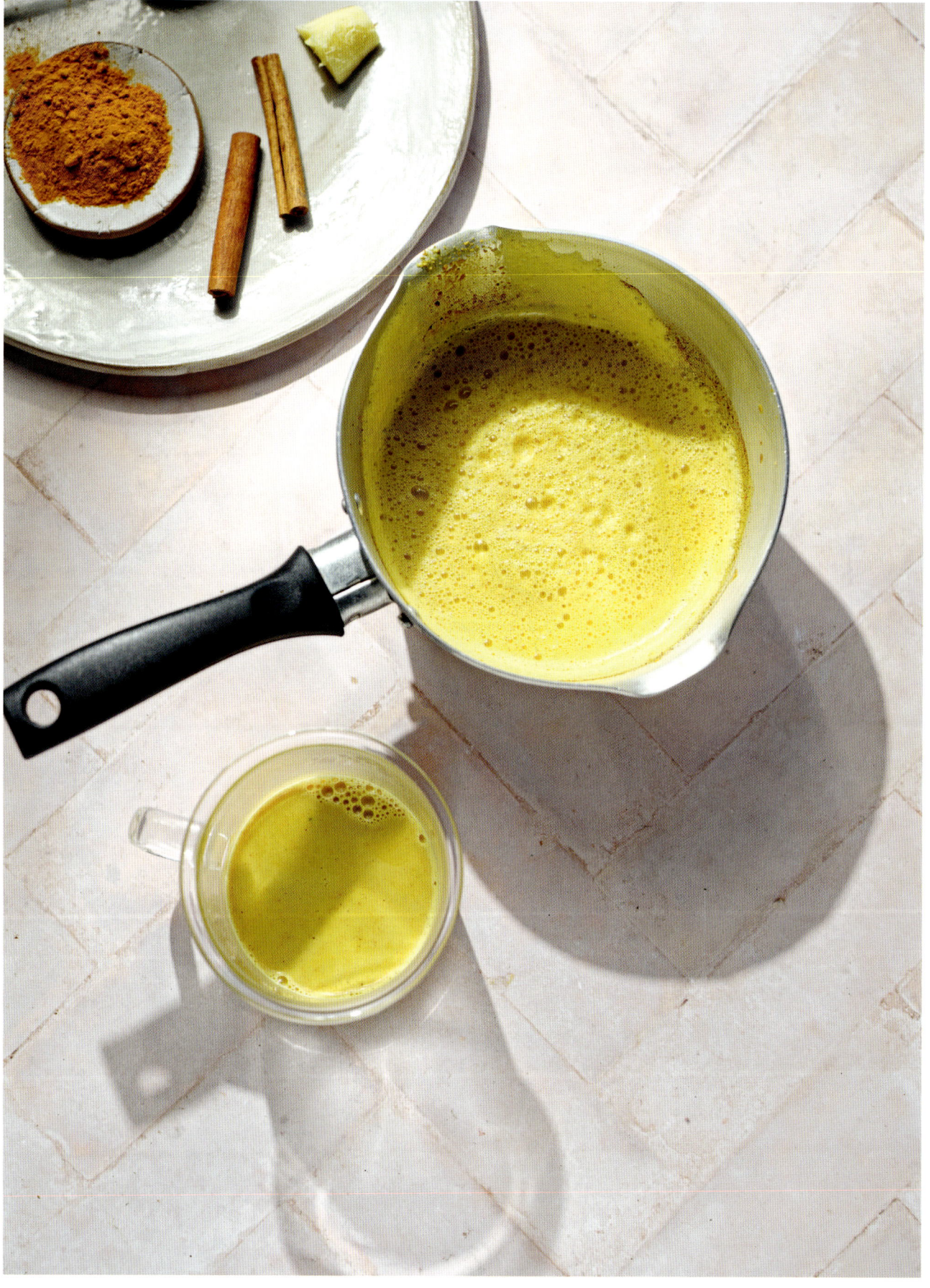

Organic Soy Golden Milk

250ml organic soy or oat milk

1 tsp good-quality vanilla essence

½ tsp ground ginger or grated fresh ginger

½ tsp Ceylon cinnamon

½ tsp cardamom powder

½ tsp turmeric

ground black pepper

1 tsp maple syrup

1 tsp almond butter (optional, see p170)

SERVES: 1

Comforting and creamy, this health-promoting drink is full of warming spices like ginger, turmeric, cardamom and cinnamon. It is a nice alternative to herbal tea in the evening.

1. Add all the ingredients to a saucepan and heat until warm, but not boiling.
2. Pour the mix into a blender and blitz for a few seconds to froth.
3. Pour into a large mug and enjoy.

PER 250ML PORTION

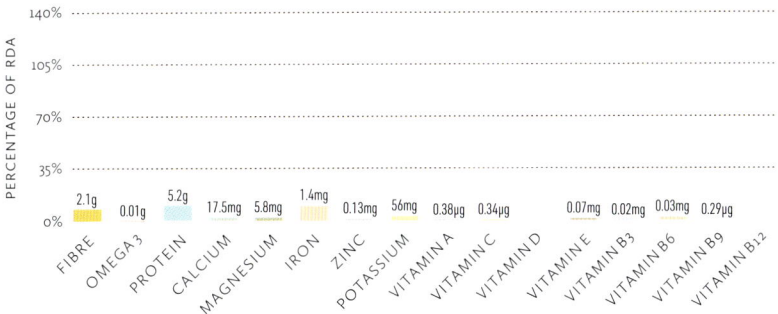

Chicory and Smashed Avo

with orange and miso dressing

GINGER MISO DRESSING

2 tbsp white miso paste

3 tbsp water

3 tbsp walnut oil

2 tsp local runny honey

1 tbsp apple cider vinegar

juice of ½ lime

a small piece of fresh ginger

CHICORY AND SMASHED AVO

2 medium-ripe avocados

Himalayan salt, to taste

1 large orange or a handful of mandarin orange segments

1 large chicory

TOPPINGS

1 tsp toasted sesame seeds

fresh chopped herbs

spring onions, finely sliced

SERVES: 4 (AS A SIDE)

This is the perfect combination of bitter foods (chicory), which support our liver detoxification processes, with the sweetness of the oranges and the healthy fats of the avocado. It can be served as part of a selection of brunch or lunch foods, or as canapés for drinks with friends.

1. Make your miso dressing by blitzing all the ingredients in a blender until smooth. Store in an airtight glass jar.
2. Remove the flesh from the avocados and place it in a bowl with a sprinkling of Himalayan salt. Mash together for a rustic texture.
3. Next, segment your orange. Using a sharp knife, remove the skin, then cut between the white pith line to get a clean segment. Repeat until you have segmented the whole orange. Alternatively, use mandarin orange segments.
4. Take a chicory leaf, spoon in the smashed avocado, top with a segment or two of orange, and drizzle with miso dressing. Arrange all the leaves on a large plate, sprinkled with the suggested toppings.

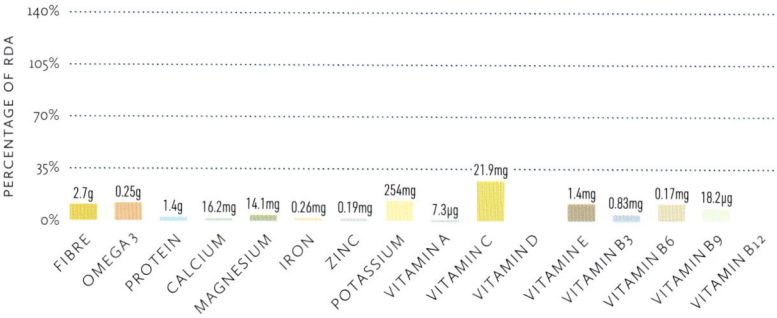

PER 100G PORTION

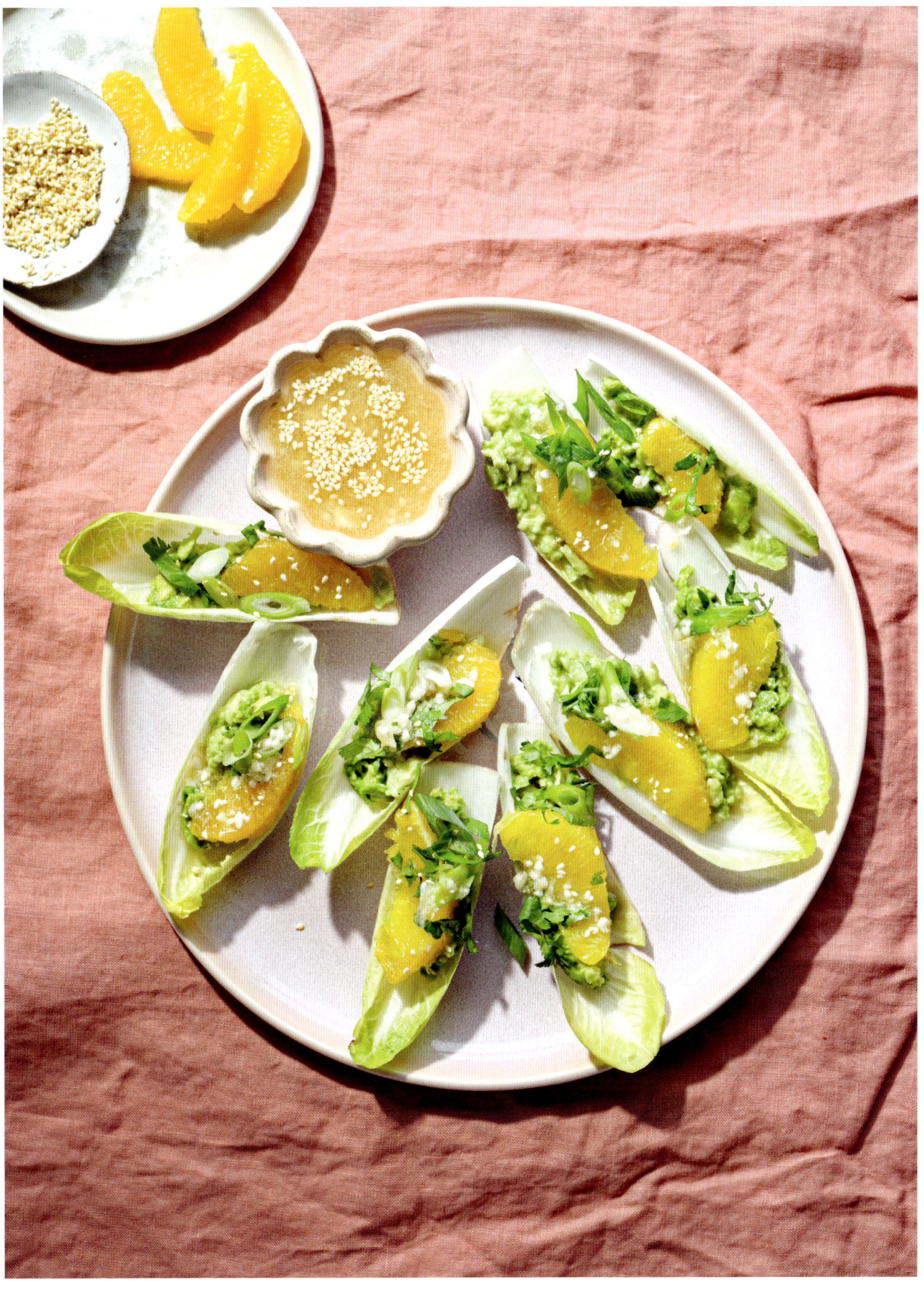

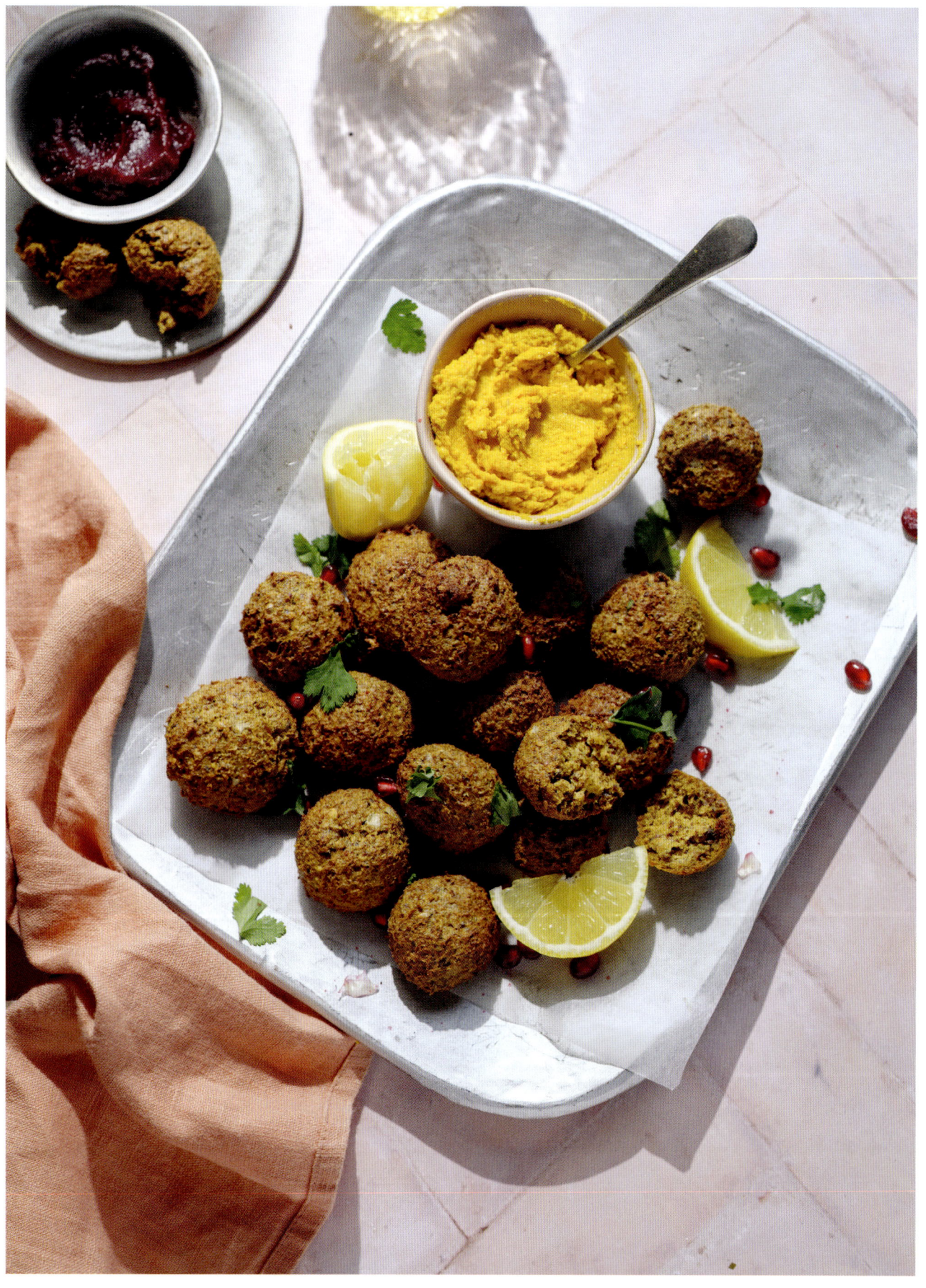

Falafels

240g sunflower seeds, soaked for 4–6 hours

200g carrots, grated

4 celery sticks

50g ground flaxseeds

juice of 1 lemon

good handful of parsley leaves

1 tsp parsley gremolata (p195)

3 tbsp liquid aminos or soy sauce

75g pitted Medjool dates

2 tbsp tahini

2 tbsp ground cumin

1 tbsp garlic powder

MAKES: ABOUT 30 PORTIONS

Home-made falafels taste far better than the shop-bought variety. You'll need a bit of time for soaking and baking, but these freeze well so they can be prepared in advance.

1. Preheat the oven to 80°C.
2. Combine the sunflower seeds, carrots and celery in a food processor, and blend to a paste.
3. Add the remaining ingredients, and pulse until everything is broken down and the mixture is well combined.
4. Using your hands or a spoon, gather a small amount of the mixture (approximately 30g) and roll it in your palms to form a ball. Repeat with the rest of the mixture.
5. Arrange the falafel balls on parchment paper on a baking tray and put in the oven for 4–5 hours. Turn them after 2 hours to enable them to cook evenly. Then turn off the oven and allow them to cool inside.
6. You can store the falafels in an airtight container in the fridge for up to 10 days. When you want to eat them, warm them in the oven or a pan, or eat them cold.

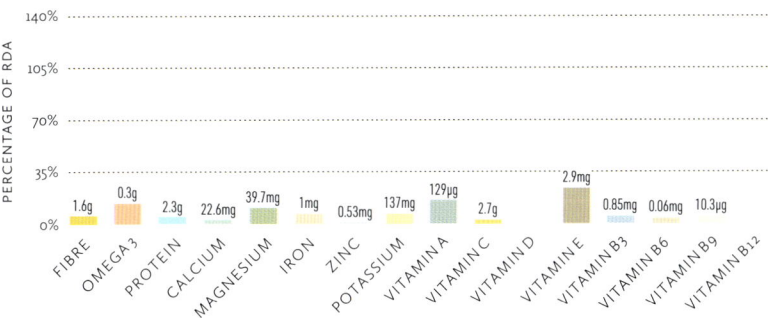

PER 30G PORTION

2. Fibre

Including fibre-rich foods in your diet will provide a variety of health benefits, including helping to lower cholesterol levels and blood pressure, and improving blood-sugar control – which in turn reduces the risk of type 2 diabetes, one of the 'Big Four' health risks for women in menopause. Eating plenty of fibre will also lead to improved digestive health and can aid in maintaining a healthy weight, as it can promote feelings of fullness and help to reduce overall calorie intake.

This section contains predominantly vegan recipes, and I hope it will confirm that you don't have to be vegan to enjoy vegan food!

Porridge Bread

360g organic porridge oats

20g flaxseeds/oat bran

50g mixed seeds (flax, chia, pumpkin and sunflower)

1 tsp pink Himalayan salt

1 organic egg

80ml olive oil

200g live probiotic yoghurt (or coconut yoghurt [see p253] for a dairy-free option)

200ml oat milk (dairy-free option)

mixed seeds to decorate

MAKES: 1 LOAF

If you want to bake your own bread, this is a great recipe, since it requires no proving or kneading. Porridge bread is full of heart-healthy fibre, and it tastes great toasted, spread with almond butter and topped with a sliced banana.

1. Preheat the oven to 180°C.
2. Put all the dry ingredients (oats, flaxseeds/oat bran, mixed seeds and salt) in a large mixing bowl.
3. In a separate bowl, mix the egg, olive oil, yoghurt and milk.
4. Add the wet mix to the dry mix and combine well.
5. Put a loaf tin liner in your bread loaf tin and spoon the mix into it, filling to the top. Sprinkle the mixed seeds on top.
6. Bake for 40–45 minutes. Check halfway and turn the tray around so the loaf browns evenly.
7. Insert a knife into the centre of the loaf: if it comes out clean, it is baked.
8. Leave to cool completely before slicing. The loaf can be cut in half, wrapped in greaseproof paper and stored in a resealable bag in the fridge. It also freezes well.

PER 80G PORTION

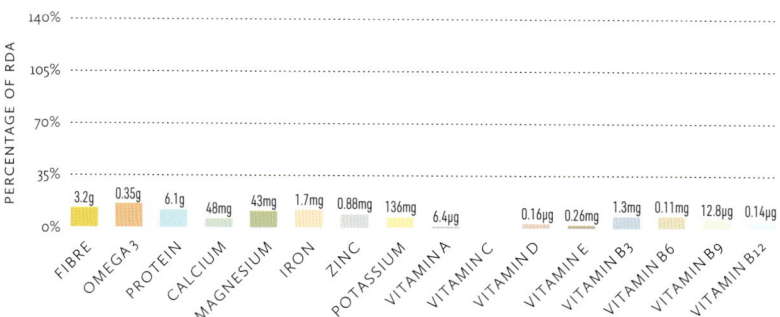

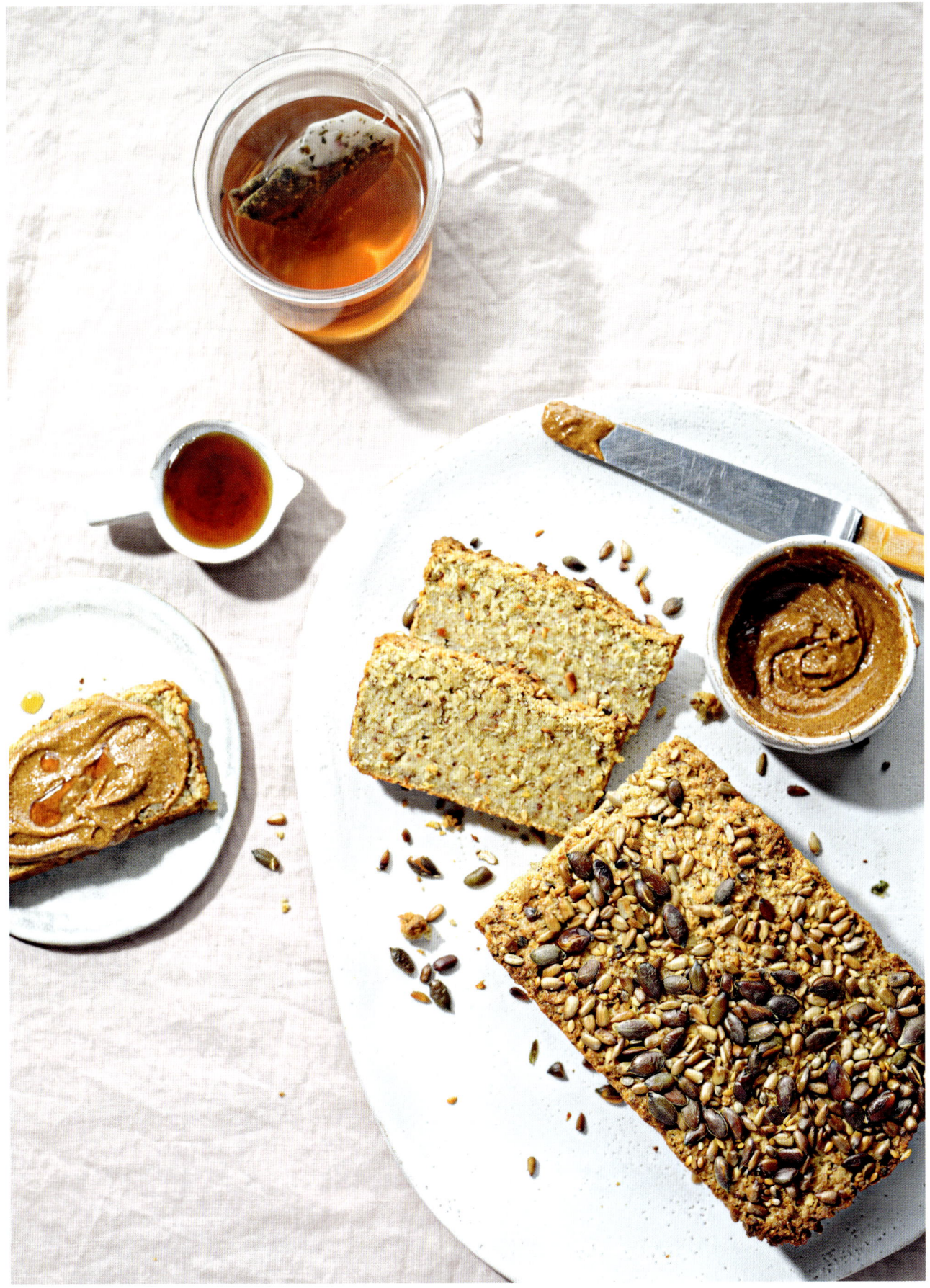

Spirulina, Lime and Mint Overnight Oats

160g rolled oats

4 tbsp sprouted milled flaxseeds

100g frozen banana, cut into pieces

1 kiwi, peeled and diced

200g ripe avocado, cut into pieces

30g fresh baby spinach leaves

300g organic soya milk/oat milk

½ tsp spirulina powder

2 tbsp desiccated coconut

zest and juice of 1 lime

handful of mint leaves

8 tbsp live probiotic yoghurt

handful of fresh blueberries

quinoa pops (optional)

1 tsp maple syrup (optional)

MAKES: 4 LARGE PORTIONS

This recipe packs in a lot of goodness for a heart-healthy start to the day. You can make it in advance for a grab-and-go breakfast.

1. Take four glass jars with airtight lids, weigh 40g of oats into each and add in 1 tablespoon of flaxseed. Mix and set aside.
2. Put the banana, kiwi, avocado, spinach leaves, soya milk, spirulina powder, coconut, lime zest and juice and mint leaves in a blender. Blend until smooth.
3. Divide the mixture (it should be quite liquid) between the four glass jars. Mix well to combine them, then put the lids on and leave to rest in the fridge overnight (or for 2–3 hours).
4. When rested, top with live probiotic yoghurt and blueberries, plus quinoa pops and maple syrup (if using).

PER 265G PORTION

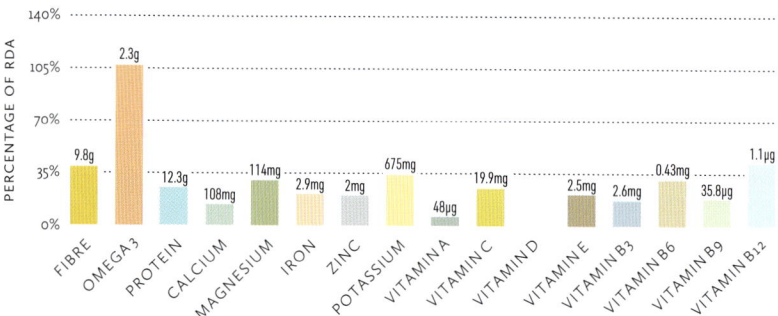

Oat and Flaxseed Porridge with Blueberry Compote

125g frozen blueberries
80g organic porridge oats
1 tbsp ground flaxseeds
1 tbsp milled organic chia seeds
½ tbsp wheat germ
500ml organic soya milk

TOPPING
2 tsp maple syrup or chicory root syrup (optional)

SERVES: 2

Full of fabulous fibre, this porridge is a great way to fill up on heart-friendly and digestive-health-supporting nutrients at breakfast. It is also perfect as a fast, easy meal at any time of the day.

1. Put the blueberries in a pot with a splash of water and cover. Place on low heat, allowing them to defrost and warm (about 10 minutes).
2. Make your porridge mix by adding all the dry ingredients to a saucepan with your choice of plant milk – I like to use organic soya milk, but you could also use oat milk.
3. Place on low heat and stir gently until cooked (at least 8 minutes). Check the consistency of the porridge and add a little extra milk if it is too thick.
4. When ready, divide the porridge between two bowls and top it with the warm blueberry compote.
5. If you're using maple or chicory root syrup, add a teaspoon to each bowl.

PER 435G PORTION (INCL. 125G COMPOTE)

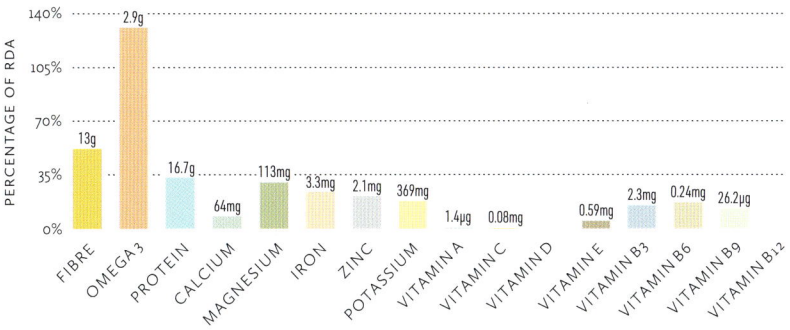

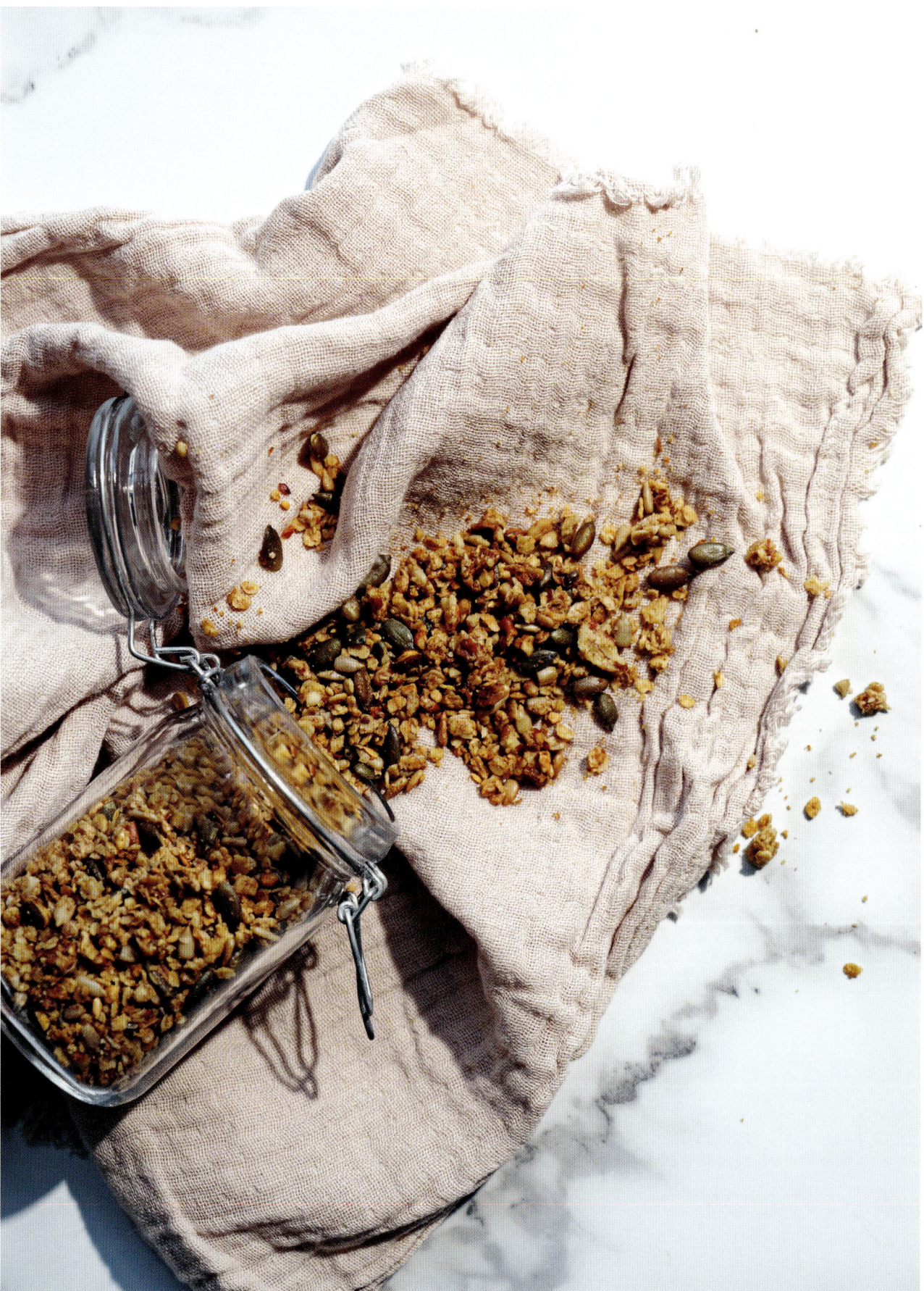

Pecan Cinnamon Granola

200g almonds

200g pecans

400g organic porridge oats

120g pumpkin seeds

120g sunflower seeds

120g mixed seeds (sesame, flaxseeds, hempseed, etc.)

40g cacao nibs

40g quinoa pops

2 tbsp Ceylon cinnamon

240ml olive oil

180ml organic maple syrup

MAKES: AROUND 17 PORTIONS

An easy, delicious and nutritious recipe, with no refined sugar. This granola will keep for several weeks (if it lasts that long!) and is great sprinkled over porridge, pancakes and yoghurt.

1. Preheat the oven to 180°C.
2. Line two baking trays with parchment paper or a silicone sheet liner.
3. Put the almonds and pecans separately into a food processor and pulse them for a few seconds to break them down into smaller pieces. The almonds are harder and will take a little longer than the pecans.
4. Put the nuts in a large bowl, add the rest of the dry ingredients (including the cinnamon) and mix well.
5. Pour the olive oil and maple syrup over the dry ingredients in the bowl and mix thoroughly.
6. Empty the contents of the bowl onto the baking trays and place in the oven for about 20 minutes. Don't overfill the trays or the granola will steam rather than roast.
7. When the mixture is golden and toasted, it's ready. (Beware: it burns easily, so keep an eye on it.)
8. Remove from the oven and allow to cool. It will go crunchy as it cools.
9. Store in an airtight 1.5-litre glass jar (you will need two for this amount) in the cupboard.

PER 85G PORTION

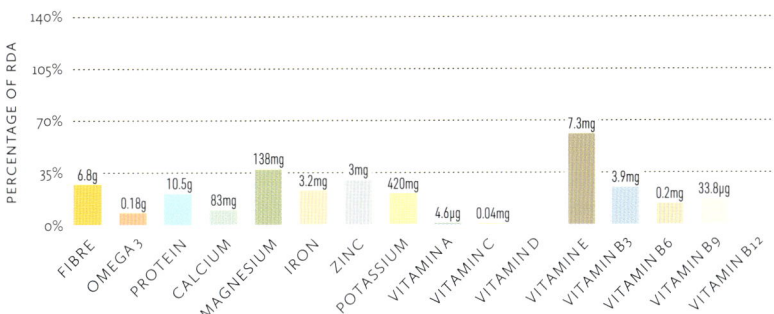

Oat and Hemp Seed Porridge

with rhubarb, pear and apple compote

80g organic porridge oats

1 tbsp cold-milled organic hemp seeds

500ml organic soya milk

2 heaped tbsp rhubarb, pear and apple compote (see p128)

TOPPING

2 tsp maple syrup

handful of chopped walnuts

1 tbsp cacao nibs

SERVES: 2

This porridge contains a good helping of plant protein, thanks to the cold-milled hemp seeds, which are also full of fibre. Topped with stewed fruit, it is easily digestible and tastes great, too.

1. Put the porridge oats and hemp seeds in a saucepan with the organic soya milk (or your plant milk of choice).
2. Place on low heat and stir gently until cooked (at least 8 minutes). Check the consistency of the porridge and add a little extra milk if it is too thick.
3. When ready, divide up between two bowls and top each with a heaped tablespoon of compote.
4. Add a teaspoon of maple syrup per bowl, plus the walnuts and cacao nibs for additional nutrient benefits.

PER 410G PORTION (INCL. 100G COMPOTE)

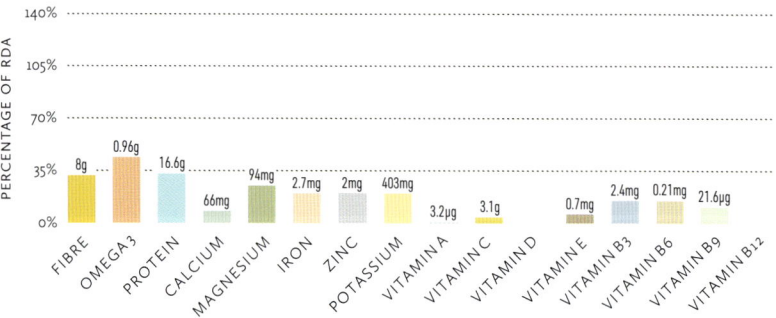

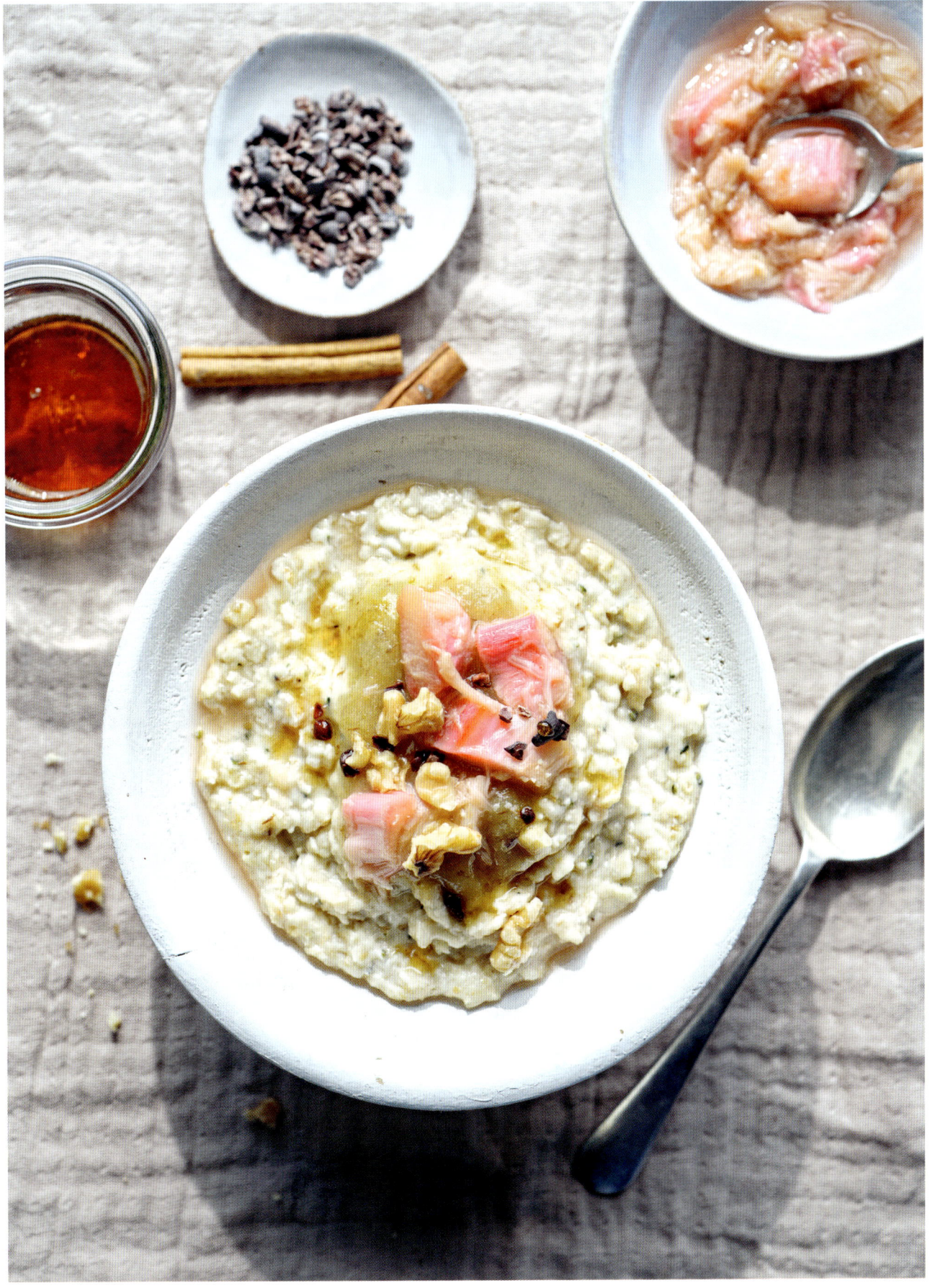

Sweet Potato and Apple Breakfast Cookies

100g rolled oats

55g coconut flakes

40g chia seeds

65g sweet potato purée

65g rhubarb, pear and apple compote (see p128)

80ml maple syrup

75g almond butter or other nut butter of choice (see 170)

1 tbsp mixed spice (I use ¾ cinnamon and ¼ clove powder)

1 tsp baking powder

¼ tsp salt

1 tsp vanilla extract

50g dark chocolate chips (85% cocoa chocolate chopped small)

50g goji berries

MAKES: 6 LARGE COOKIES

Tasty and filling, these cookies are a great snack for any time of the day – perfect with a juice or smoothie. They will keep in an airtight container for up to a week and can also be frozen.

1. Preheat the oven to 180°C.
2. Pulse the oats, coconut flakes and chia seeds in a food processor until mixed (but not milled into flour).
3. Put the sweet potato purée and fruit compote in a bowl, then add the maple syrup, nut butter, spice mix, baking powder, salt and vanilla extract. Mix well.
4. Add the oat mix to the wet mix, along with the dark chocolate chips and goji berries. Combine well.
5. Using a large ice-cream scoop, take a portion of the cookie mix and place it on a lined baking sheet. Press down with a plastic pastry scraper to flatten and shape the cookies. (If you wet the scraper, it won't stick to the mix.) Repeat for all six cookies.
6. Bake for 25 minutes, until the cookies are golden around the edges.
7. Remove from the oven and allow to cool on a wire rack.

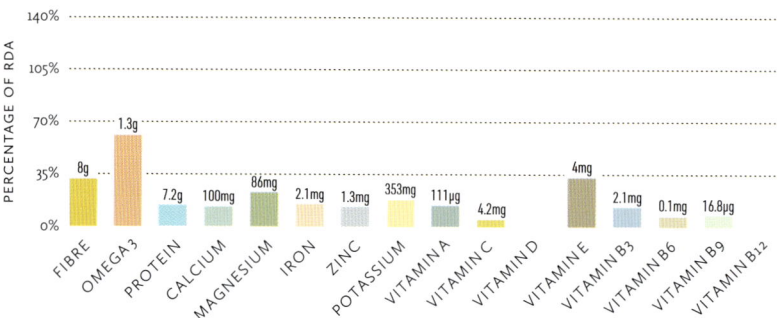

PER 90G PORTION

110 NOURISH FOR MENOPAUSE

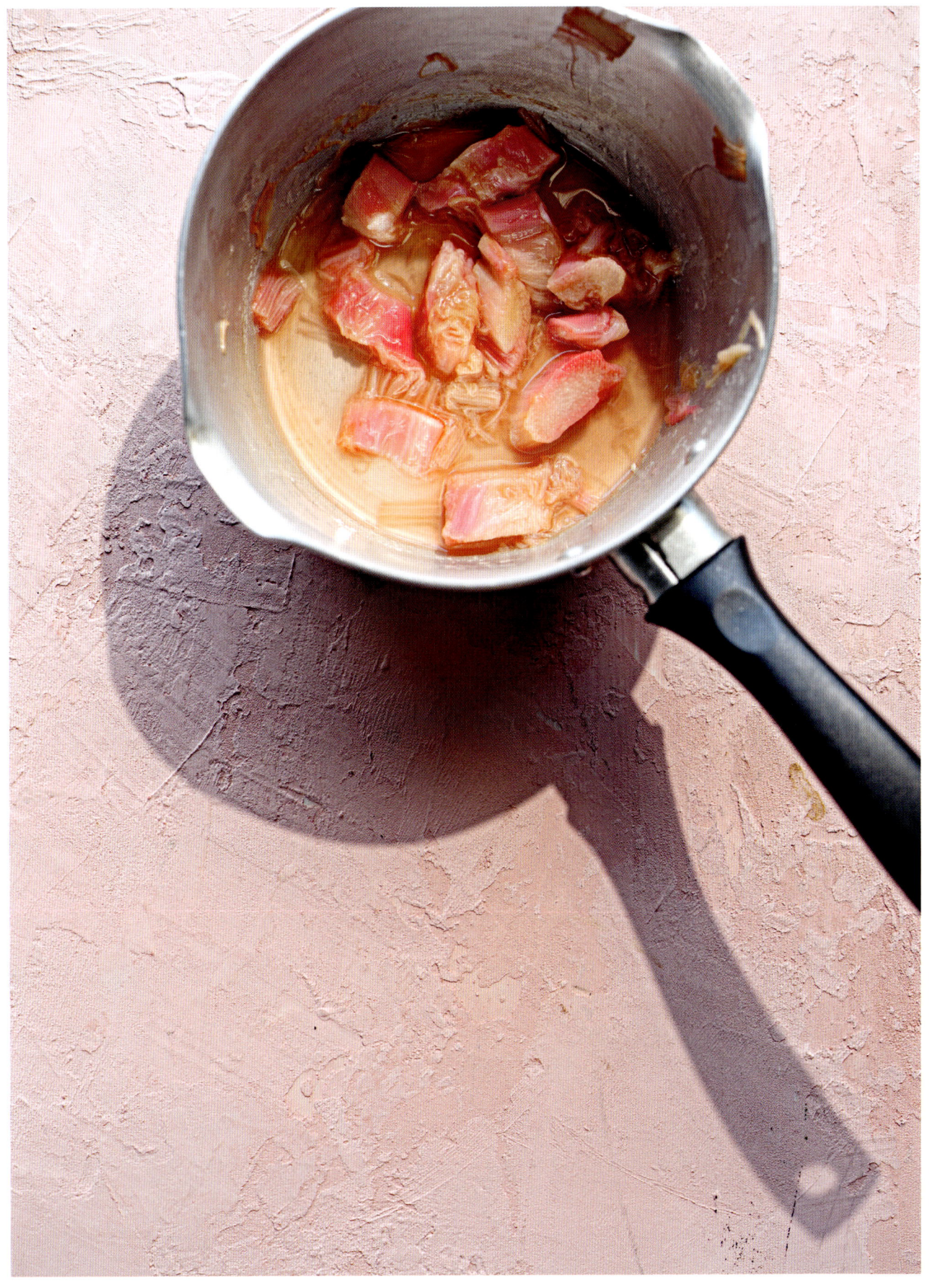

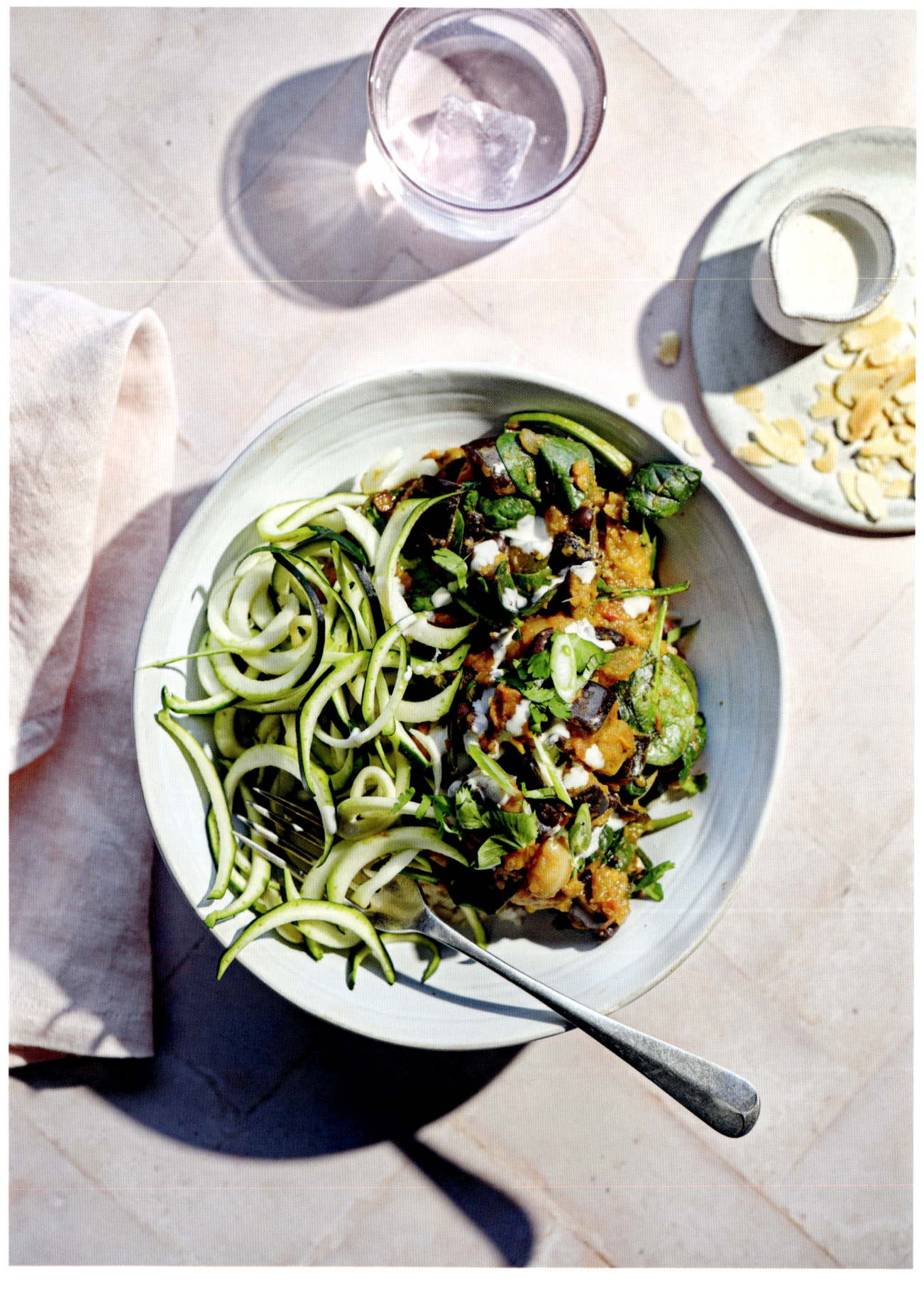

Vegan Power Bowl

with cashew cream

Full of beneficial fibre, B vitamins and complex carbs, this tasty one-pot meal will set you up for a day of activity.

500g aubergines (approx. 2), diced

40ml olive oil

1 tsp smoked paprika

1½ tsp pink Himalayan salt plus extra, to taste

2 pinches of ground black pepper

125g onions, finely chopped

75g carrots, finely chopped

75g celery, finely chopped

1 tsp ground cumin

1 tsp ground cinnamon

1½ tbsp tinned harissa paste

1 tsp veg stock powder

400g tinned chopped tomatoes

200g sweet potatoes, peeled and diced

150g courgettes, diced

240ml water (optional)

400g tinned cannellini beans, drained

400g tinned black beans, drained and rinsed

125g fresh baby spinach

clove of garlic

1 tbsp maple syrup (optional)

CASHEW CREAM

clove of garlic

50g cashew nuts

10ml olive oil

175g organic soya milk (or oat milk)

1 tsp lemon juice

pinch of pink Himalayan salt and black pepper

TO SERVE

1 tbsp chopped parsley/coriander/chives

100g wholegrain brown basmati rice or Moroccan quinoa (see p226) per person

spiralised courgettes (optional)

SERVES: 6+

1. Preheat the oven to 180°C.
2. Add the aubergines and 25ml of olive oil to a mixing bowl with the smoked paprika, ½ teaspoon of salt and a pinch of pepper. Stir to coat and transfer to a large, lined baking tray.
3. Bake the aubergines in the oven until soft (25–30 minutes).
4. Meanwhile, make your cashew cream by chopping the garlic and the cashews together in a blender, then adding them to a pan with 10ml of olive oil. Gently cook for 2 minutes, then add the plant milk and warm through.
5. Put this mixture back into the blender, along with the lemon juice, a pinch of salt and black pepper. Blend until smooth, then transfer to a small serving bowl and set aside.
6. In a separate large casserole pot, put the rest of the olive oil, chopped onions, carrots and celery. Sauté for 5 minutes on a low heat to soften. Place the lid on the pot.
7. Add the cumin, cinnamon and harissa paste. Mix well and sauté for a further few minutes.
8. Add the stock powder, tomatoes, sweet potatoes, courgettes, 1 tsp of salt and a pinch of black pepper. If the mixture seems very dry, add some water as needed. Add all the beans and cook for 30 minutes, or until the sweet potatoes are soft.
9. Mix in the baby spinach leaves and the baked aubergine. Grate in a clove of fresh raw garlic and mix through.
10. Season again and add maple syrup (if using), then serve with your preferred accompaniments and a drizzle of cashew cream.

PER 400G PORTION

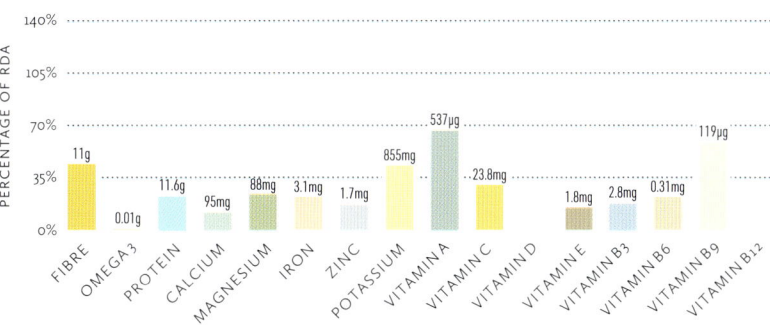

Apple Doughnuts

1 organic Pink Lady apple, cored

1 heaped tbsp almond butter (see p170)

1 tbsp desiccated coconut

1 tbsp goji berries

MAKES: 2 PORTIONS

These are great for a child's lunch box or as a handy mid-morning or mid-afternoon snack for a grown-up. The combination of the protein in the almond butter with the fibre in the apple will help balance your blood sugars and keep you full for longer.

1. Slice the cored apple horizontally, so you end up with rings.
2. Spread almond butter on each ring with a teaspoon or palette knife.
3. Sprinkle with desiccated coconut and goji berries.

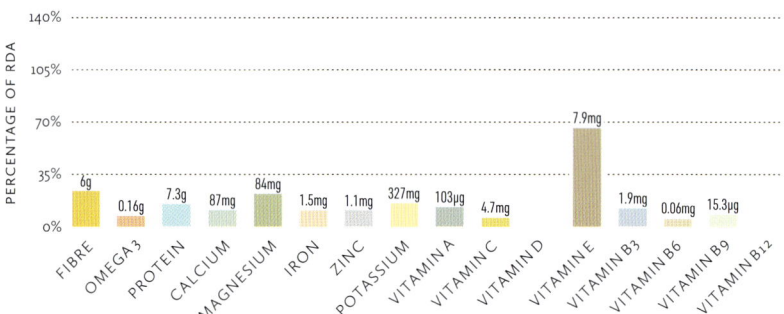

PER 65G PORTION

NOURISH FOR MENOPAUSE

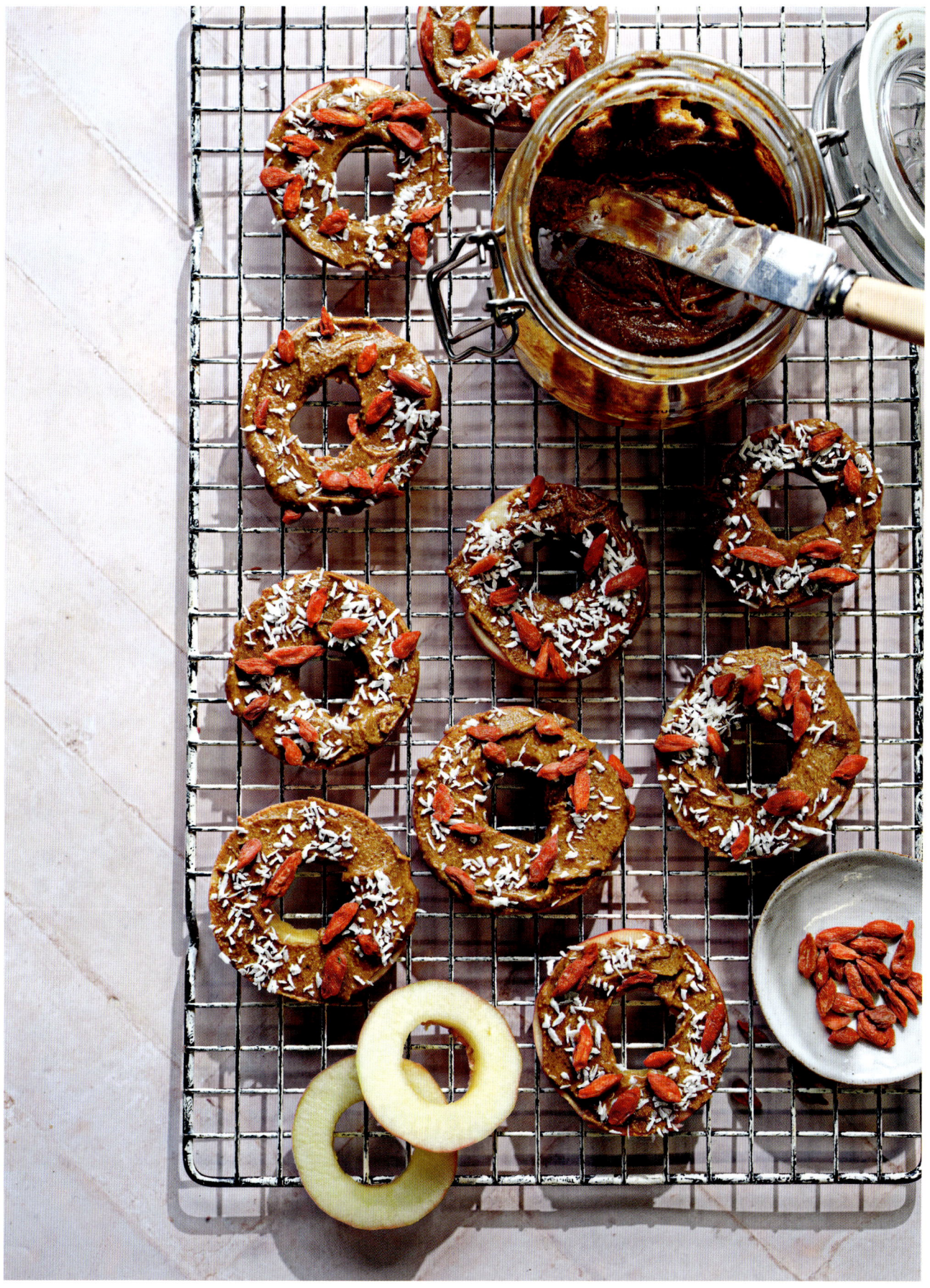

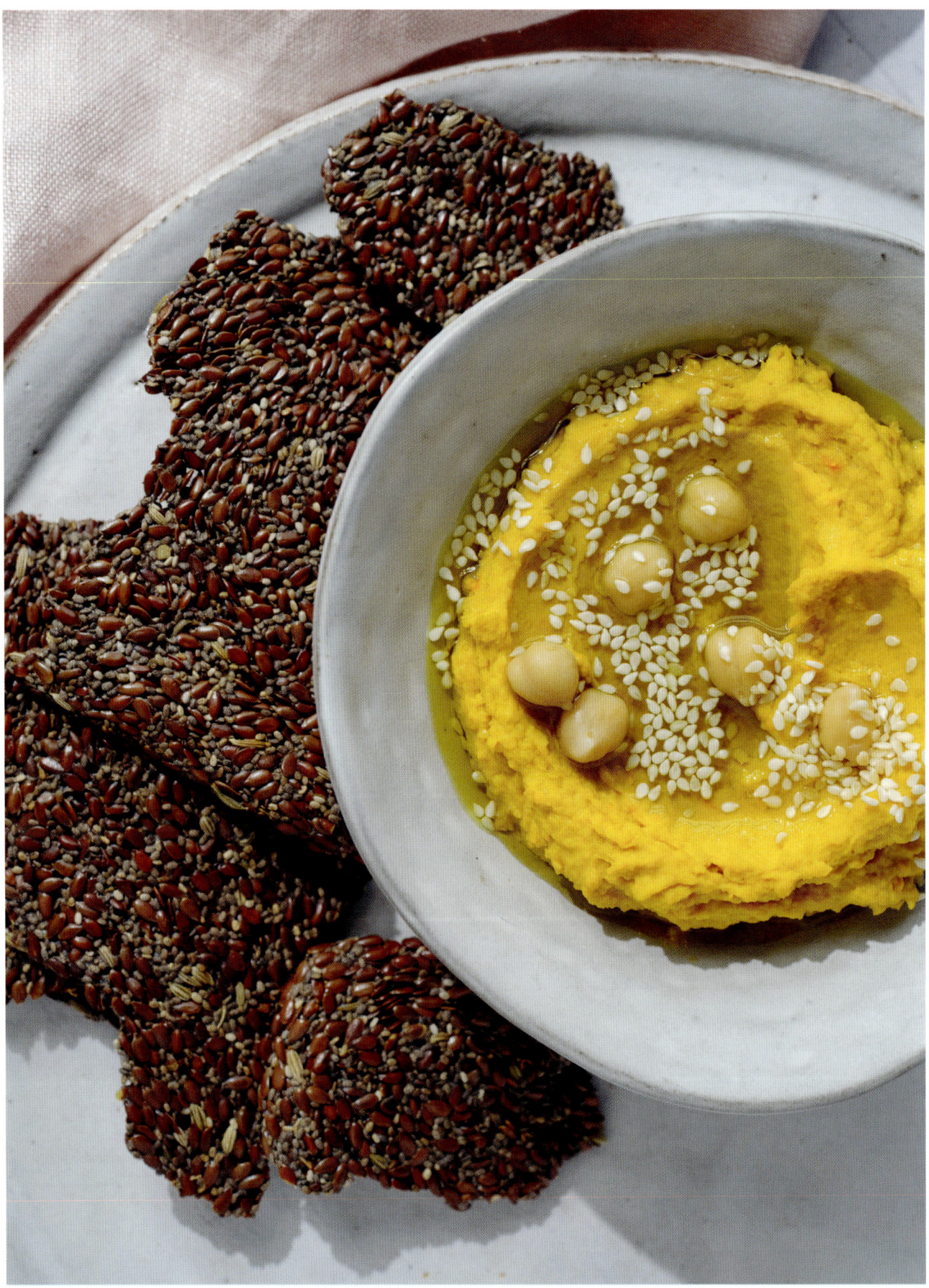

Roasted Carrot and Yellow Pepper Hummus

1 carrot, peeled and chopped into small chunks

olive oil

pink Himalayan salt, to taste

1 yellow pepper

400g tinned chickpeas, rinsed and drained

2 large tbsp tahini

2 large cloves of garlic

1 tsp organic turmeric powder or 1 piece of fresh root turmeric

juice of 1 large lemon

ground black pepper, to taste

handful of chickpeas (optional)

sprinkling of sesame seeds (optional)

MAKES: 6–8 PORTIONS

A great source of protein, calcium and fibre, hummus is ideal for wraps. It can also be used as an alternative to mayonnaise.

1. Preheat the oven to 180°C.
2. Put the carrots in a mixing bowl. Drizzle with a little olive oil and season with salt. Mix well and transfer to a lined baking sheet. Place the whole pepper beside it and roast in the oven for 40 minutes, or until the carrots are soft and the pepper is browned.
3. Remove the pepper from the oven, place it in a bowl and cover it with a lid. Allow to cool for up to an hour. (Covering the pepper like this makes the skin easier to remove.)
4. If the carrots need a little longer, cook for a further 10 minutes.
5. When ready, deseed and remove the skin from the pepper.
6. Put the flesh from the roasted pepper and the carrots in a food processor.
7. Add the remaining ingredients to the food processor and blitz on high until smooth.
8. Adjust the seasoning to taste. Besides salt and pepper, it may need a little more oil or lemon juice. If using, top with chickpeas and a sprinkling of seasame seeds for decoration.

PER 95G PORTION

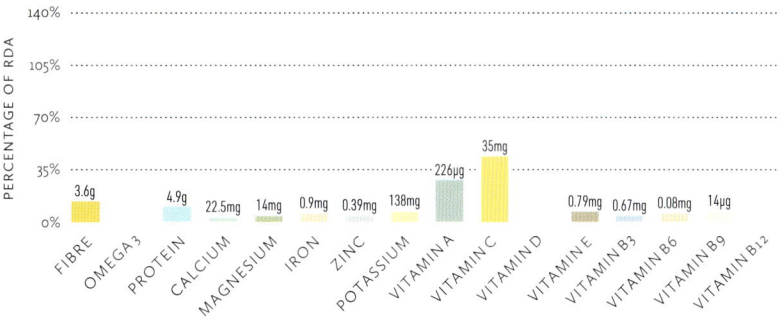

Sage and Date Hummus

400g tinned chickpeas

1 large tbsp tahini, preferably runny

1 tbsp walnut butter (see p170)

1 large clove of garlic, crushed

juice of ½–¾ lemon

1 tbsp olive oil

handful of fresh sage leaves (about 10 leaves), finely chopped

2 Medjool dates (or 3 dried dates steeped in hot water to soften), finely chopped

240ml plant milk (such as oat or organic soya milk)

1 tsp salt and black pepper

MAKES: 8 PORTIONS

This delicious hummus is mildly sweet, thanks to the dates, which taste amazing paired with the fresh sage leaves and garlic. Serve it with vegetable sticks or flaxseed crackers (see p143), as part of a salad bowl or on a veggie burger instead of mayonnaise.

1. Place all the ingredients in a food processor and blend until smooth. If the mixture seems too thick, adjust the consistency with a little extra plant milk.
2. Store the hummus in a flip-top jar with a rubber seal in the fridge. This is best eaten at room temperature, though, so take it out shortly before you plan to serve.

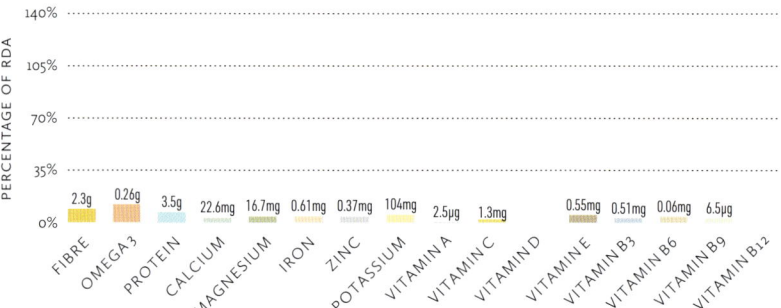

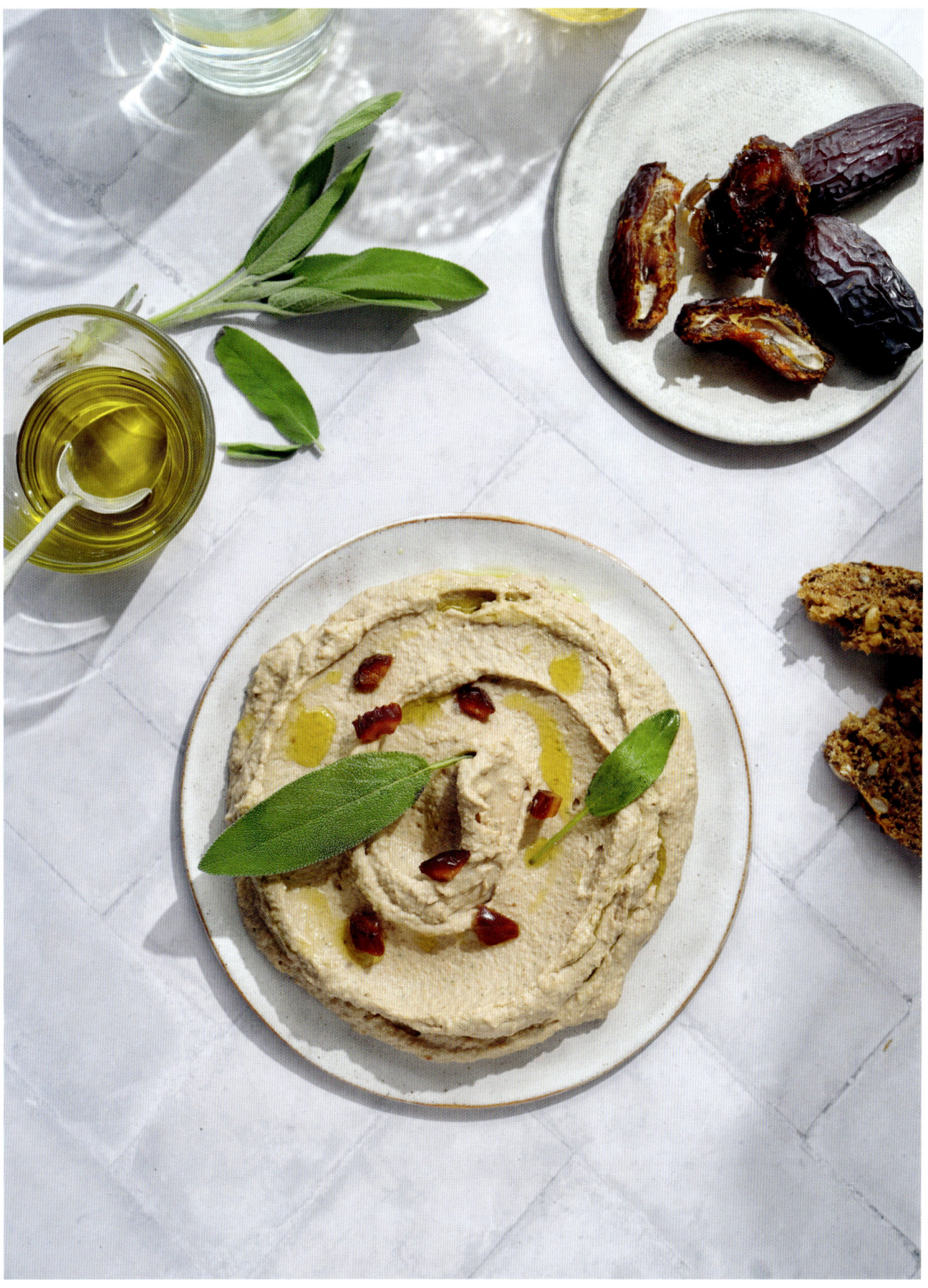

Avonaise

3 ripe avocados
1 tsp Dijon mustard
1 tbsp nutritional yeast flakes
2 tbsp olive oil
2 tsp apple cider vinegar (see p255)
2 tbsp lime juice
½ tsp pink Himalayan salt
1 tsp garlic powder

MAKES: 500G

High in heart-healthy monounsaturated fats, this is a good alternative to mayonnaise, with none of the saturated fat, additives or sugar. Add it to salads as part of the dressing, spread it on a sandwich or use it as a condiment with grilled meat or fish.

1. Scoop out the flesh of the avocados into a food processor or blender.
2. Add in the other ingredients and blitz on high until perfectly smooth.
3. Store it in an airtight glass jar in the fridge for a week or more.

PER 30G PORTION

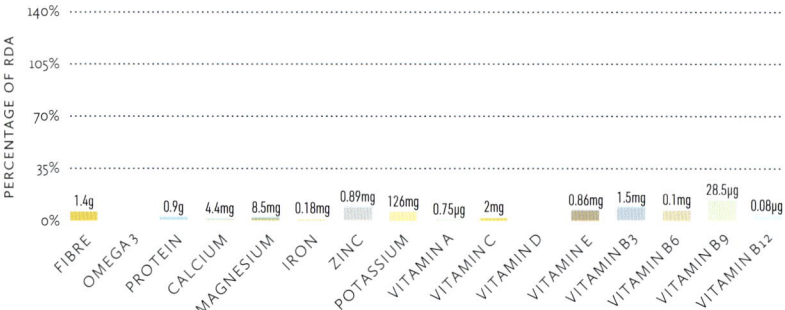

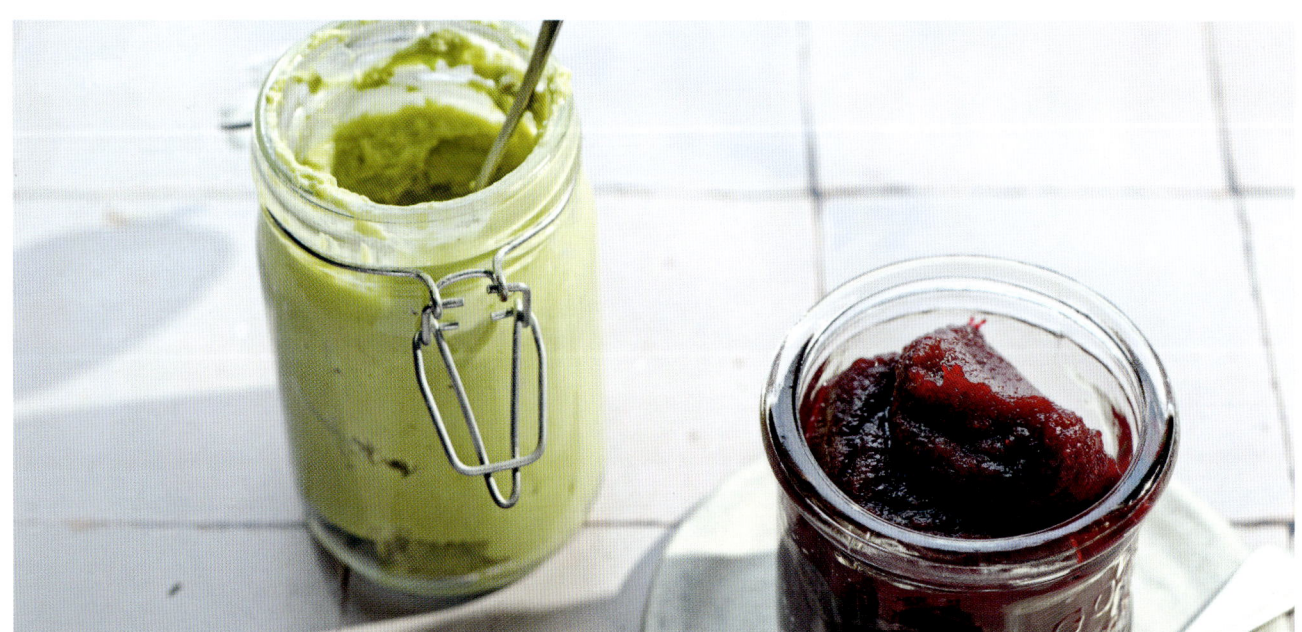

Beetroot Ketchup

500g raw beetroots
1½ tbsp balsamic vinegar
28 dates, pitted
½ tsp clove powder
½ tsp smoked paprika
1 tsp fresh ginger
1 tsp celery salt
1 large clove of garlic
1 tsp pink Himalayan salt
few grinds of black pepper
pinch of dried red pepper flakes (optional)

MAKES: 500G

This is great with veggie burgers or falafels, spread on a sandwich or served as a dip with sweet potato fries or veg sticks. It will keep for a couple of weeks in an airtight glass container in the fridge. It also freezes well.

1. Add the raw beetroots to a pot of water. If they are very big, cut them in half and remove the tops. Boil until soft (about 30–40 minutes).
2. Drain the beetroots and leave them to cool. Once cool, remove the skins with a paring knife.
3. Put all the ingredients into a high-speed blender or food processor, and blitz until perfectly smooth.
4. Taste and adjust the seasoning if necessary.

Tip: You will need to soak regular dates in boiling water for an hour in advance. If you're using Medjool dates, you can halve the quantity, and there is no need to pre-soak.

PER 40G PORTION

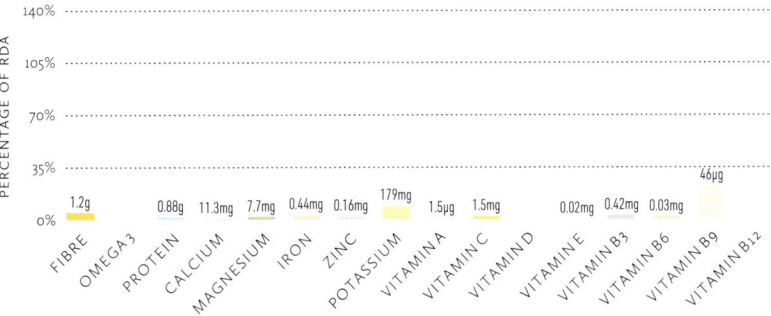

Savoury Granola

3 tbsp fresh rosemary
1 tbsp fresh sage leaves
35g hazelnuts, roughly chopped
50g walnuts, roughly chopped
100g oat flakes
100g rye flakes
100g raw buckwheat flakes
70g pumpkin seeds
70g sunflower seeds
30g sesame seeds
zest of 1 orange
1 tbsp nutritional yeast
1 tsp pink Himalayan salt
120ml extra virgin olive oil
2 tbsp wholegrain Dijon mustard
1 tbsp maple syrup
juice of 1 orange

MAKES: 500G

This is a great topping for salads or veg – it really elevates simple ingredients, while adding lots of beneficial fibre, protein and healthy fats. You can store it in a clip-top glass jar for up to a month.

1. Preheat the oven to 180°C and line a baking sheet with greaseproof paper.
2. Finely chop the herbs in a food processor and transfer them to a large mixing bowl.
3. Add the rest of the dry ingredients to the bowl (this is everything except the olive oil, mustard, maple syrup and orange juice).
4. Mix all of the wet ingredients in a separate bowl.
5. Combine the wet and dry ingredients and mix well.
6. Spread the granola out in a single layer on a tray and bake for 15–20 minutes, or until crunchy and golden. You can stir it from time to time to ensure it doesn't burn.
7. Remove from the oven and set aside to cool.

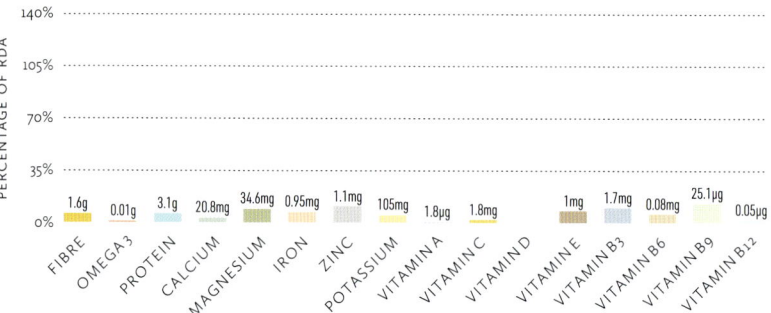

PER 30G PORTION

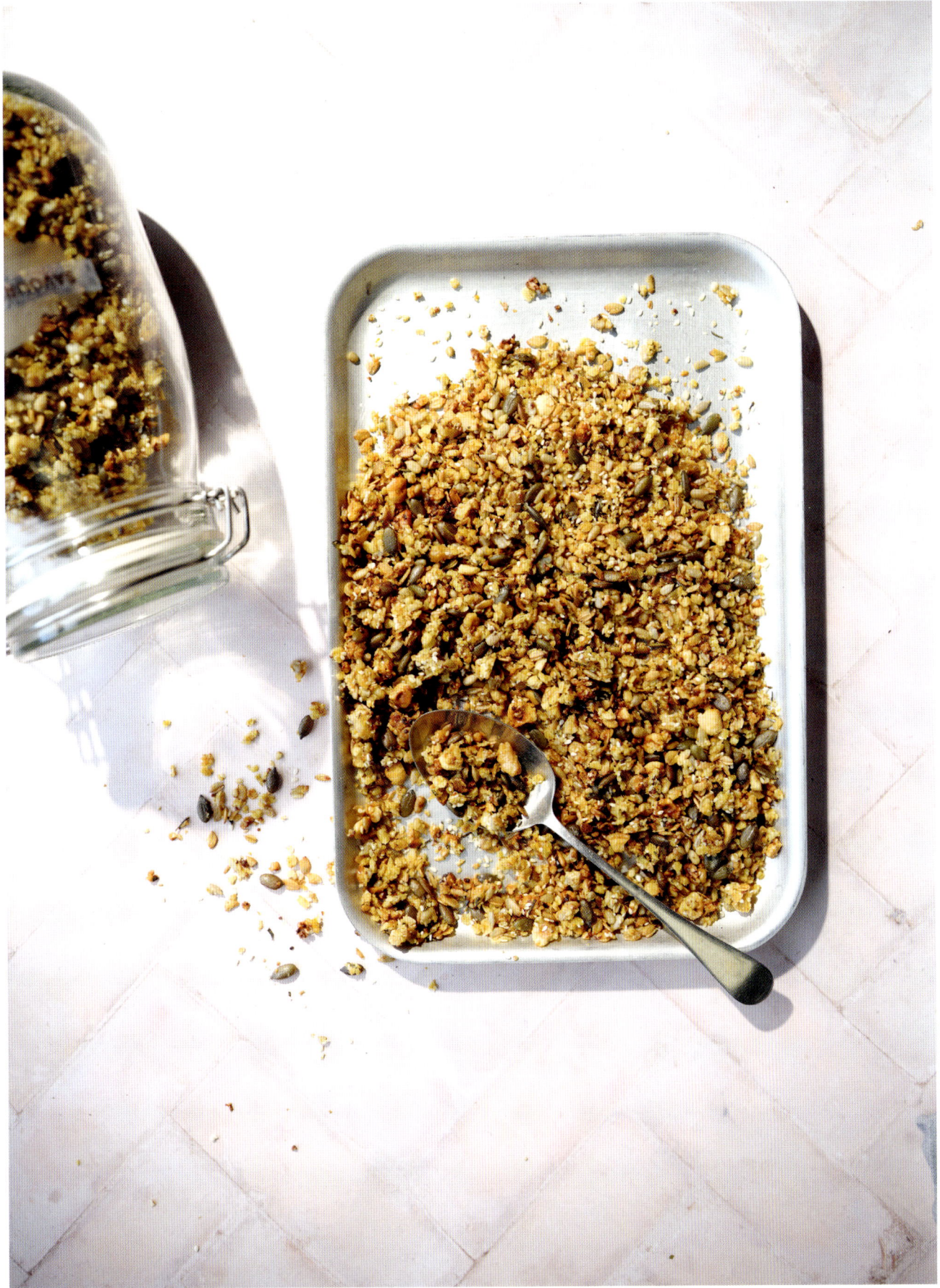

Date and Ginger Caramel

25–30g ginger, peeled and chopped into small chunks

300g dates, pitted

MAKES: 385G

This is great as a topping for porridge, with yoghurt and granola, or as part of a dessert. Dates are very high in fibre and antioxidants, while ginger is a natural anti-inflammatory food. This will keep well for a couple of weeks in an airtight container in the fridge.

1. Blitz the ginger in a high-speed blender with the dates (and soaking water, if using regular dates rather than Medjool, as these will need to be pre-soaked).
2. Scrape down the sides of the blender and blitz again. Repeat this a few times until you have a paste.
3. Adjust the flavour with more ginger if desired.

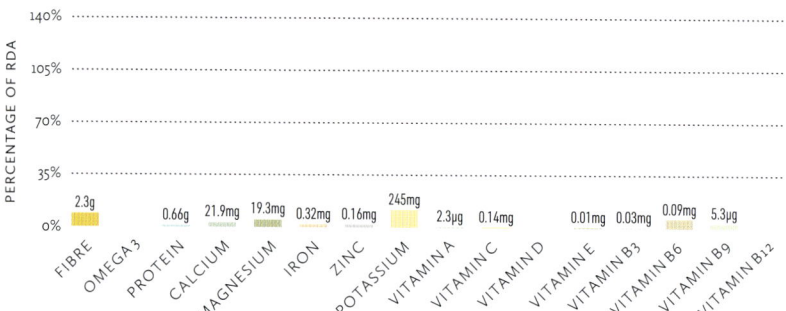

Pear Tart with Date and Ginger Caramel

4 pears, halved and cored (unripe Conference pears work best)

1 tsp vanilla extract

220g almonds

220g walnuts

1 tsp pink Himalayan salt

1½ tbsp olive oil

1 large thumb of ginger, sliced

4 whole star anise

1 tsp raw cane sugar

125ml water

2 tsp vanilla paste or essence

385g date and ginger caramel (see p124)

SERVES: 6

This delicious dessert contains lots of good-for-you ingredients. Pears and dates contain soluble fibre, which helps to improve digestion, so poached or stewed fruit can help with heartburn, indigestion and reflux. The tart is also gluten-free, with healthy fats and no refined sugar. Just add a spoon of gut-loving probiotic Greek-style yoghurt and enjoy!

1. Preheat the oven to 180°C.
2. Place the pear halves face down in a medium to large pot. Cover with water, add a teaspoon of vanilla extract and put a lid on. Bring the water to a boil, then immediately turn the heat down low. Let the pears simmer gently for 10 minutes, or until they are soft (but not falling apart).
3. Remove the pears with a slotted spoon and leave to cool. Once cool, slice each pear half lengthways and set aside until you are ready to assemble the tart.
4. Make the base by putting the nuts into the food processor and blitzing until they resemble breadcrumbs. Slowly add the salt and olive oil while continuing to blitz the nuts. Turn off the food processor and test to see if the mixture sticks when pressed together between your fingers. If not, slowly add more oil – but be careful: it can get very oily very quickly.
5. When you are happy with the consistency, spoon the mix into a 22cm (9in) loose-bottomed cake tin and press down firmly. Put in the oven for 5–8 minutes until lightly brown and you can smell the nuts roasting. Remove and allow to cool, then place in the fridge to firm up.
6. Make a ginger glaze by putting the ginger slices, star anise and raw cane sugar in a small pot with the water. Place on a high heat and bring to the boil. The goal is to infuse the water with the ginger and star anise and reduce it to syrup. After 15–20 minutes, remove from the heat and add a good-quality vanilla bean paste or essence. Store any leftover glaze in a small glass Kilner jar in the fridge.
7. To assemble the tart, remove the base from the fridge and carefully open the tin by releasing the sides. Spread your date and ginger caramel on the base, then arrange the poached pears on top in whichever pattern you like. >

8   Spoon over some of the ginger glaze and serve with a dollop of Greek-style natural yoghurt and some cocoa powder. This tart will keep for 3–4 days in the fridge.

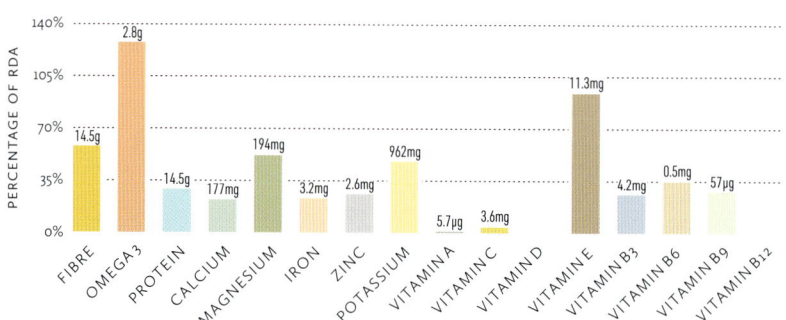

PER 270G PORTION

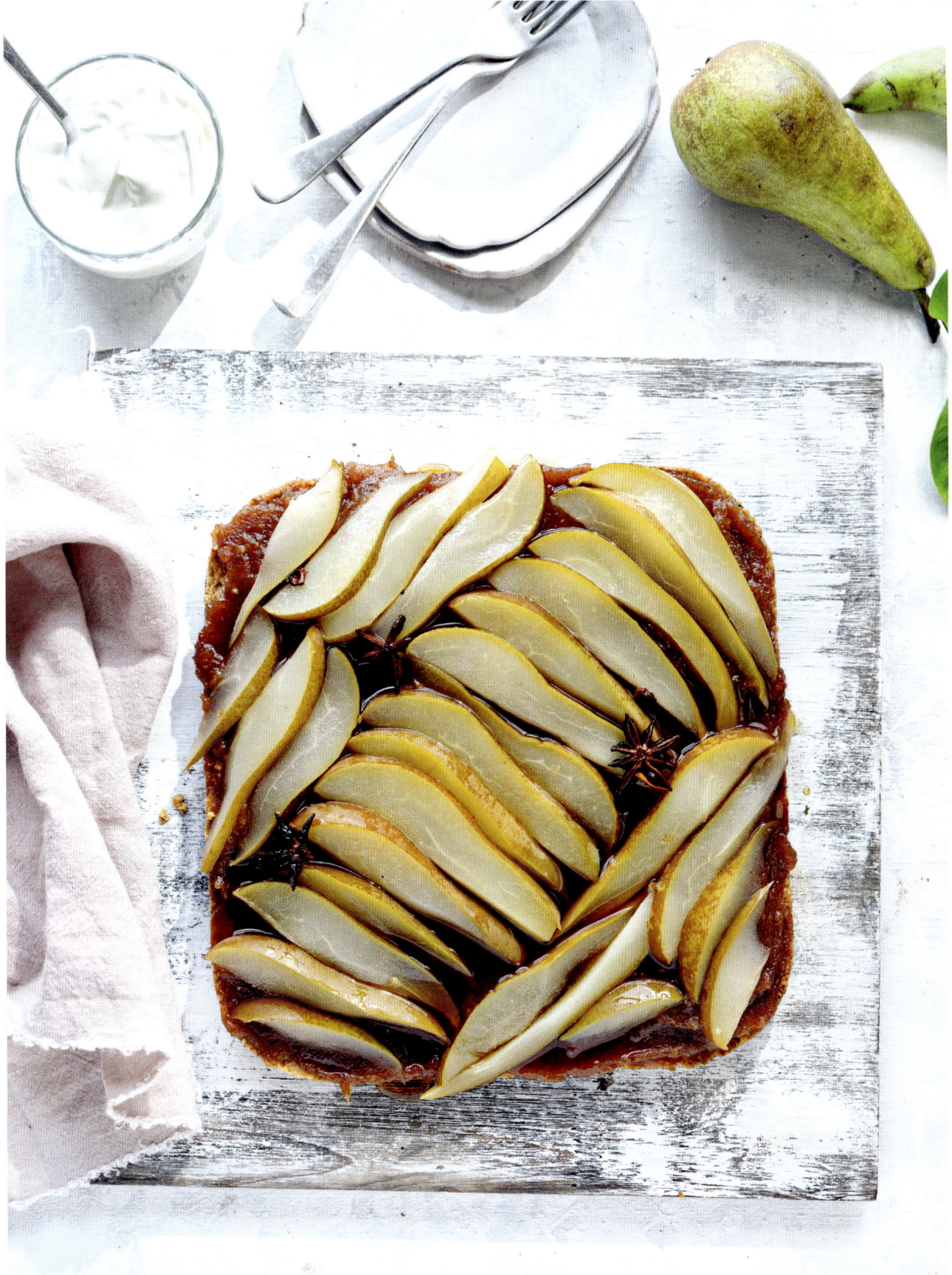

Rhubarb, Pear and Apple Compote

big bunch of rhubarb, washed, peeled and chopped into bite-sized chunks

3 eating apples, peeled and chopped

3 pears, rinsed and chopped

2 tsp vanilla essence

2 tbsp maple syrup

MAKES: 500ML

The combination of the three fruits in this compote delivers a good amount of fibre. You can add this to porridge for a delicious warming breakfast, or serve it with live probiotic yoghurt and berries.

1. Put the rhubarb in a large saucepan with a splash of water.
2. Add the apples to the pot.
3. Add the pears (you can leave the skin on).
4. Place the pot on low heat with the lid on. Cook for 15–20 minutes, or until the fruits have completely softened. Remove and allow to cool.
5. Blitz the mixture until smooth, adding the vanilla essence and maple syrup.
6. Put half the compote in the fridge to use and freeze the rest.

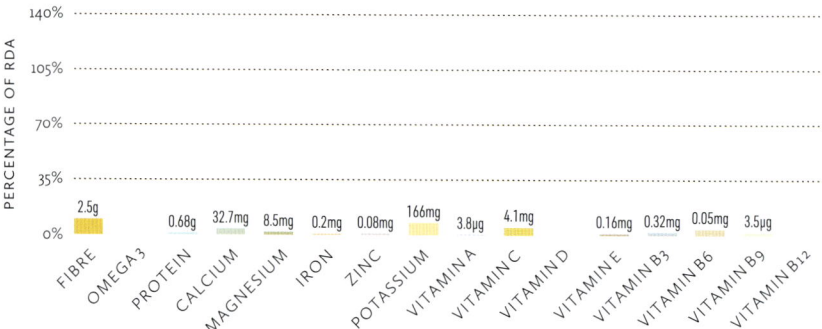

PER 135G PORTION

Carrot Cake Squares

with lemon cashew cream frosting

Gluten-free, dairy-free and refined-sugar-free, these fibre-rich squares are ideal if you want a little treat – without doing any damage.

CARROT CAKE

- 200ml olive oil
- 200ml organic maple syrup
- 4 organic eggs
- 1 tsp vanilla extract
- 2 bananas, cut up into pieces
- 300g carrot pulp/grated carrot
- 360g ground almonds
- 150g ground walnuts, plus extra walnut chips for decoration
- 2 tsp baking powder
- pinch of pink Himalayan or sea salt
- 100g raisins

LEMON CASHEW CREAM

- 280g raw, unsalted cashews, soaked and softened
- 120ml maple syrup
- 1 tbsp vanilla extract
- zest and juice of 1 lemon

MAKES: 40 PORTIONS

1. Preheat the oven to 180°C.
2. Mix the olive oil, maple syrup, eggs, vanilla extract and bananas together in a blender until you have a smooth mix. Transfer this to a large bowl.
3. In a separate bowl, combine the rest of the carrot cake ingredients.
4. Add these dry ingredients to the wet blend and mix well.
5. Line a medium-sized (34 x 24cm) baking tin with greaseproof paper and pour in the mixture.
6. Bake for 30–35 minutes.
7. While the cake mix is baking, make the cashew cream by combining all ingredients in a food processor or blender. Blend on high until perfectly smooth.
8. Adjust your cream with a little more lemon zest, juice or maple syrup to taste, and chill in the fridge until ready to use.
9. Check that the cake is baked by inserting a wooden skewer into the mix: if the skewer comes out clean, it is ready. Remove the cake from the oven and leave it to rest for a while. Then, lift it out of the tin using the excess paper around the sides and place it on a wire cooling rack. It will feel very soft, but this is normal. Allow to cool for at least an hour.
10. When cooled, lift the cake and place it on a wooden board to cut into squares. Before you start cutting, decide whether you are going to serve half and freeze the rest, since this will affect your cashew cream decoration plans.
11. Spread the cashew cream across the whole cake (or half the cake) and slice it into squares. If you have any walnuts or lemon zest left over, you can use these to top each individual square.
12. You can store these in a glass container (with a clip-side lid) in the fridge. I suggest keeping half in the fridge and freezing the rest for another day's enjoyment. >

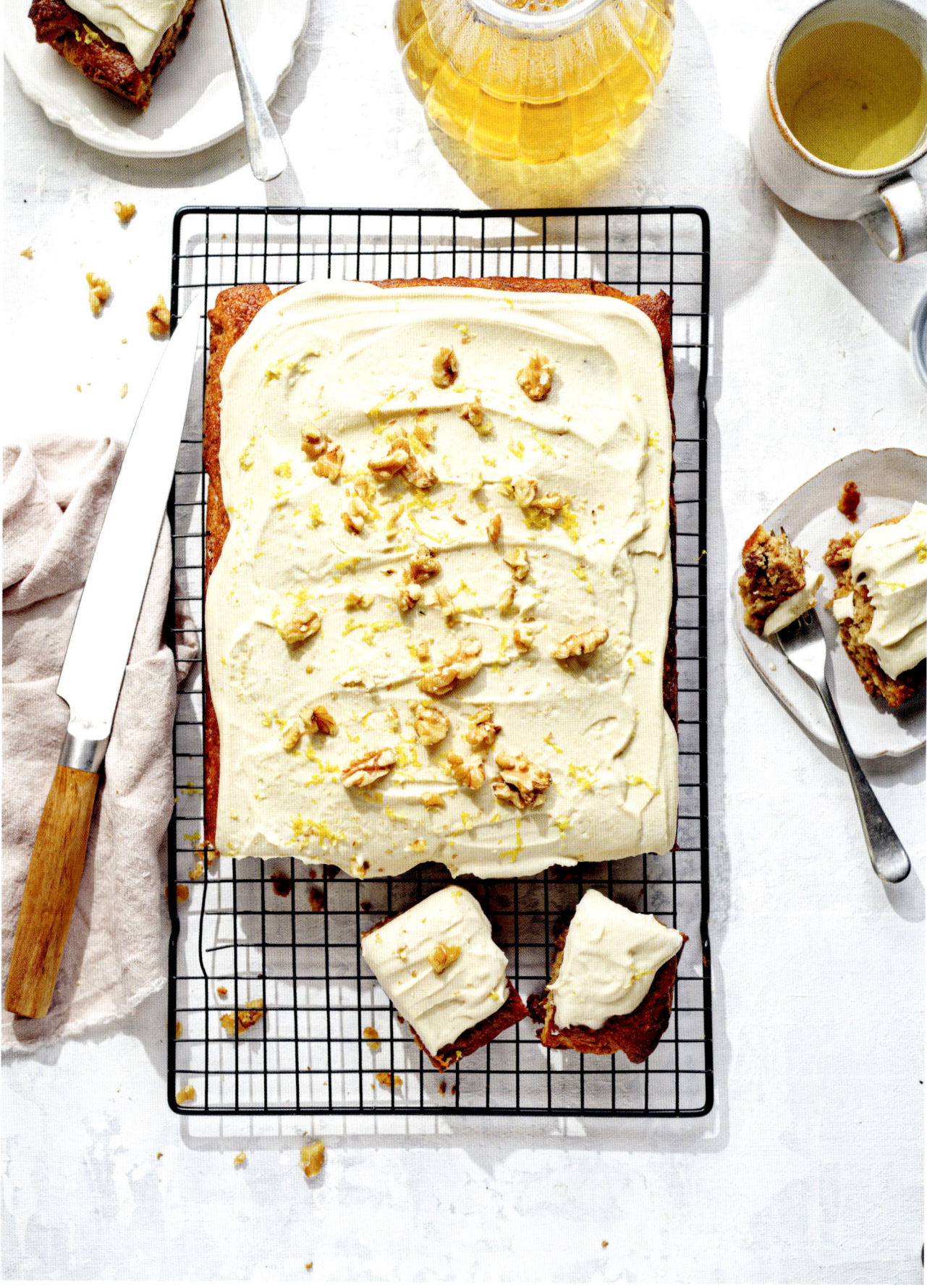

Tip: To make sure your cashews are fully softened, they'll need to be soaked for at least three hours. You can do this by placing the nuts in a bowl and covering them with boiling water.

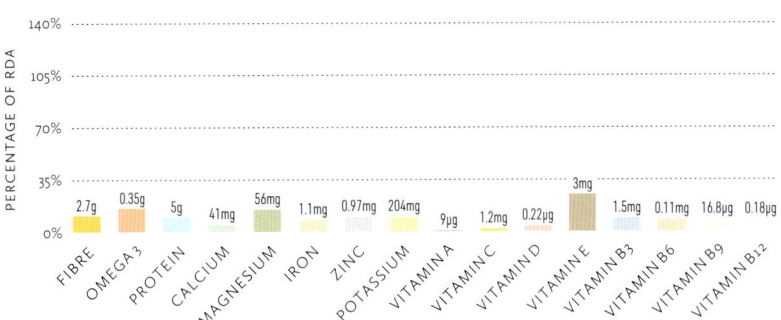

3. Omega-3

Omega-3 essential fats are called essential for a reason – because we have to get them from dietary sources; we cannot produce these ourselves. They're important for the structure of our cells and for hormone production and play a key role in brain health: they've been shown to improve cognitive function and memory and to have a positive effect on mood, reducing symptoms of depression and anxiety.

This section contains some of my favourite recipes – the Mediterranean bouillabaisse is like a seafood hug in a bowl, and the lime chia pudding is my go-to omega-3-rich breakfast option. I hope you enjoy them too!

Lime Chia Pudding

with raspberry mousse

CHIA PUDDING

3 tbsp whole chia seeds

250ml plant-based milk (oat or organic soya milk)

zest of 1 lime

1 tsp vanilla essence

½ tsp of fresh ginger, grated

RASPBERRY MOUSSE

100g frozen raspberries, slightly thawed

2 large Medjool dates, stone removed and chopped small

½ large ripe avocado, flesh scooped out

1 tbsp chopped fresh mint

SUGGESTED TOPPINGS

goji berries

desiccated coconut

pecan cinnamon granola (see p107)

roasted pistachios, chopped

MAKES: 3 PORTIONS

High in protein, fibre and omega-3 essential fats, this is so tasty, it almost feels like a dessert! I make these in Kilner jars, and they keep well in the fridge for several days. They're perfect for breakfast or as a snack.

1. Make the chia pudding by combining all the ingredients. Mix well to prevent the chia seeds from clumping together.
2. For the raspberry mousse, put all the ingredients in a food processor and blend until everything is well combined, smooth and thickened.
3. To serve, scoop 2–3 spoons of chia mix into a glass container or bowl, add the same amount of raspberry mousse and finish with the suggested toppings.
4. If you want to keep until later, cover the pudding and mousse and refrigerate. Add the toppings when you are ready to eat.

PER 125G PORTION

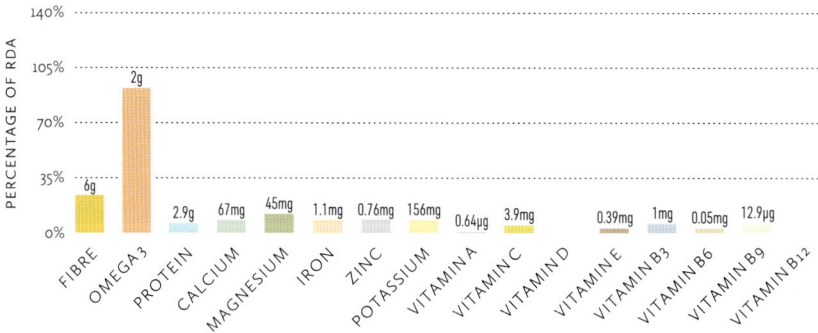

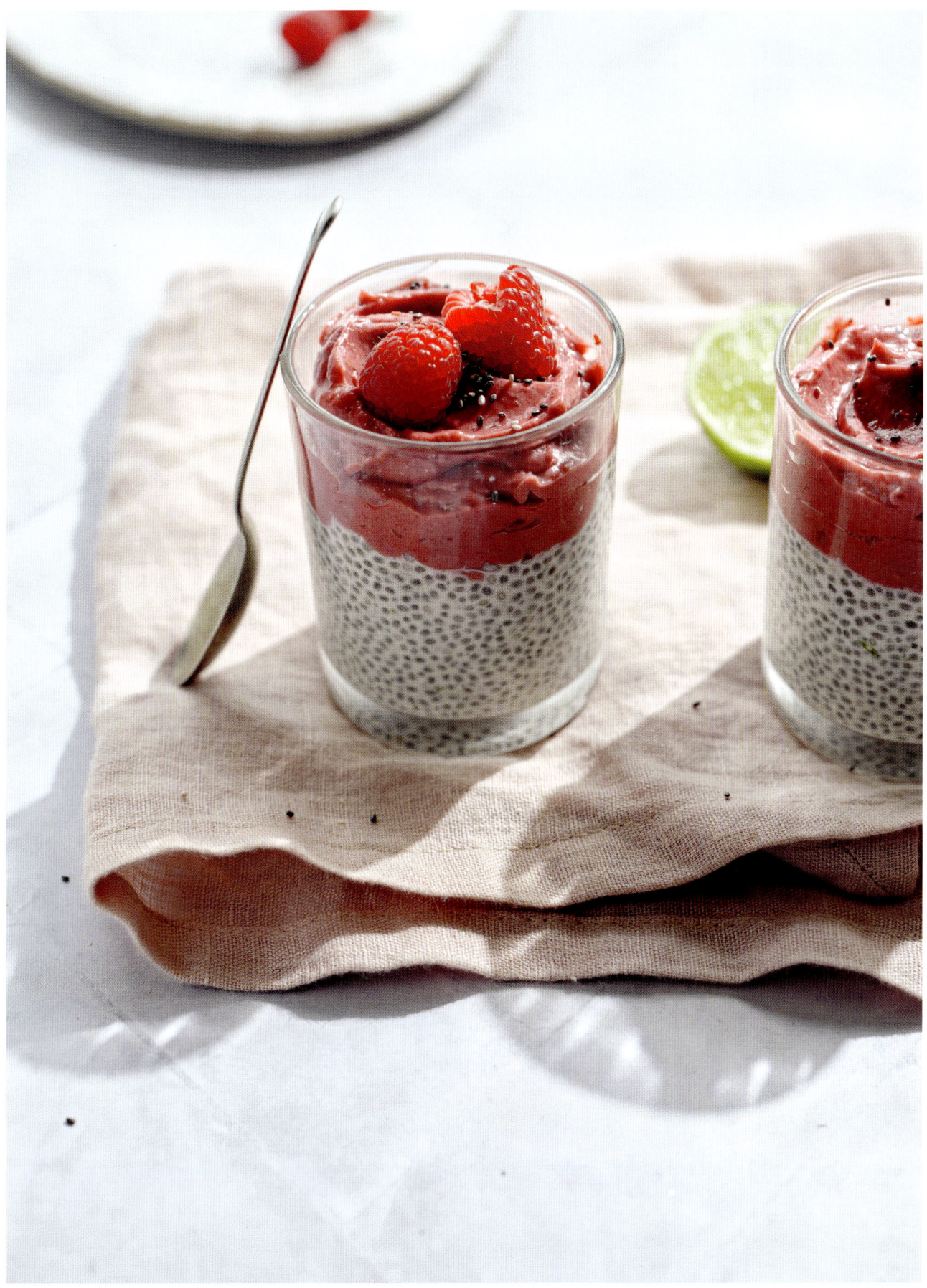

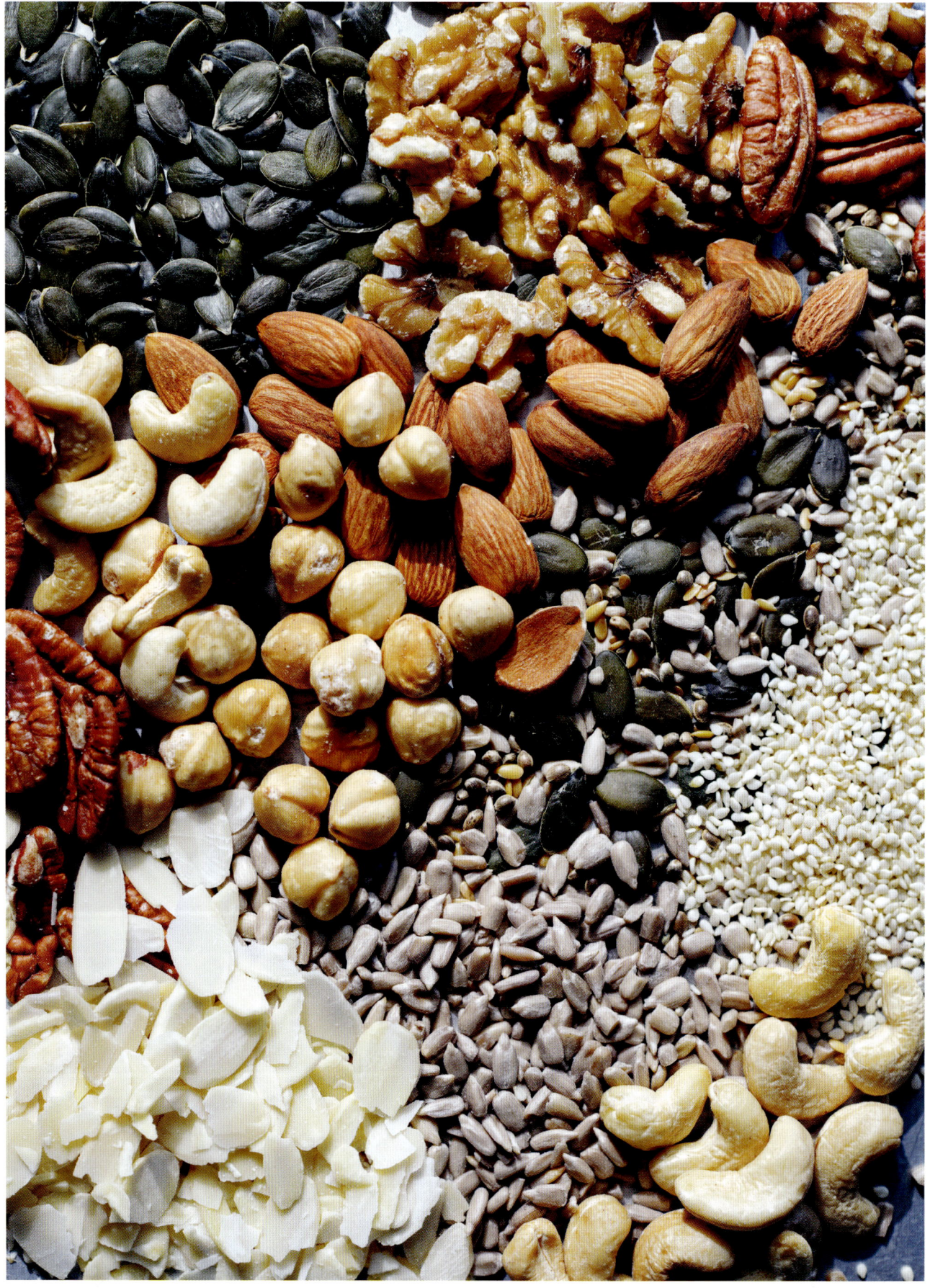

The Nutrient Powerhouse Smoothie Bowl

100g frozen blueberries

½ small frozen banana, cut into pieces

½ courgette, cut into pieces

15g almonds

15g pumpkin seeds

15g ground flaxseeds (Menoligna)

125g live probiotic yoghurt

50ml water

½ tbsp hemp seeds

½ tbsp chia seeds

½ tbsp cacao nibs

½ tbsp vanilla protein powder

SERVES: 2

This delicious smoothie bowl – packed with quality protein, fibre and healthy fats, plus gut-loving ingredients – is a great way to start your day or refuel after exercise.

1. Put all the ingredients in a high-speed blender, and blitz until smooth.
2. Serve immediately – I like to top this with chopped walnuts and fresh blueberries or blackberries.
3. This will keep in the fridge in an airtight glass container for up to 3 days – consume within 24 hours for optimum flavour, colour and nutrient benefit.

PER 225G PORTION

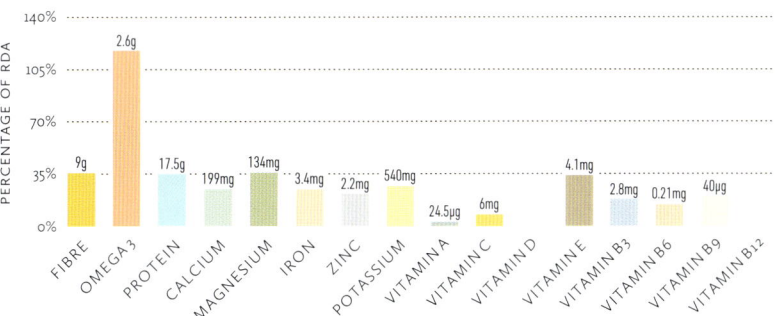

Mediterranean Seafood Bouillabaisse

This delicate, filling and nutritious meal is packed with fibre and vitamin C, with the shellfish providing plenty of protein and key minerals.

Ingredients
1 tbsp olive oil
1 onion, chopped
½ celery stick, diced
½ fennel bulb, diced
1 medium carrot, diced
½ leek, finely sliced
½ tsp turmeric
2 cloves of garlic, minced
35g dried red lentils
1 bay leaf
300ml fish stock
6 plum tomatoes
1 tbsp tomato purée
1 tsp pink Himalayan salt
ground black pepper
225g mixed seafood (salmon, white fish, smoked fish)
16 large mussels
4 large premium prawns, raw
2 tbsp flat-leaf parsley, finely chopped

TO SERVE

1 tsp parsley gremolata (see p195)

100g cooked wholegrain rice per person

SERVES: 4

1. Gently heat the oil in a large saucepan and sauté the onion until soft (about 3 minutes).
2. Add the celery, fennel, carrot and leek, then the turmeric and half the garlic. Cook for about 7 minutes.
3. Pour boiling water over the plum tomatoes. Allow them to rest for a while, then remove the skins. Cut the tomatoes in half, remove the seeds and chop the flesh into quarters.
4. Add the red lentils, bay leaf, fish stock, plum tomatoes, tomato purée and the rest of the minced garlic to the pot. Season with salt and pepper, then cover and allow to simmer gently for 15+ minutes, or until the lentils are soft and have thickened the sauce. If needed, add an extra 50ml of water.
5. Cook the rice separately, according to the instructions on the packet.
6. Towards the end of the rice cooking time, add the mixed seafood, mussels, prawns and chopped parsley to the bouillabaisse pan. Replace the lid and allow to cook on a low heat for 8–10 minutes, or until the mussels have opened.
7. Serve with rice and a dollop of gremolata.

PER 670G PORTION (INCL. 100G RICE)

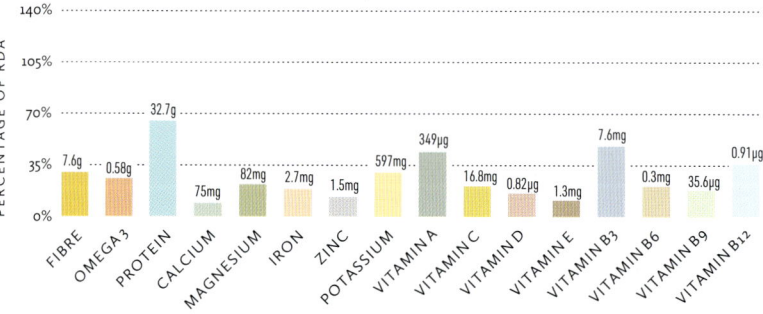

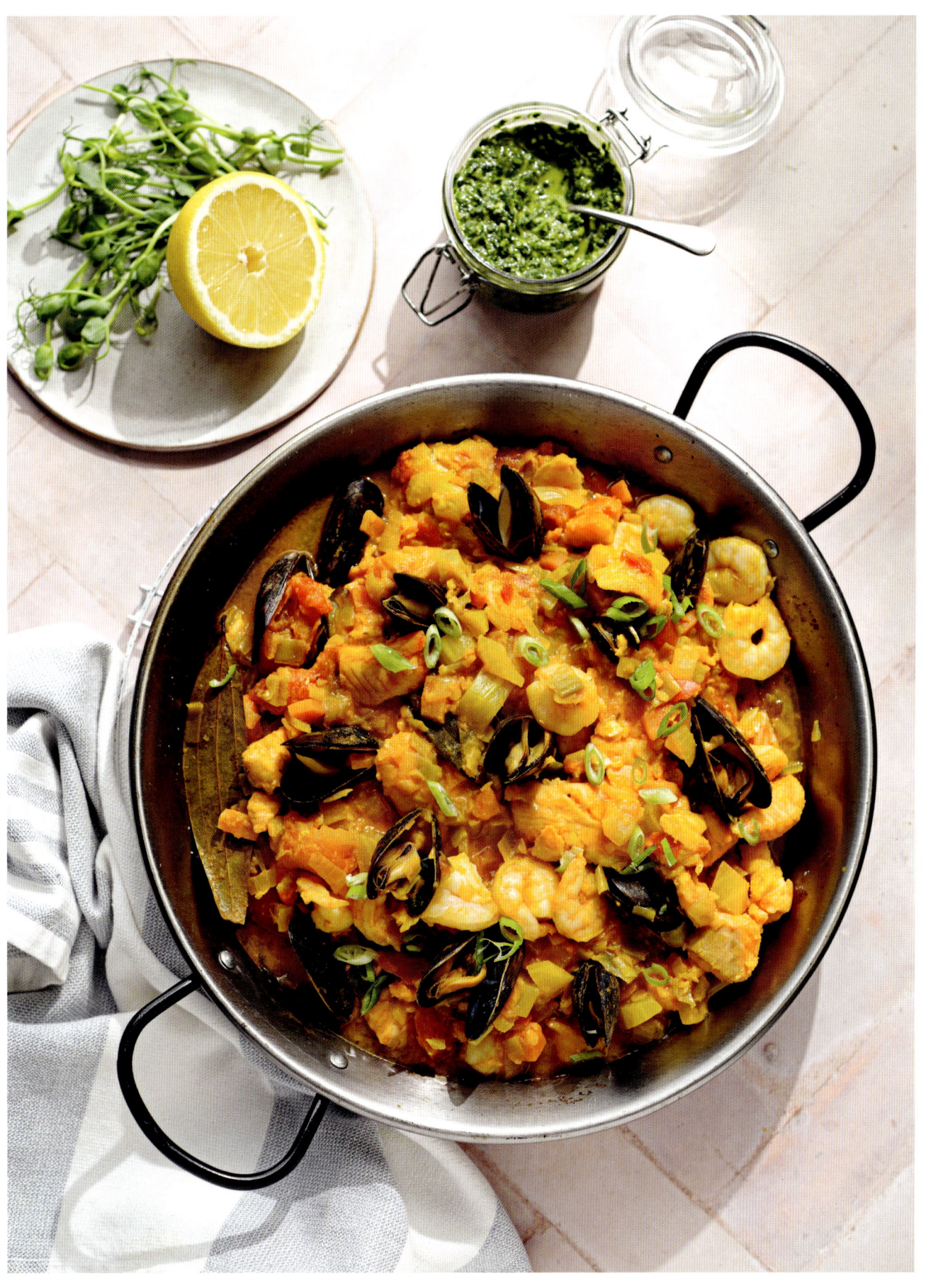

Harissa Charred Salmon

with papaya, mint and avocado salsa

4 fresh salmon fillets, skin removed

1 heaped tsp harissa paste

SALSA

4 spring onions, finely sliced

8 mint leaves, finely chopped

1 medium-sized ripe avocado, diced

1 papaya, seeds removed and diced

1 passion fruit

zest and juice of 1 lime

pink Himalayan salt, to taste

1 tbsp olive oil

1 tbsp sesame oil

½ bunch of chives, finely chopped

SERVES: 4

The heat of the harissa combines well with the freshness of the mint and lime in this recipe. Light and healthy, this is the perfect summertime dinner.

1. Pat dry the salmon fillets and cover them in the harissa paste. Store in the fridge until ready to use.
2. For the salsa, put the spring onions and mint leaves in a bowl.
3. Add the avocado and the papaya.
4. Cut open the passion fruit and spoon out the contents into the bowl.
5. Zest the lime and squeeze the juice into the bowl, then season with salt.
6. Add the olive oil and mix until everything is well combined; you can mash a little to blend the flavours.
7. Heat the sesame oil in a frying pan, then add the marinated salmon fillets. Allow to brown for a few minutes until crispy, then turn over and cook the other side for 1 minute.
8. Remove from the heat.
9. Put the pan-fried salmon fillet on a warmed plate, topped with 2 tablespoons of salsa and some chives to decorate.

PER 315G PORTION

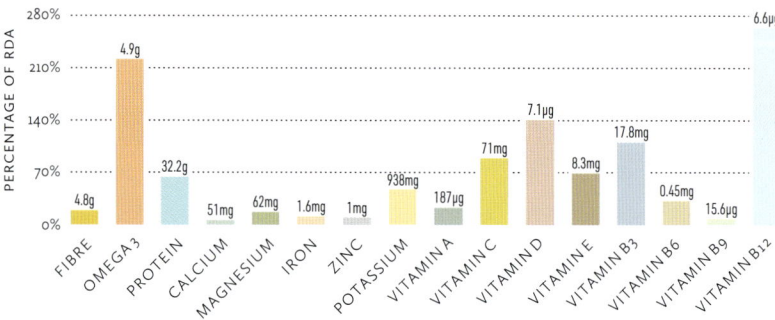

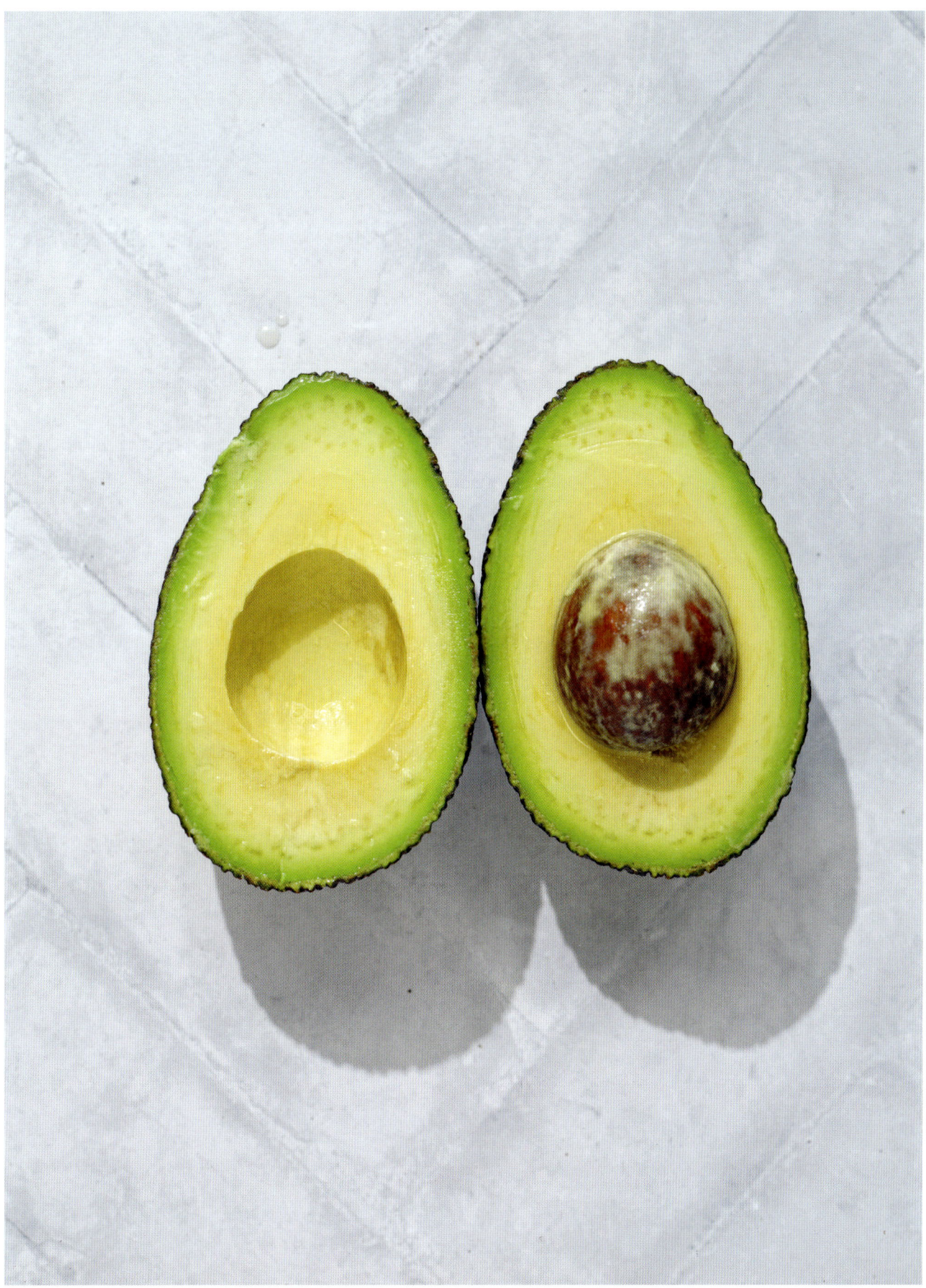

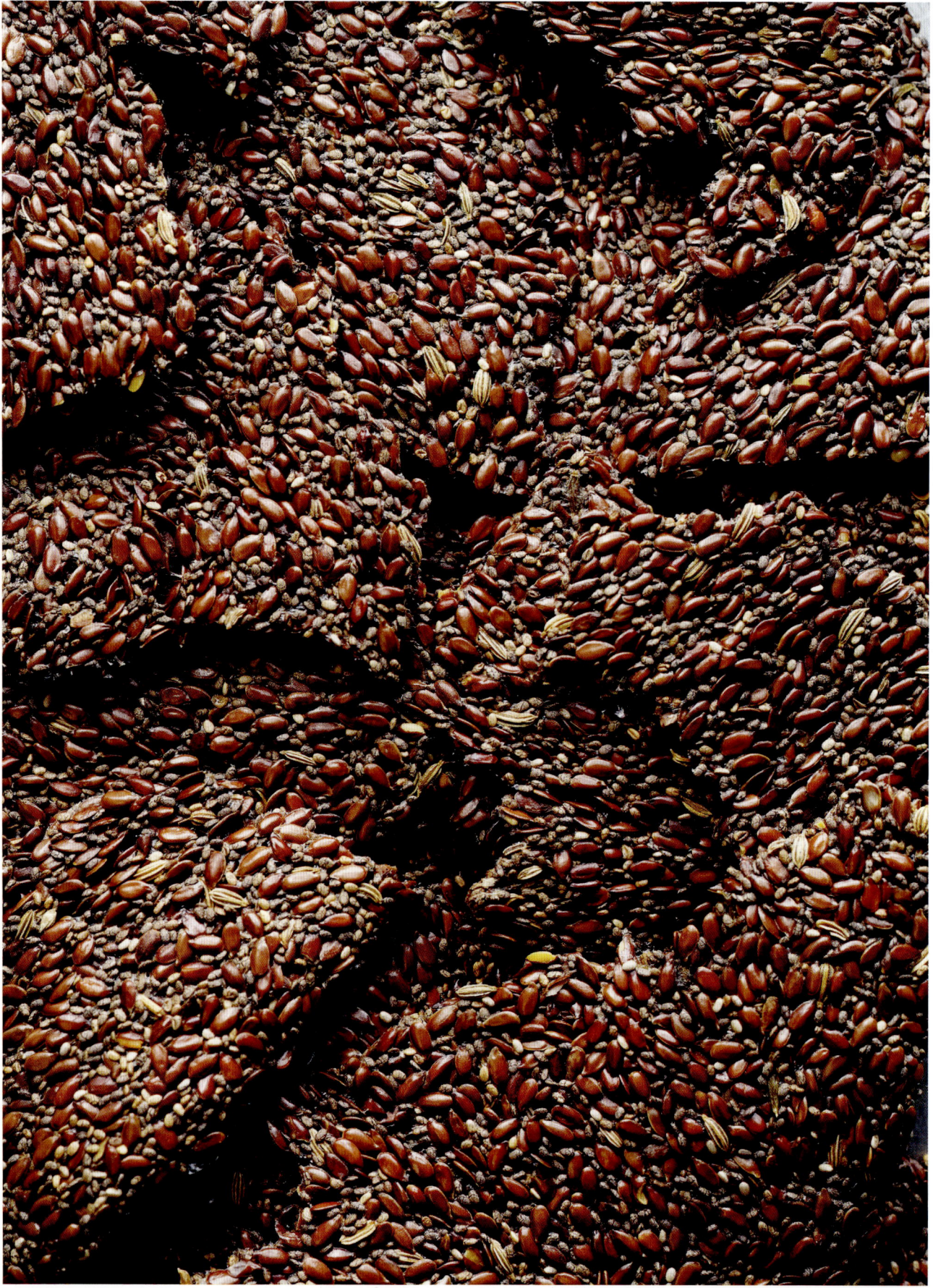

Flaxseed Crackers

110g whole flaxseeds

40g chia seeds

1 tbsp fennel seeds

1 tbsp sesame seeds

1 tsp pink Himalayan salt

360ml filtered water

MAKES: 8+ PORTIONS

These tasty, fibre-rich crackers are also a great source of protein and omega-3. Enjoy them instead of bread, or serve them with hummus or other dips. You can store them in an airtight container at room temperature for several weeks.

1. Preheat the oven to 80°C and line a baking tray with a silicone sheet.
2. Put all the ingredients together in a bowl, and mix well. Set aside for 1 hour, until the mixture has formed a gel.
3. Spread the flaxseed gel out on the baking tray as thinly and evenly as possible to cover the entire surface.
4. Bake for 2 hours, then turn the flaxseed mixture over. Remove the tray from the oven, place a second silicone sheet over the flaxseed mixture and flip the whole sheet over on to the other side. Carefully peel off the original silicone sheet and return the flaxseed mixture to the oven for a further 30 minutes to 1 hour, or until it is dry and brittle, and turning up at the corners.
5. Remove from the oven and allow to cool completely, then break up into smaller pieces.

PER 65G PORTION

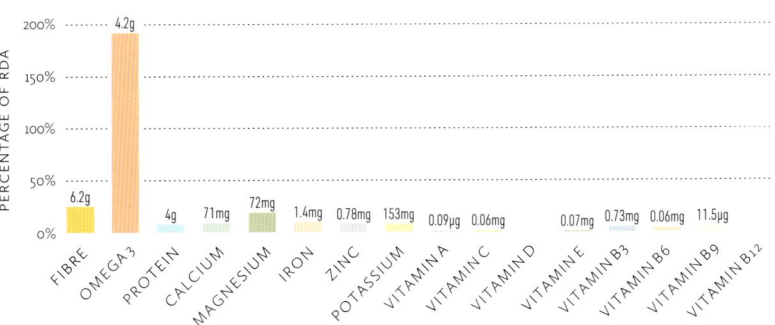

Balsamic Dressing

350ml extra virgin olive oil

150ml aged balsamic vinegar

75ml maple syrup

2 tbsp Dijon mustard (smooth)

½ tsp pink Himalayan salt

MAKES: 1,200ML

This is my go-to everyday dressing, which is rich in heart-healthy monounsaturated fatty acids (MUFAs). Use the best olive oil you can get and a good balsamic vinegar, too, for a smooth taste. There is no need to refrigerate this dressing; it keeps well in the cupboard.

1. Combine all the ingredients in a glass jar with a tight-fitting lid.
2. Mix with a fork to start with, then put the lid on tightly and shake like a cocktail until everything is smooth and combined.
3. Store in a flip-top glass bottle in the cupboard.

Note: This balsamic dressing is rich in heart-healthy monounsaturated fats, thanks to oleic acid in the extra virgin olive oil, and contains trace amounts of my 16 tracked nutrients, which was difficult to show accurately to scale for a single serving (40ml). It is a good source of calcium, magnesium and potassium, and is extremely useful as a daily salad dressing.

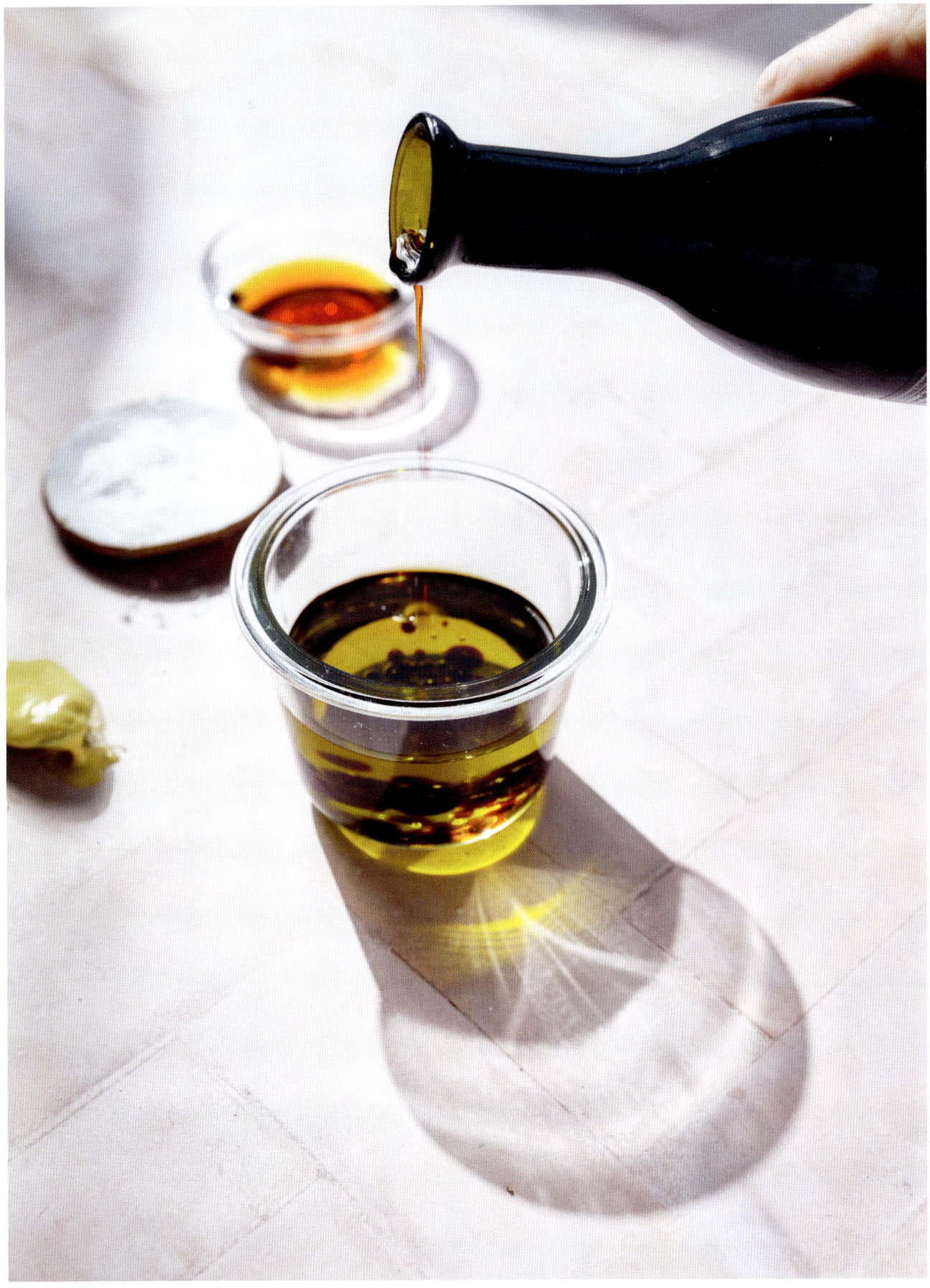

Smoked Mackerel Pâté

2 cooked fillets of smoked mackerel, skin removed

400g tinned cannellini beans or butter beans, drained and rinsed

handful of parsley, finely chopped

handful of dill fronds, finely chopped

juice of ½ lemon

1 clove of garlic (optional)

pink Himalayan salt, to taste

ground black pepper

1 tbsp extra virgin olive oil

MAKES: 6 PORTIONS

A delicious way to get omega-3-rich, oily fish into your diet, this pâté is also dairy-free, since I use cannellini beans instead of cream cheese. Serve it as a dip with veg sticks and flaxseed crackers.

1. Blitz all the ingredients together in a food processor until smooth.
2. Store in an airtight glass container in the fridge.

PER 100G PORTION

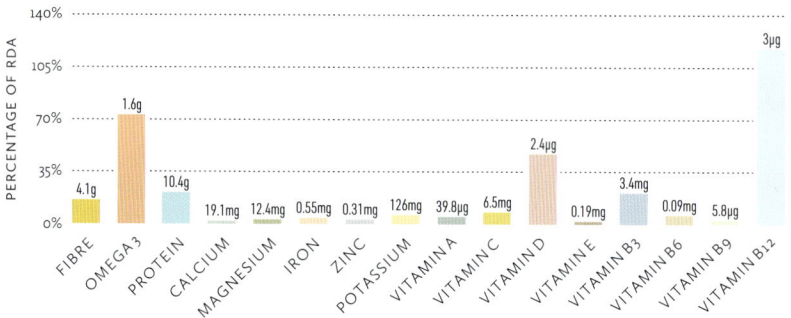

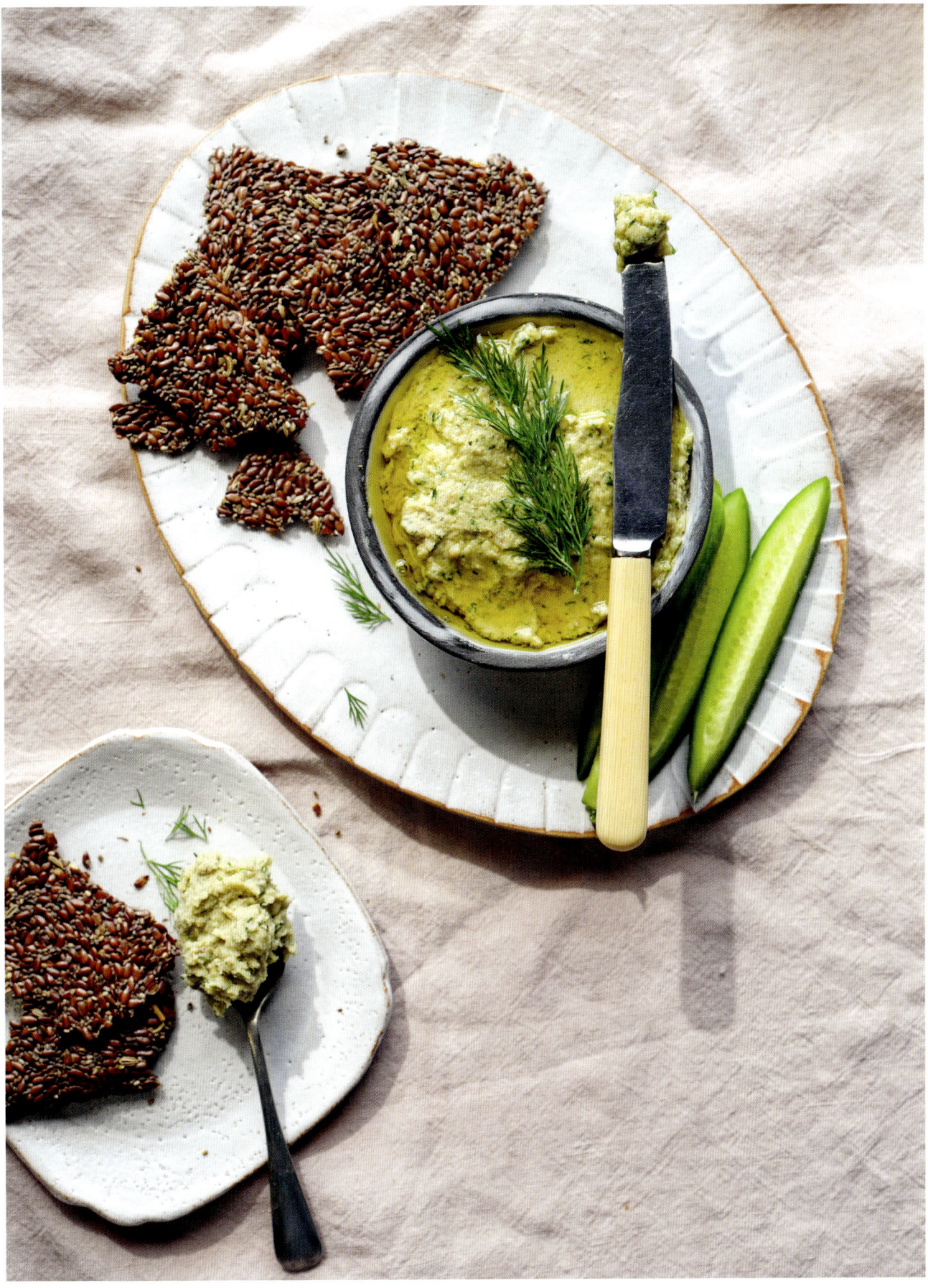

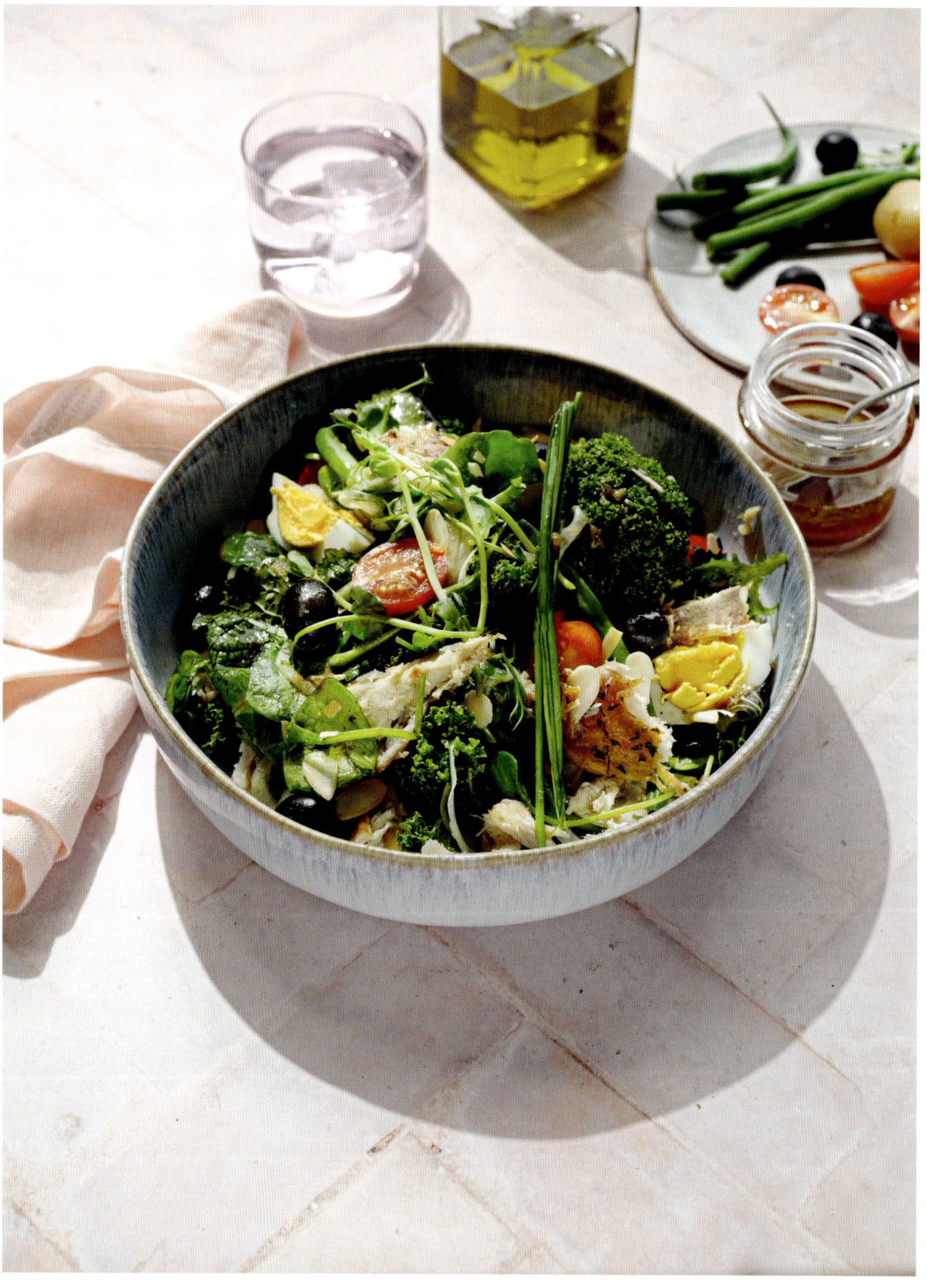

Mackerel Niçoise Salad

220g French beans, trimmed

2 mackerel fillets

2 large handfuls of mixed green leaves (e.g. spinach, rocket, chicory), washed and spin-dried

4 baby salad potatoes, cooked and quartered

1 red onion, finely sliced

6 cherry tomatoes, halved

handful of black olives, stones removed

2 boiled eggs, sliced

FRENCH DRESSING

3 tbsp olive oil

1 tbsp red wine vinegar

1 tsp wholegrain Dijon mustard

1 clove of garlic, crushed

salt and pepper, to taste

1 tbsp honey

TO SERVE

handful of fresh chives, chopped

handful of flaked almonds, toasted

SERVES: 2

This is a variant of the classic Niçoise salad, with tuna replaced by mackerel, which contains more beneficial omega-3 fatty acids.

1. If using raw mackerel fillets, preheat the oven to 180°C.
2. Blanch the French beans in boiling water for 2–3 minutes, until just tender. Strain and allow to cool.
3. Prepare the mackerel fillets. If using pre-cooked, simply remove the skin and flake the mackerel in large chunks, ready to add to the salad. If using raw fillets, pan-fry skin-side down on a high heat until crispy, then finish in the preheated oven for 5 minutes. Allow to cool.
4. Blend all the dressing ingredients with a whisk. Set aside.
5. Start to assemble the salad. Place the leaves, French beans, cooked salad potatoes and red onion in a large mixing bowl with half of the dressing. Mix well.
6. Divide the mix between two salad bowls, top each with a mackerel fillet, along with the cherry tomatoes, black olives and a sliced boiled egg.
7. Drizzle the remaining dressing on top and add some chopped herbs – for example, chives – and some toasted flaked almonds.

PER 395G PORTION

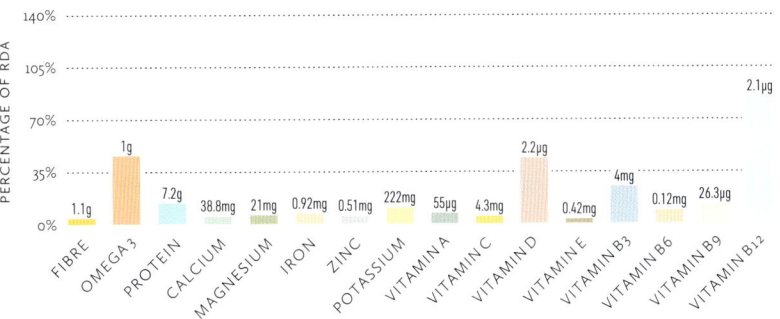

Summer Rolls

with prawns and ginger miso dipping sauce

4 small (22cm) round rice paper sheets

1 medium carrot, cut into sticks

½ small red pepper, cut into sticks

2 spring onions, finely sliced

8 mangetout, finely sliced

large handful of salad leaves, finely sliced

edible flowers, such as nasturtiums (optional)

75g cooked king prawns, halved lengthways, tails removed

handful of coriander leaves

handful of toasted cashews, chopped

handful of toasted sesame seeds

TO SERVE

ginger miso dressing (see p96)

MAKES: 4 ROLLS

Delicious and fresh, these summer rolls are packed with prawns, fresh coriander, toasted cashews and crunchy veg. Two large rolls are an ideal portion per person.

1. Place a rice paper sheet in a shallow bowl of warm water and allow it to soften for 20 seconds. Remove it from the water and place it on a clean plastic chopping board.
2. Starting with the vegetables and flowers (if using), pile all the ingredients in the centre of the sheet. Be careful not to overfill.
3. Fold the left side of the sheet over the filling, followed by the right side and the bottom piece. Roll it tightly over the filling and roll forward. Cut off any excess with a sharp knife. You should see all the brightly coloured vegetables and flowers through the sheet.
4. Serve with a heaped tablespoon of ginger miso dressing, used as a dipping sauce.

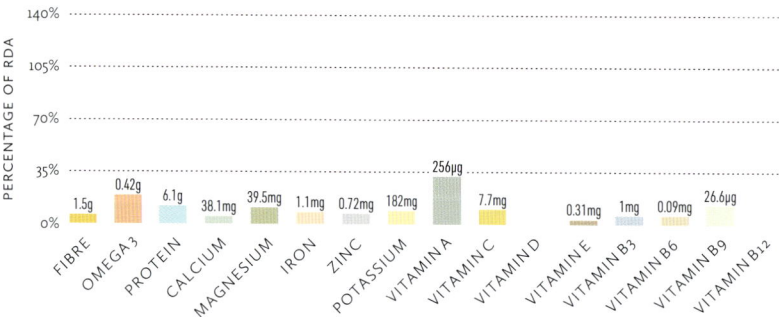

85G PORTION

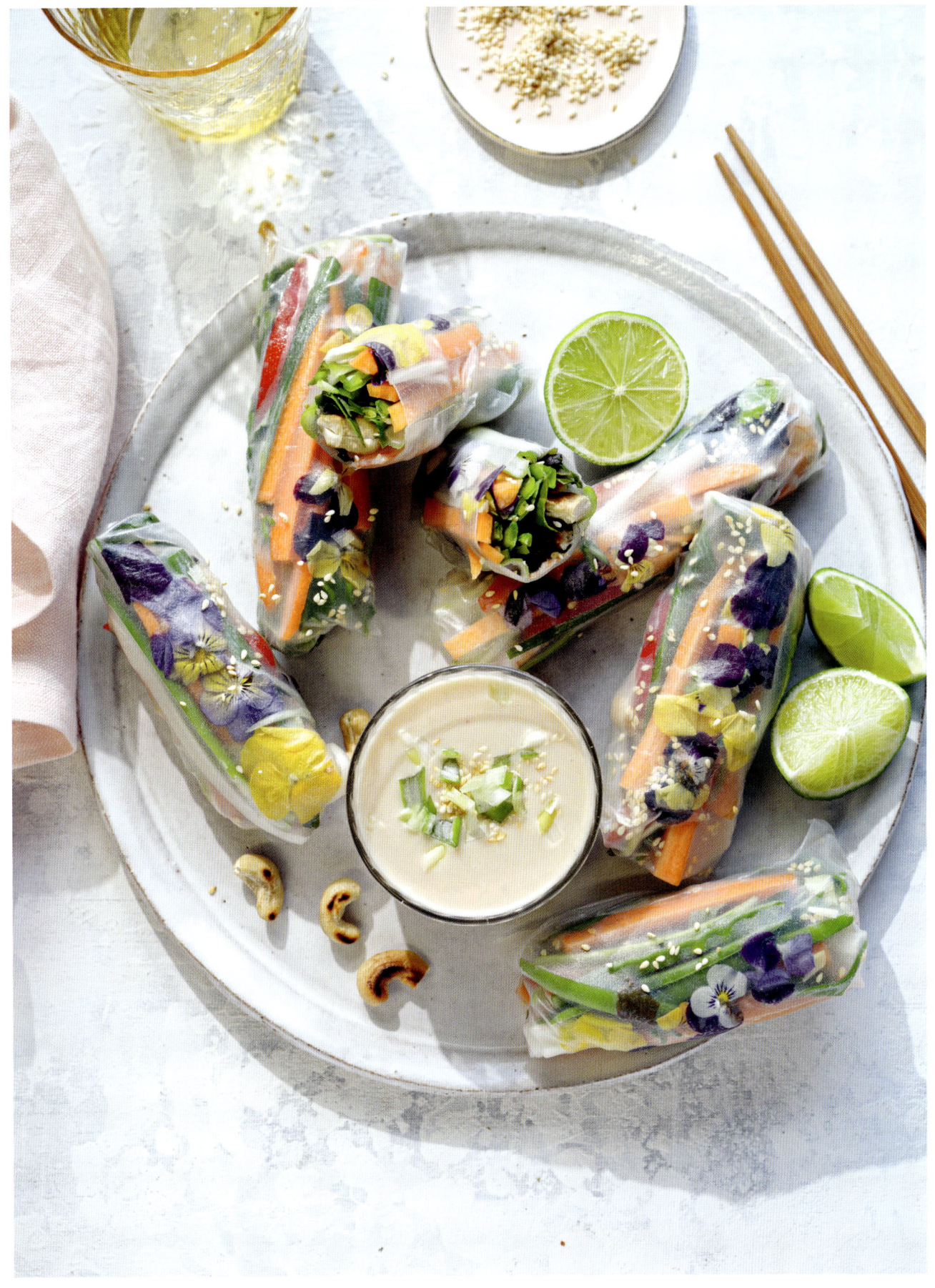

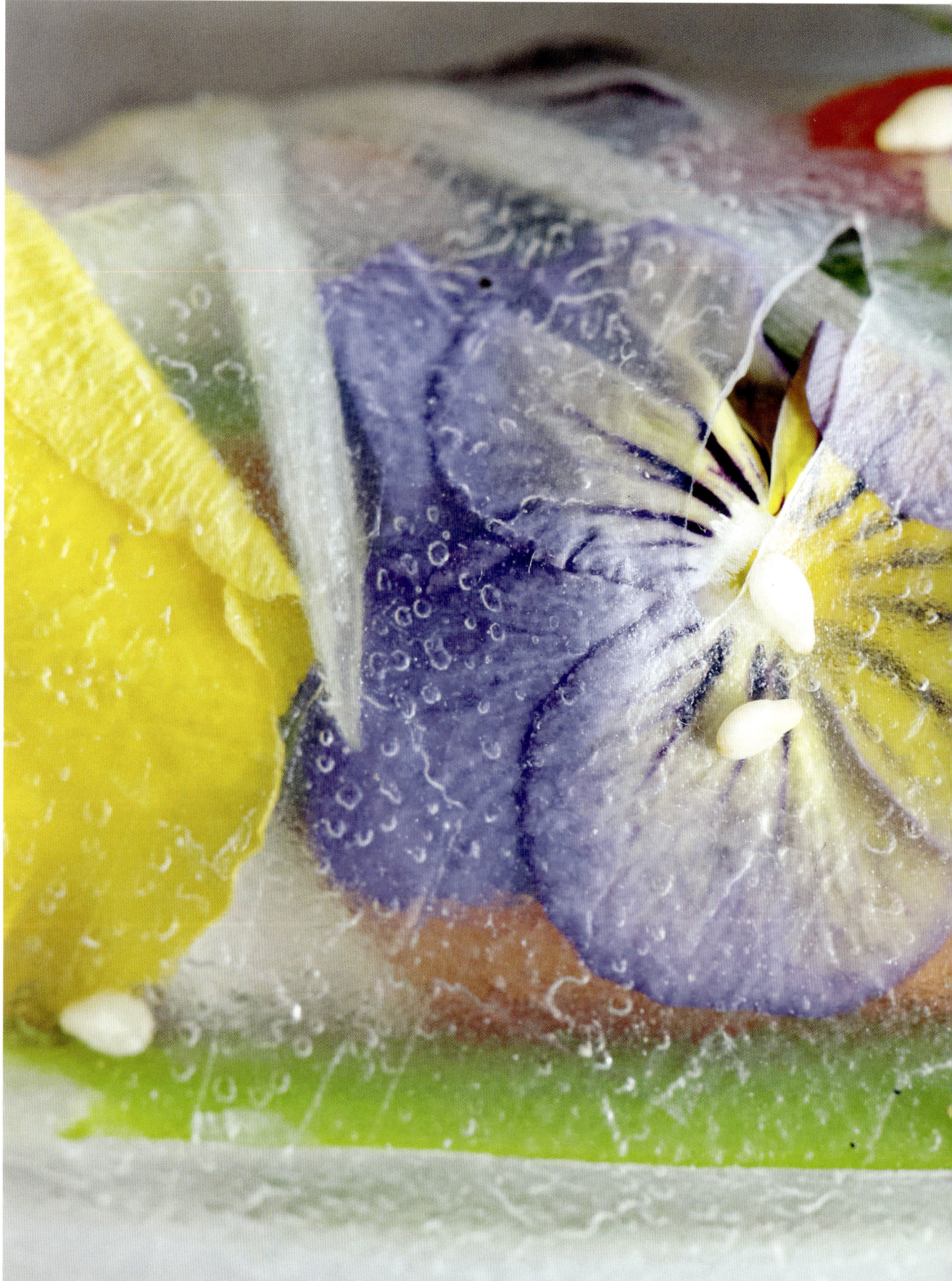

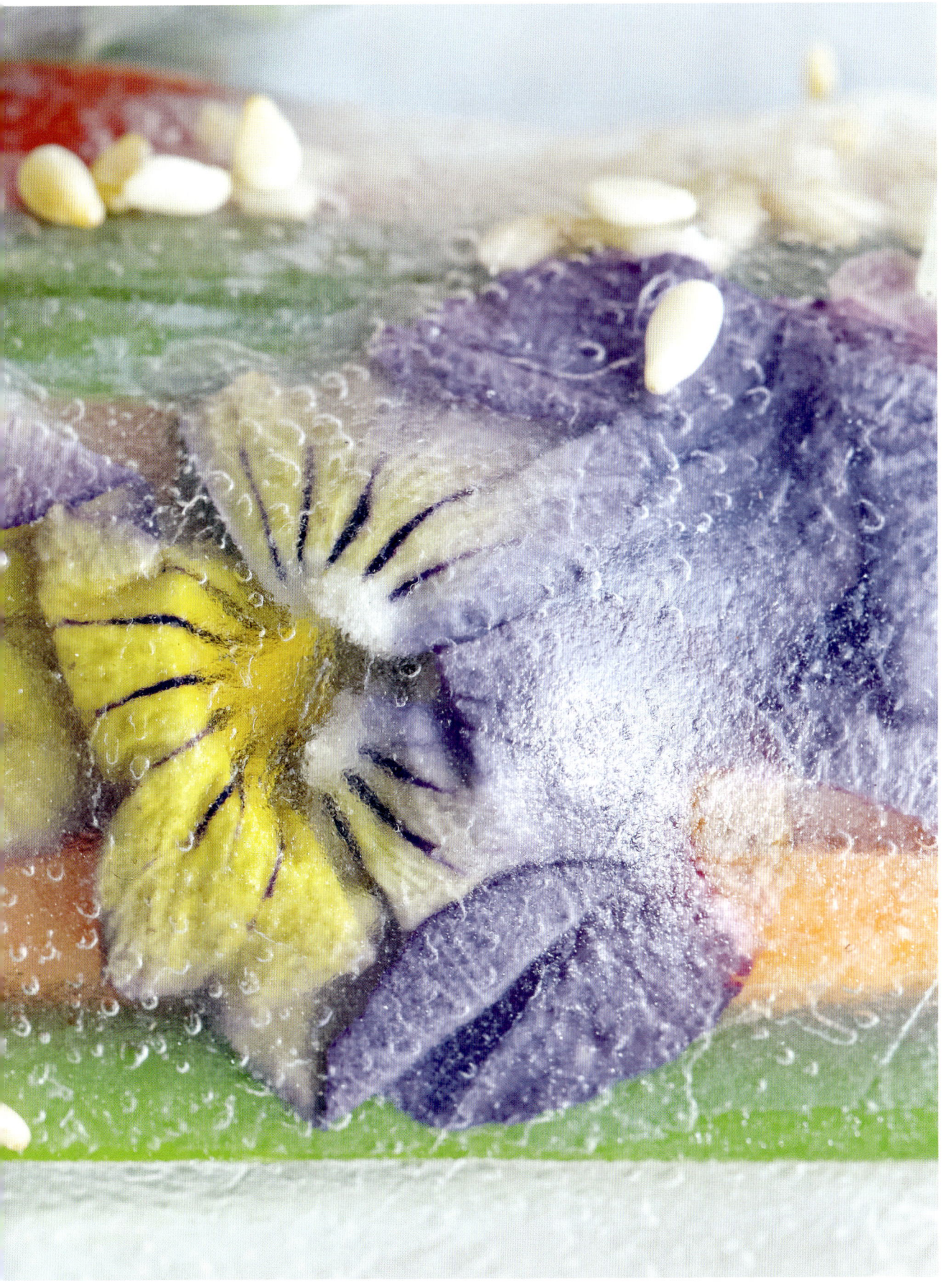

Salmon Kedgeree

1 tsp veg stock powder
450ml boiling water
250g fresh salmon fillets
2 tbsp fresh dill, chopped
1 tbsp olive oil
1 medium onion, finely chopped
1 tsp curry powder (madras)
½ tsp turmeric powder
175g wholegrain rice
70g frozen peas
3 spring onions, finely sliced
1 tbsp lemon juice
200g smoked salmon, sliced
2 hard-boiled eggs, quartered
handful of chopped parsley
handful of broccoli sprouts
ground black pepper

SERVES: 4

Perfect for a weekend brunch, this dish is also a great option for dinner. If you don't fancy salmon, it can also be made using mackerel or trout.

1. Put the stock powder and the water in a medium saucepan, and bring to the boil.
2. Reduce the heat to a simmer and add the fresh salmon. Poach for 6–8 minutes.
3. Carefully remove the salmon with a slotted spoon, reserving the stock water.
4. After removing the skin from the poached salmon, flake it into a bowl with the chopped dill.
5. Put the olive oil in a large saucepan and fry the onion until soft, then stir in the spices.
6. Add the rice and fry for a minute, then pour in the stock.
7. Bring to a boil, cover with a lid and simmer for 10–12 minutes, or until the rice is cooked. Remove the pan from the heat, add the frozen peas and put the lid on to steam.
8. Divide the rice between two plates and add the spring onions, lemon juice and salmon pieces (fresh and smoked). Garnish with the eggs, some chopped parsley and broccoli sprouts.

PER 350G PORTION

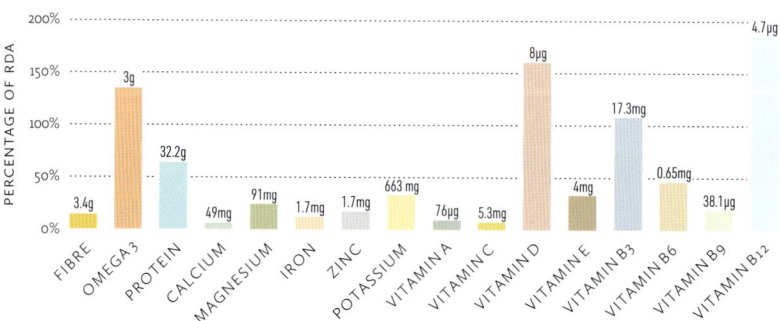

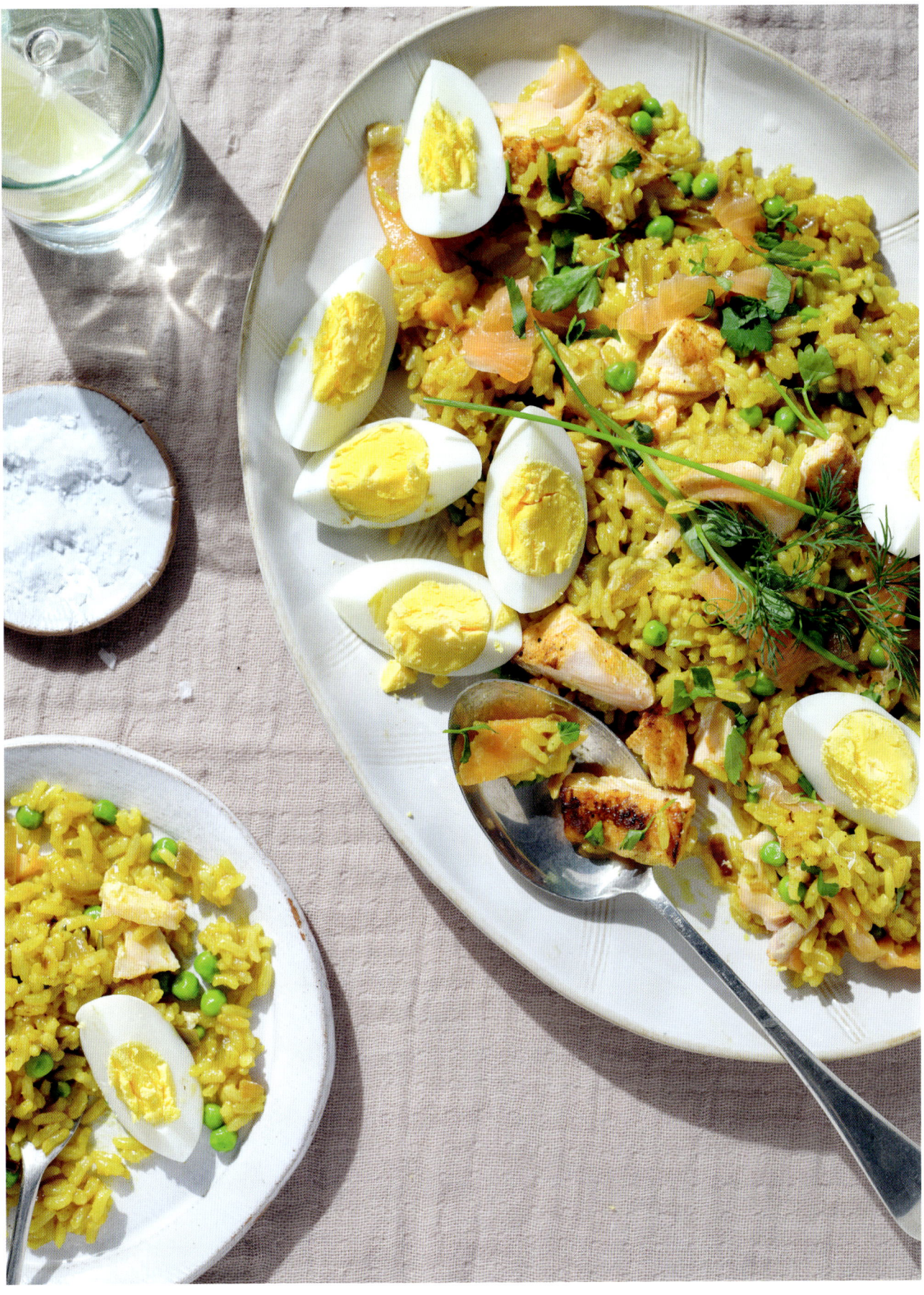

4. Calcium and Magnesium

Calcium and magnesium are both classed as major minerals that we need in optimum doses at this life stage. They are important for heart health – as they can help to lower blood pressure and reduce the risk of heart disease – and are also essential for building and maintaining strong bones. Magnesium has also been shown to improve sleep quality and reduce insomnia during menopause.

One of the highlights of this section is my nut butter recipe; I've detailed the steps to make almond butter, but you can make any nut butter (such as walnut or hazelnut butter) using the same method.

The Recovery-Boosting Salad in a Jar

8 tbsp French dressing (see p149)

65g black-eyed beans, cooked

½ small fennel bulb, finely sliced

80g wholegrain basmati rice, cooked

½ courgette, spiralised

1 small raw beetroot, finely sliced

1 boiled egg, sliced

6 cherry tomatoes, quartered

1 spring onion, sliced

1 tbsp feta cheese, crumbled (omit if you prefer a dairy-free option)

big handful of leaves of choice (such as baby spinach leaves or rocket leaves)

2 radishes, finely sliced

handful of fresh pomegranate seeds

2 tbsp savoury granola (see p122)

pink Himalayan salt and black pepper, to taste

SERVES: 2

With complex carbs, plant protein, antioxidant-rich raw veggies and essential fats in the form of olive oil and toasted seeds, this is the perfect post-workout salad. It will keep for a couple of days in the fridge, so make two portions and eat it on the go, straight out of the jar.

1. Make the French dressing, then divide it between two medium-sized wide-mouth glass jars with rubber-sealed lids.
2. Spoon in the beans on top of the dressing, followed by the fennel, rice and spiralised courgette.
3. Arrange the beetroot slices around the inside of the jar.
4. Add half a sliced egg to each jar, followed by the cherry tomatoes, spring onions and feta cheese.
5. Finish with the spinach or rocket leaves and radish slices, then top with pomegranate seeds and savoury granola.
6. Place the jars in the fridge. When you are ready to eat your salad, remove it from the fridge and allow it to come to room temperature (the dressing will coat the ingredients more easily then). Turn the jar upside down and gently shake the salad to make sure all the veggies are well coated.

PER 380G PORTION

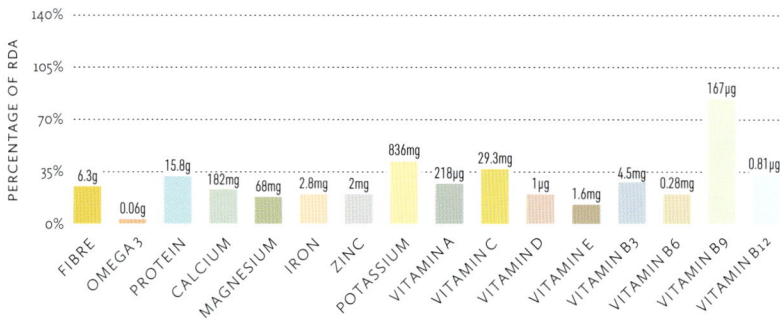

158   NOURISH FOR MENOPAUSE

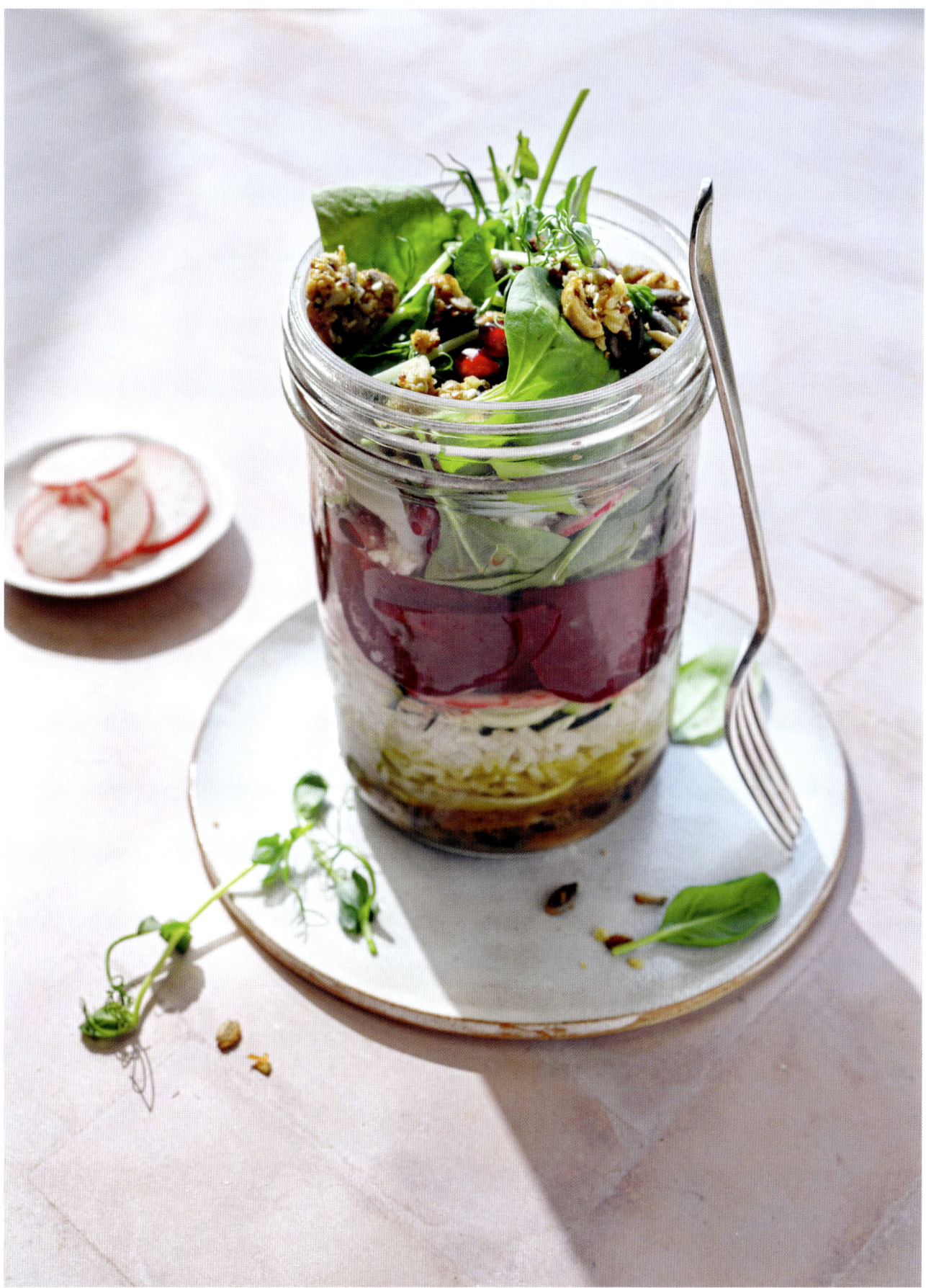

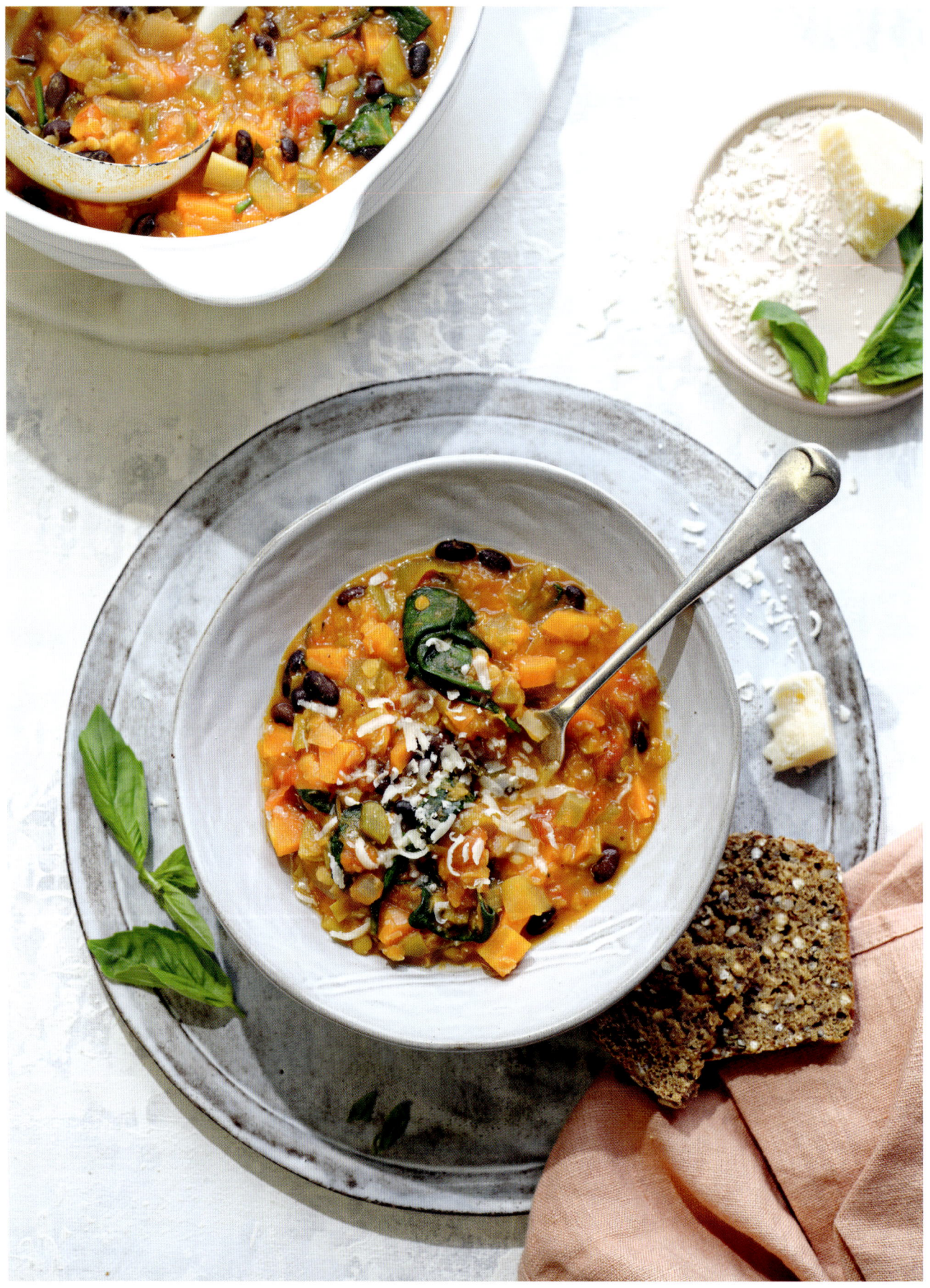

Minestrone Bean Stew

1 tbsp olive oil

1 large onion, finely chopped

4 cloves of garlic, grated

1 leek, finely sliced

2 celery sticks, chopped

2 sprigs of rosemary

handful of organic red chard or baby spinach leaves

handful of organic kale, de-stemmed and chopped

4 organic carrots, cleaned and chopped

4 plum tomatoes, skins removed

190g dried red lentils

400g tinned kidney beans, rinsed

400g tinned cannellini beans, rinsed

1.5 litres chicken bone broth (see p235) or veg stock

2 large bay leaves

salt and pepper, to taste

6 tsp parsley gremolata (see p195)

SERVES: 6+

This is my spin on the traditional Italian recipe – without pasta. It is still filling, thanks to the beans and legumes, and it has the added bonus of containing home-made chicken bone broth. However, you can also use vegetable stock.

1. Put the olive oil in a large stockpot, and add the onion, 3 garlic cloves, the leek and the celery.
2. Allow to sweat gently with the lid on until softened.
3. Add in the rest of the ingredients, except the remaining garlic clove, stirring gently. If you are using spinach leaves instead of chard, add these at the very end.
4. Cook on a low heat for 45 minutes until the vegetables are tender.
5. Adjust the seasoning if necessary. I like to grate the last garlic clove in at this stage to enhance the flavour, or you can top the stew with some parsley gremolata.

PER 347G PORTION

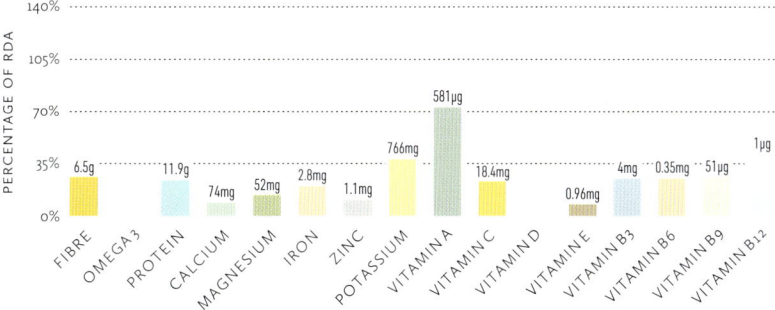

Red Lentil, Turmeric and Kale Hotpot

1 tbsp olive oil

1 large red onion, finely chopped

2 sticks of celery, finely chopped

1 leek, finely chopped

1 carrot, finely chopped

260g dried red lentils

2 tsp organic turmeric powder

2 litres vegetable stock

350g kale, de-stemmed and chopped

salt and black pepper, to taste

½ bunch of fresh chopped parsley

1 tbsp parsley gremolata (see p195)

SERVES: 6

Filling and nourishing, this fast-to-make soup is ideal for either a substantial lunch or a light supper. The addition of the kale provides a good calcium boost.

1. In a large stockpot with a drizzle of olive oil, add the onion, celery, leek and carrot. Allow to sweat gently with the lid on until softened.
2. Add the red lentils, turmeric and vegetable stock.
3. Cook on a low heat for 20 minutes, or until the vegetables are tender and the lentils have softened and swelled.
4. Stir in the kale and cook for a further 5 minutes.
5. Taste and adjust the seasoning if necessary. If it's too thick, add more water.
6. Add the parsley at the end, before serving in warmed bowls with a teaspoon of gremolata.

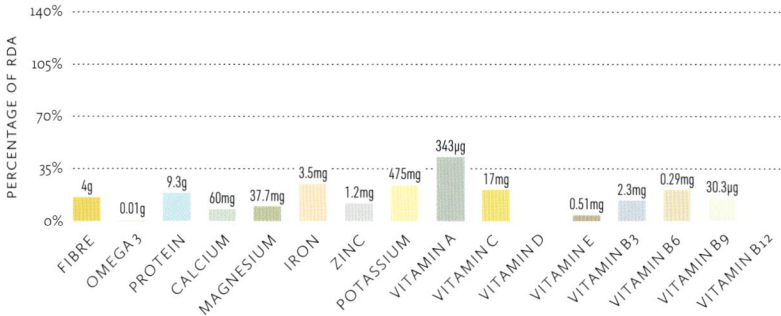

PER 375G PORTION

Kale Quinoa Wraps

140g white quinoa
230ml water
60ml oat milk
70g kale leaves, de-stemmed and chopped
1 tsp salt
1 tbsp nutritional yeast flakes
1 tsp walnut oil

MAKES: 8 PORTIONS

These four-ingredient wraps are easy to make and much healthier than the shop-bought kind. They can be made in advance, then stored in the fridge or frozen. See the falafel wrap recipe (p223) for serving suggestions.

1. Soak the quinoa for 4–6 hours or overnight. Rinse and add to a high-speed blender with the water. Blitz on high until you have a smooth batter.
2. Add the oat milk, kale leaves, salt and yeast and blitz again until perfectly smooth. The batter mix should be runny and not too thick – add some water if necessary.
3. Brush a crêpe pan with a little walnut oil and heat. Add one ladle of batter mix to the pan and spread out by tilting the pan and using the back of a spoon. Once set and cooked on one side, flip over with a spatula and brown on the other side.
4. Once browned on both sides, remove the wrap from the pan and cool on a wire rack. Repeat the process until all of the batter has been used – this quantity will yield approximately 8 wraps.
5. Place a small sheet of parchment paper between each wrap and store in an airtight glass container in the fridge, or freeze.

PER 80G PORTION

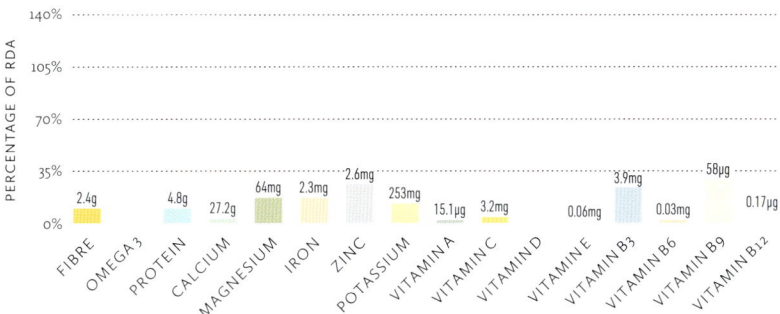

Grilled Baby Gem Caesar Salad

2 baby gem lettuces, washed, spin-dried and halved (or quartered if very large)

olive oil for brushing

pink Himalayan salt and pepper, to taste

fresh Parmesan cheese, shaved

2 handfuls of pine nuts, toasted

handful of chives, chopped

DRESSING

1 clove of garlic, grated

zest of half a lemon and 1 tbsp juice

2 tsp Dijon mustard

2 tsp Worcestershire sauce

1 tbsp runny tahini

90ml extra virgin olive oil

pink Himalayan salt and pepper, to taste

pinch of sesame seeds, to garnish

SERVES: 2

This is a great make-ahead salad to bring to a party, as it looks impressive. It also works for a family meal with roast chicken or grilled fish. The dressing keeps well and can be used with other salads.

1. Brush the baby gem lettuces with olive oil, season with salt and pepper, and set aside.
2. Make the dressing by putting all the ingredients in a bowl and whisking until well combined. Taste and adjust the seasoning, if necessary, by adding salt, pepper or a little Worcestershire sauce. Garnish with sesame seeds and set aside.
3. Place the baby gem cut-side down on a hot griddle pan to sear. Turn over after 1–2 minutes using tongs. You may have to cook the lettuce in batches.
4. When all are done, start assembling the salad on a large flat salad plate.
5. Put a spoon or two of dressing on the plate and move it around to coat. Add the grilled baby gem with another drizzle of dressing on top and Parmesan shavings.
6. Finish with a grind of black pepper, some toasted pine nuts and chopped fresh chives.

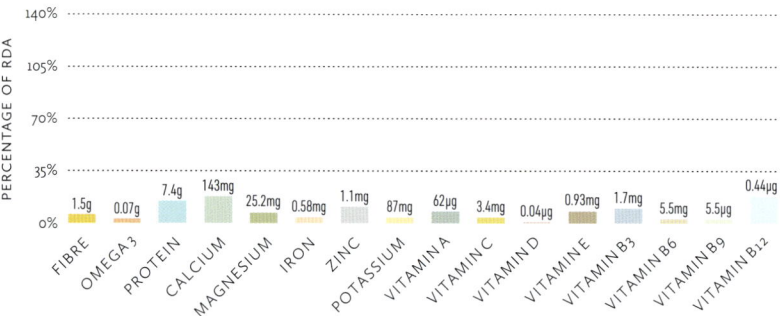

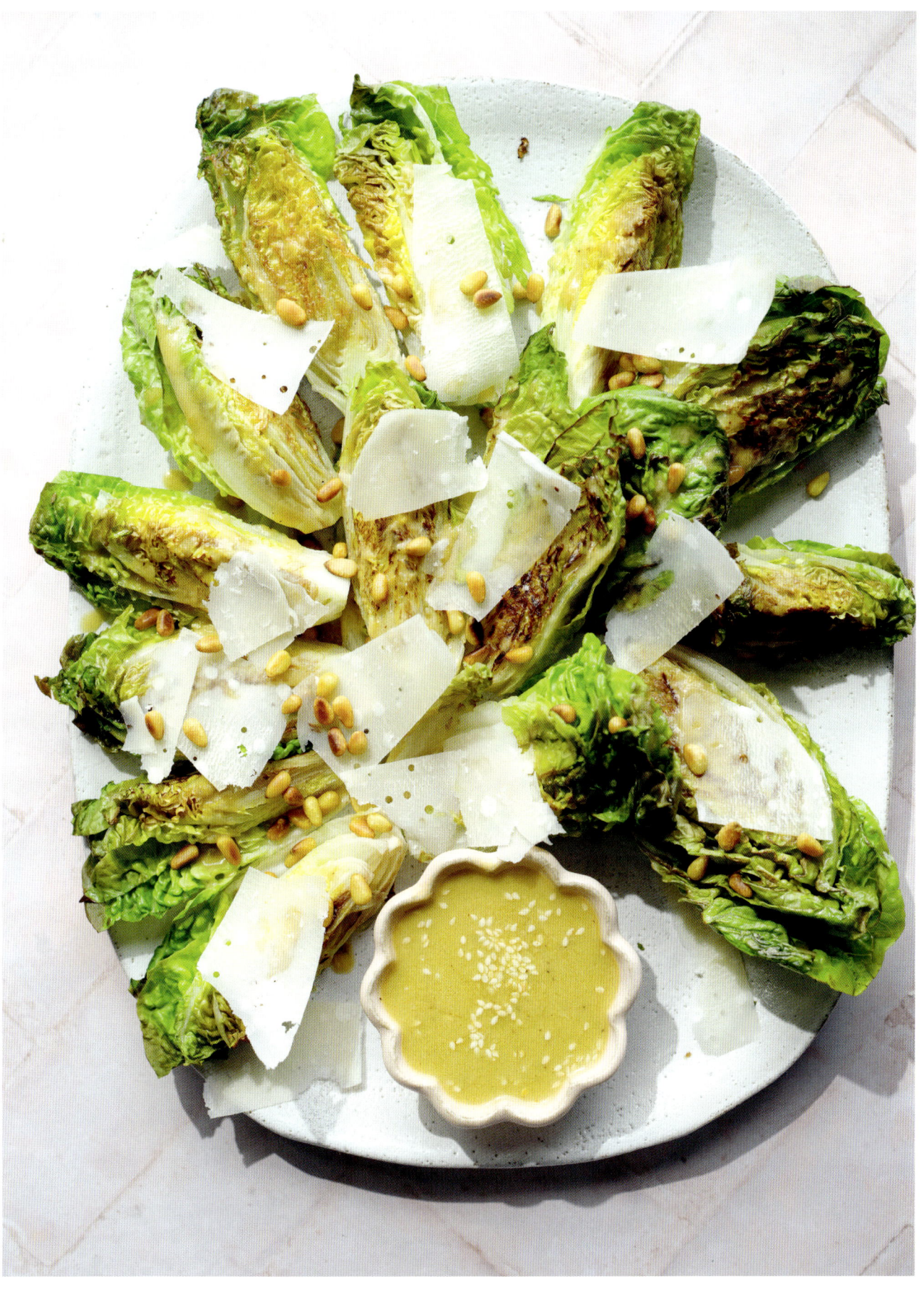

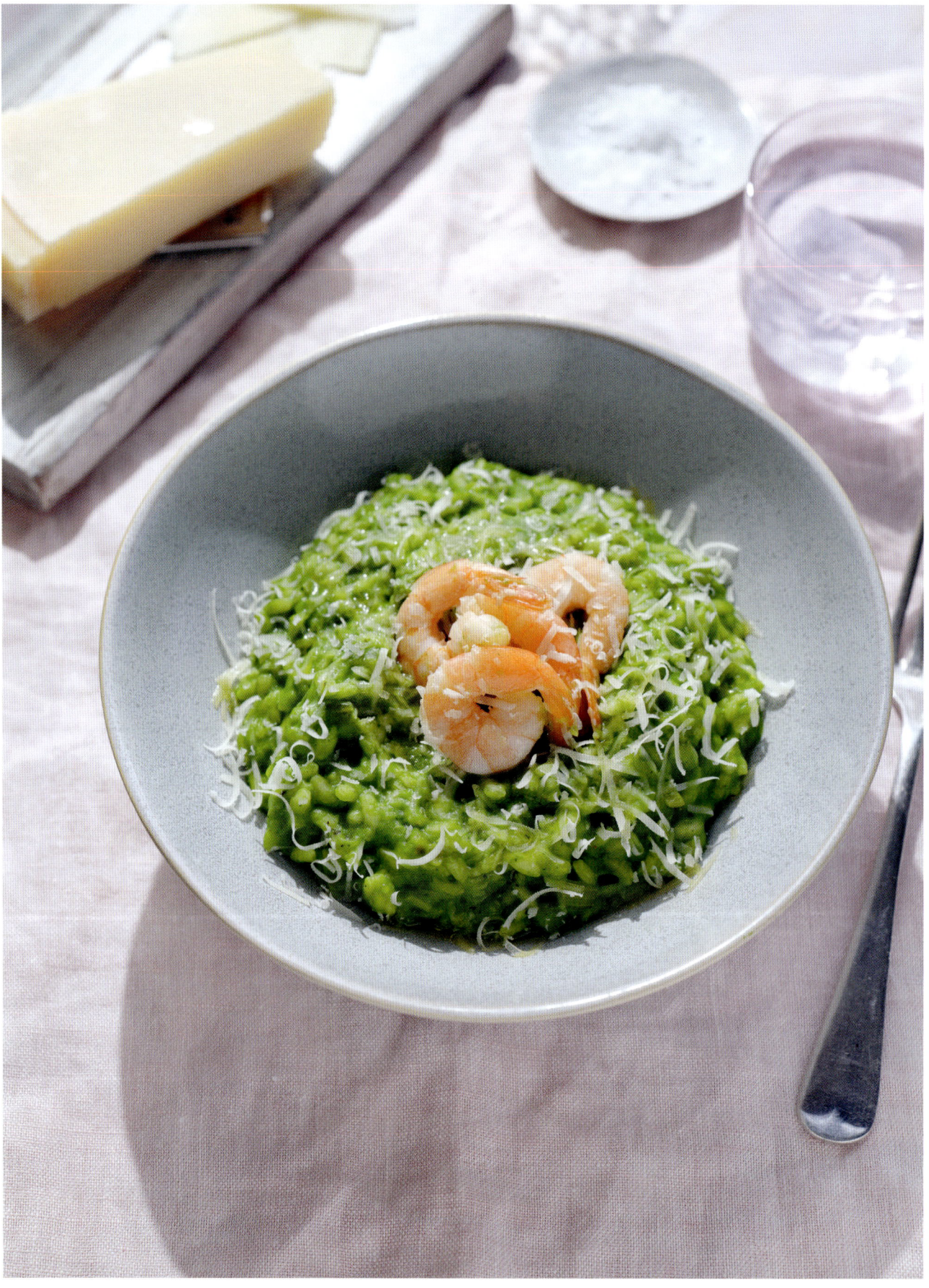

Spinach, Pea and Mint Risotto with Roasted Asparagus and Prawns

250g frozen garden peas

200g baby leaf spinach

handful of fresh mint leaves

2 white onions, finely chopped

2 celery stalks, finely chopped

5 tbsp olive oil

300g risotto rice

1 fat clove of garlic, minced

1 litre veg stock

1 bunch of green asparagus

pink Himalayan salt, to taste

1 tbsp sesame oil

200g fresh prawns (3–4 per person), marinated in garlic, lemon and ginger

75ml white wine or prosecco

2 tbsp Parmesan cheese, grated

1 tbsp crème fraiche (optional)

salt and pepper, to taste

fresh parsley, chopped

SERVES: 4+

An elaborate recipe, but this risotto is so tasty and fresh (not to mention packed full of beneficial nutrients) that it is really worth the effort. Speak to your fishmonger to get the most succulent jumbo king prawns.

1. Bring a large pot of water to the boil. When simmering, add in the frozen peas and spinach leaves. Allow to cook for 1–2 minutes, then quickly drain in a colander. Keep the cooking water.
2. Add the greens to a blender along with the fresh mint, and blitz until smooth. Keep this green mix warm and to one side.
3. Preheat the oven to 160–180°C.
4. Start making the risotto. Blitz the onions and celery in a food processor.
5. Heat 4 tablespoons of olive oil in a heavy-based large saucepan on a low heat.
6. Add the onion/celery mix and allow to cook gently for 10+ minutes (with the lid on), until it softens and turns translucent.
7. Add the risotto rice and minced garlic to the pan. Mix well and cook for a minute until the rice is well coated with the onion/celery mix.
8. Add 2 ladles of hot veg stock to the pan. Stir to combine until the liquid has been absorbed; this will take a few minutes. Repeat the process until all the liquid has been absorbed and the rice is soft but still al dente (with a bite).
9. Meanwhile, put the asparagus in a roasting tin with a drizzle of olive oil and a grind of salt. Roast for 12 minutes in the oven.
10. Put some sesame oil (or nut oil of choice) in a pan and place on the heat. When the pan is hot, add the marinated prawns and pan-fry quickly for 2–3 minutes until cooked through.
11. Once your rice has fully absorbed all of the stock, add the white wine or prosecco, stir and allow that to be absorbed as well.
12. Add the green mix to the risotto pan and stir until it is well combined. >

13 Then add the finishing touches: 1 tbsp grated Parmesan, crème fraiche (if using) and some salt and pepper to taste.
14 To serve, plate up a heaped ladle of risotto into a shallow bowl. Top with roasted asparagus spears and 3-4 prawns per person, a light sprinkling of the remaining Parmesan and chopped fresh parsley.

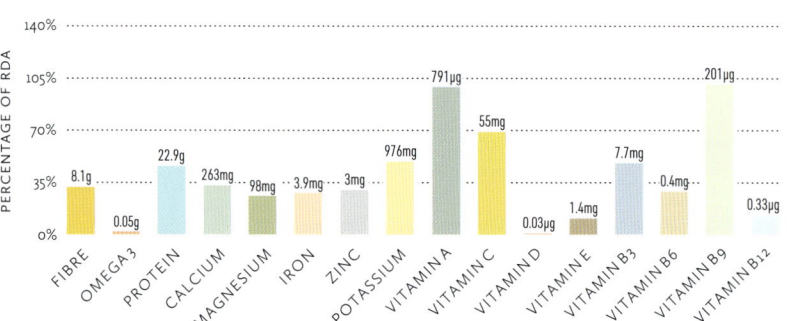

PER 620G PORTION

Nori Seaweed Hand Roll

with prawns and enoki mushrooms

4 nori seaweed sheets

2 tbsp ginger miso dressing (see p96)

4 tbsp brown rice, cooked

16 enoki mushrooms

handful of broccoli sprouts

12 small, cooked prawns

½ avocado, sliced

sesame seeds, toasted

MAKES: 4 ROLLS

These are fun to make and taste delicious. The seaweed sheets are a great source of iodine (good for thyroid function), while the enoki mushrooms are rich in niacin, vitamin C and phosphorus. Add zinc-rich prawns and liver-supporting broccoli sprouts and you have a nutrient-packed treat!

1. Take one nori seaweed sheet and cut (and discard) one-third off the length. Place the larger piece on a chopping board.
2. Put the ginger miso dressing in a small bowl and mix with the cooked brown rice.
3. Place 1 tablespoon of rice on the middle of the nori sheet and spread it across the width of the section. Top this with 3–4 enoki mushrooms, broccoli sprouts, 3 prawns, avocado slices and sesame seeds.
4. Wet the edge of the nori sheet and roll it into a cone shape. Repeat until all are made.

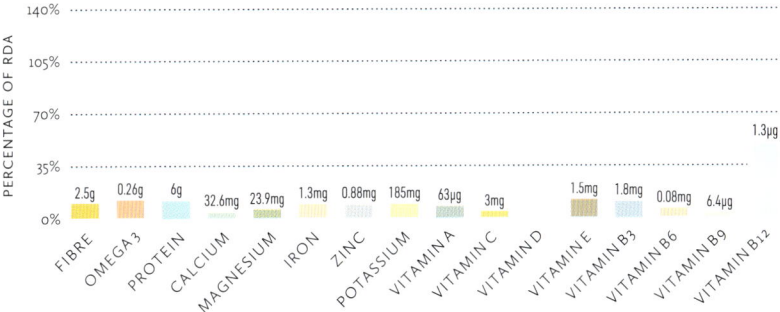

PER 80G PORTION

Almond Butter

400g raw almonds

5–6g pink Himalayan salt or sea salt

MAKES: 325G

Not only is this really easy to make, but your almond butter will also taste much better (and work out cheaper) than any shop-bought version – there is really no comparison. This method also applies to any of the other nut butters used in this cookbook; you'll need a food processor with a strong motor and an S-shaped blade, but then walnut butter and hazelnut butter are also at your fingertips. Give them a go!

1. Preheat the oven to 180–200°C.
2. Spread out the almonds on a baking tray and place in the oven for 8–10 minutes, or until they are slightly browned and you can smell the toasted almond aroma. Keep an eye on them in the oven, as they can burn quickly and easily.
3. Once the almonds are nicely toasted, remove them from the tray to a bowl or plate to cool. Don't rush this important step: if you try to process them when warm, they won't be able to release their oils to make a nice, smooth, creamy butter.
4. Once sufficiently cooled, put the almonds in the food processor along with the salt.
5. Start processing the almonds. This will happen in several stages, and you will be running the food processor almost continuously for 8–10 minutes.
   Stage 1: The almonds break down into a fine powder.
   Stage 2: The almonds start to stick together but also get compressed in the bowl of the food processor. Stop the motor, scrape down the sides and loosen the mix from the floor of the container. This makes it easier for the S-shaped blade to work effectively.
   Stage 3: The almonds start to form a ball rotating around the bowl. After a few minutes, it will loosen out as the oils release.
   Stage 4: Allow the motor to run for a few minutes to let the almond mix get loose and runny. Once it has reached the desired consistency, it is ready.
6. Store in an airtight, clip-top glass jar in the cupboard. This will keep for at least a week at room temperature – slightly longer if refrigerated. For serving suggestions, see recipes using almond butter on pp95, 114, 186, 238 and 247.

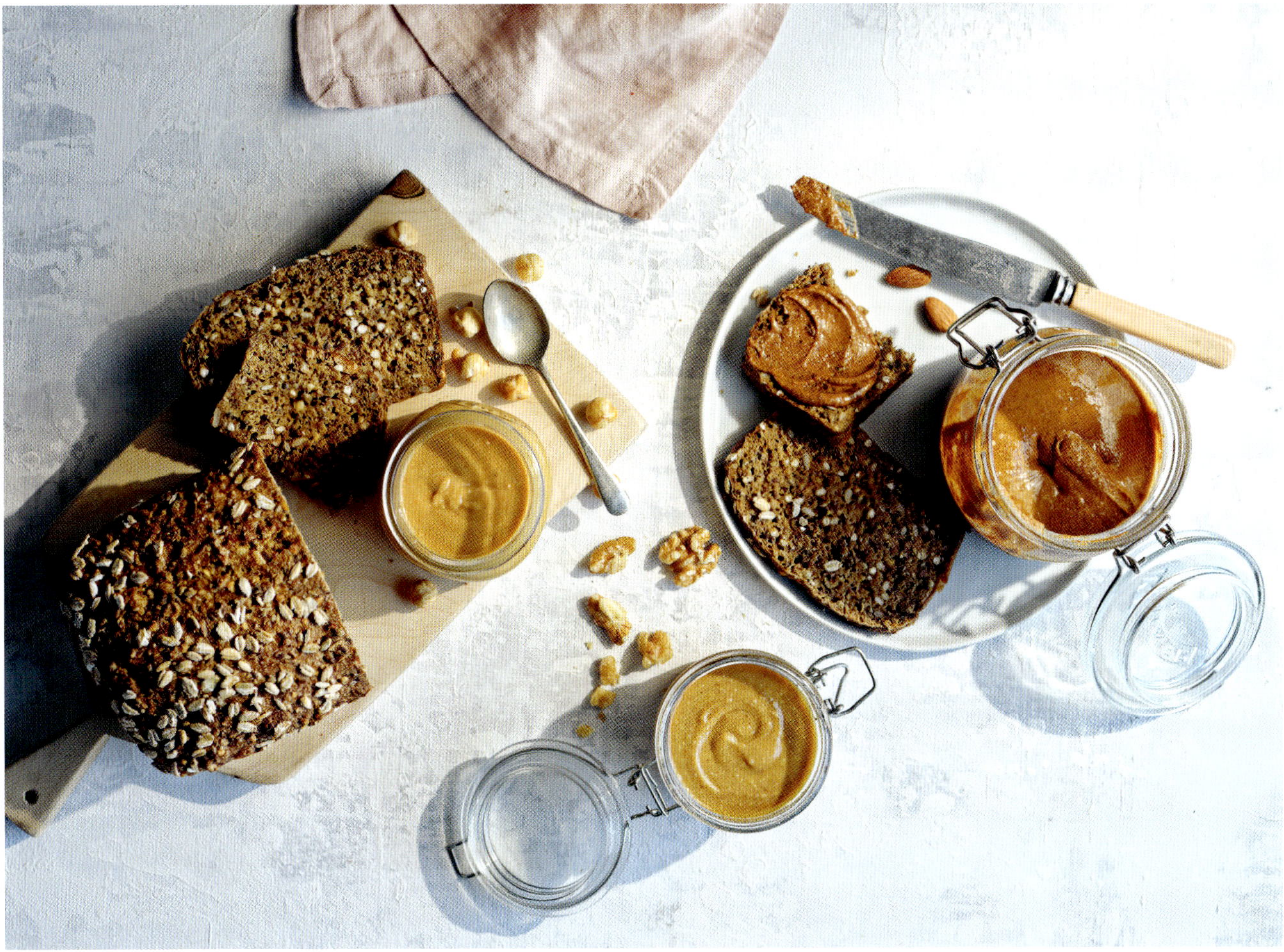

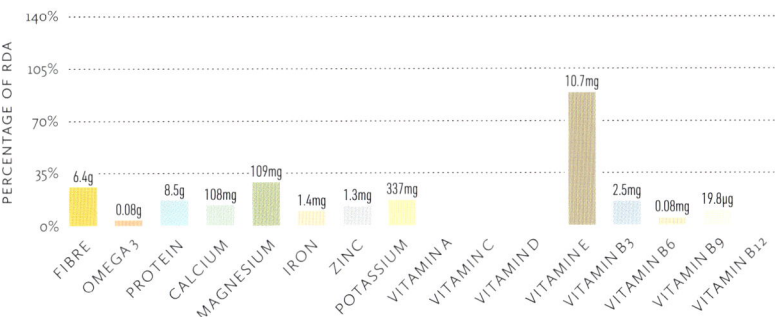

PER 40G PORTION

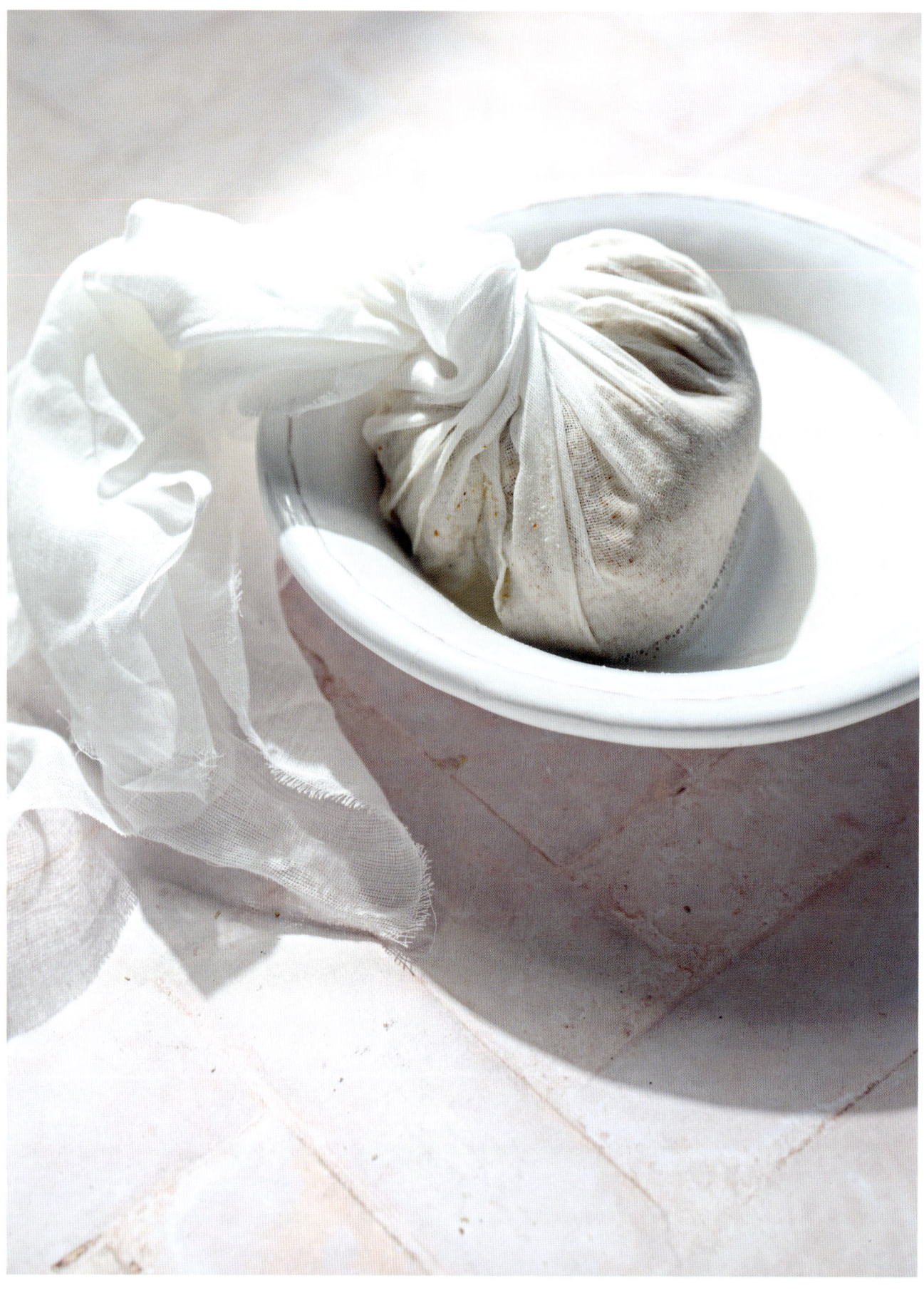

Almond Milk

300g almonds, soaked for 6–8 hours

1.5 litres filtered water

2 Medjool dates, soaked for 4–6 hours

¼ tsp pink Himalayan salt

MAKES: 1 LITRE

This recipe is suitable for all kinds of nut and seed milk, including hazelnuts, Brazil nuts, sesame seeds and pumpkin seeds. Adding Medjool dates and Himalayan salt results in a creamy, rich, slightly sweet and salty plant-based milk with no additives, thickeners or stabilisers. Both your nuts and your dates require a long soaking time, so you may want to do this overnight.

1. Rinse the almonds and add them to a high-speed blender with the water, dates and salt. Blend on high for 1 minute.
2. Strain the mixture into a bowl through a fine sieve, a nut-milk bag or a cheesecloth. If you are stuck, a pair of light-coloured (unused!) tights will also work.
3. Squeeze out all the liquid until you are left with a fine, sand-like pulp in the bag. You can keep this, dehydrate it and grind it into fine flour for use in other recipes.
4. Transfer the milk to an airtight container or bottle and store it in the fridge for up to 5 days. If it separates, simply shake it before use.

PER 185G PORTION

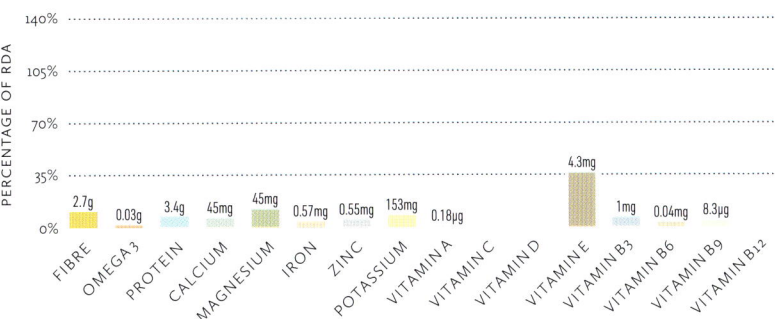

Chocolate Tahini Bliss Balls

60g porridge oats, ground into a flour
3 tbsp cacao powder
½ tsp pink Himalayan salt
120ml runny tahini paste
3 tbsp maple syrup
sesame seeds to coat

MAKES: 12–15 BALLS

These are really quick to make – and they taste delicious, thanks to the combination of raw cacao and calcium-rich tahini paste.

1 Combine the oat flour, cacao and salt in a mixing bowl.
2 Add the tahini paste and maple syrup, and mix until it is the right consistency. You should be able to shape it and roll it into small balls. Test this by squeezing some of the mix together between your fingers – if it sticks together, it is the right consistency.
3 Put a generous scoop of sesame seeds on a small plate and set aside.
4 Empty the oat mixture on to a silicone mat. Fold the edges of the mat over the mix one by one and press down until you form a square or rectangle with the mix. The goal is to be able to slice it up into even squares, and it's easier if you have a nice square shape to begin with.
5 Using a pastry cutter, cut the mix into evenly spaced columns lengthways and across, until you end up with even-sized squares.
6 Lift one square at a time and shape with your fingers into a ball, then roll gently in the palm of your hands.
7 The mix will get oily; dip into the sesame seeds to decorate.
8 Once all the balls have been rolled in the sesame seeds, refrigerate. You can enjoy them directly from the fridge, though they can also be frozen.

PER 20G PORTION

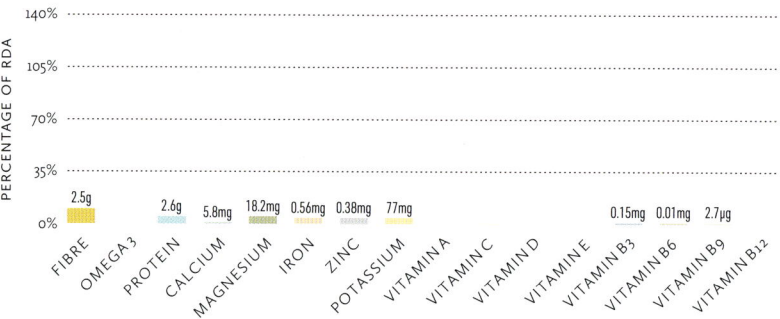

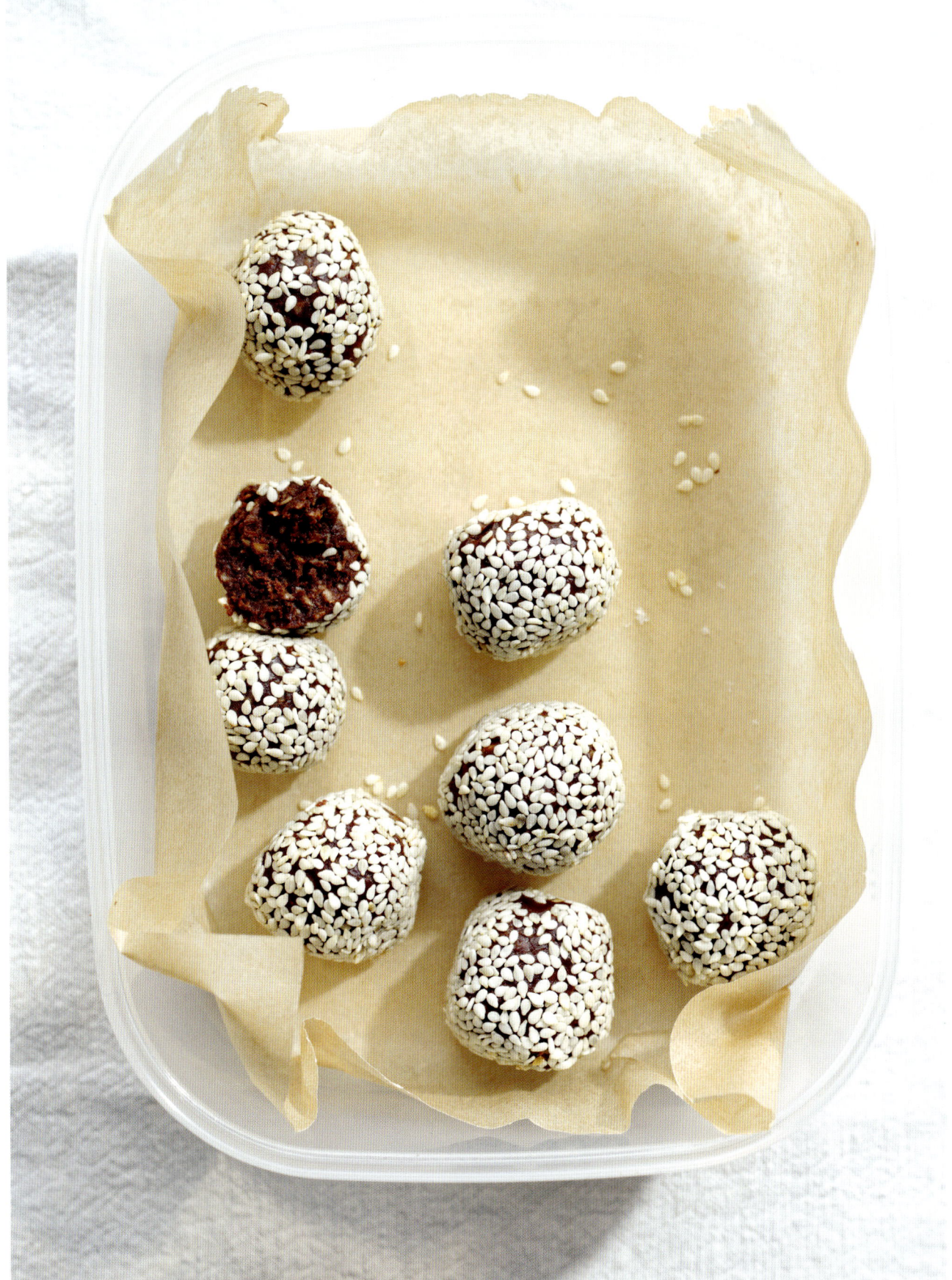

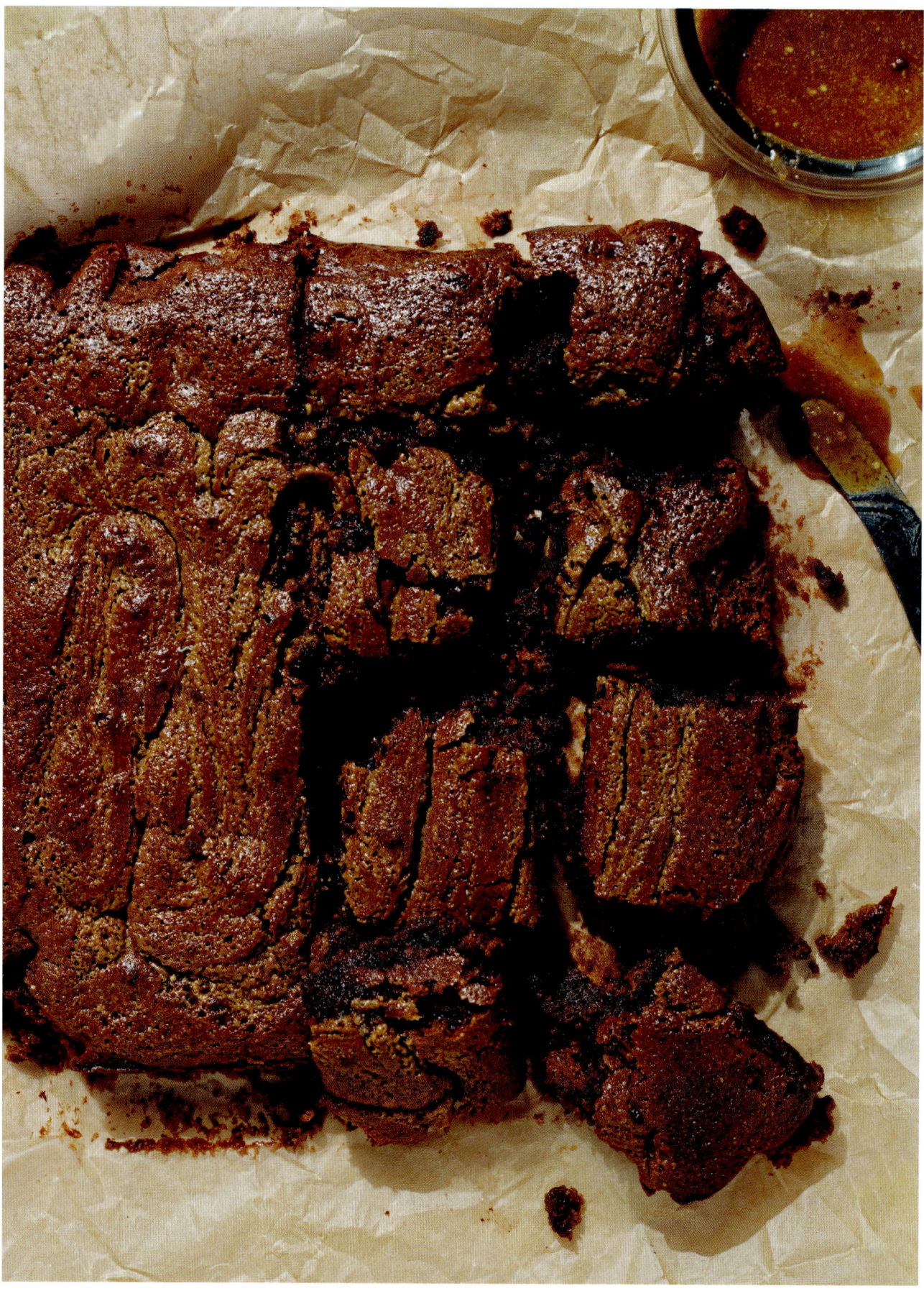

Hazelnut Butter Brownies

375g hazelnut butter (home-made yields the best results, see p170)

250ml organic maple syrup

2 organic eggs

1 tsp vanilla extract

50g raw cacao powder

1 tsp baking powder

pinch of pink Himalayan or sea salt

dark chocolate chips (optional)

MAKES: 16 PORTIONS

These are so delicious, you may have to hide them! No nasty ingredients, no refined sugar and no flour – just good fats, antioxidant-rich cacao and heart-healthy almonds. Hands down one of my favourite treats.

1. Preheat the oven to 180°C.
2. Combine the hazelnut butter and maple syrup in a bowl. Set aside about one-third of this mixture in a separate bowl until later.
3. Add the eggs and vanilla extract to the remaining two-thirds of the mixture.
4. Add the cacao powder, baking powder and salt and mix thoroughly.
5. Line a 20–22cm baking tin with parchment paper and pour in the mixture, then swirl the reserved hazelnut butter/maple syrup mixture over it. Use a cocktail stick to swirl this around, creating a pretty marbling effect.
6. Bake for exactly 22 minutes (in a fan oven) to ensure a fudgy centre.
7. Remove from the oven and leave to cool before cutting up into squares.
8. Store in a glass container (putting parchment paper between layers) and keep in the fridge. Warning: they may not last long!

PER 54G PORTION

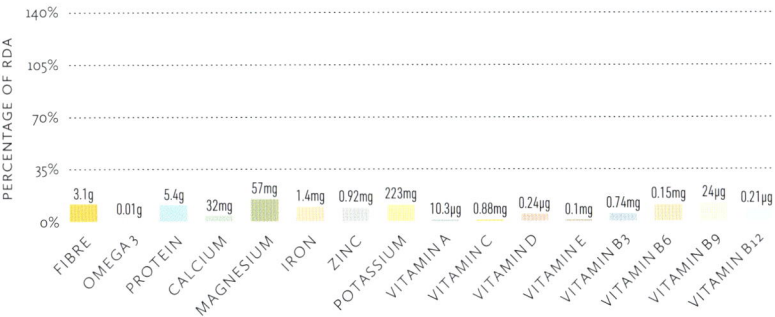

5. Antioxidants

Antioxidants are found in all brightly coloured fruit and vegetables, and they help to protect us from disease. Their other benefits include increased energy, improved skin health and a reduction in inflammation (which can manifest itself in menopausal women as joint pains or headaches).

This section is what eating in colour looks like! Every recipe is packed with powerful, antioxidant-rich phytonutrients, from the bright vegetable juices to one of my favourites, sweet potato toast. Again, I've focused on whole food, plant-based vegan recipes in the hope that I can provide some delicious options for eating more plants.

Beetroot, Ginger and Fennel Juice

400g fresh raw beetroot (heads removed), chopped small

1 whole head of broccoli, chopped small

40g fresh root ginger

2 fennel bulbs, chopped small

1 apple, chopped into chunks

1 cucumber, sliced lengthways

1½ tbsp chia seeds

MAKES: 2 LITRES

This delicious juice is rich in nitric oxide, which supports heart health and regulates blood pressure. The addition of chia seeds to this fantastic concentration of nutrients gives an extra fibre, protein and omega-3 boost.

1. Feed the vegetables through the mouth of a juicer one by one, starting with the hard ingredients – that is, beetroot, broccoli and ginger.
2. Continue with the rest: fennel, apple and, lastly, cucumber.
3. Pour the mixture into a jug and stir.
4. Add the chia seeds and mix well for a few minutes so they can absorb the liquid; keep stirring all the time to avoid the seeds clumping together.
5. You can store the juice in 250ml food-grade plastic bottles in the freezer. I keep a couple in the fridge for immediate consumption and freeze the rest for optimum freshness. (If freezing, don't fill to the top of the bottle to allow for expansion in the freezer.)

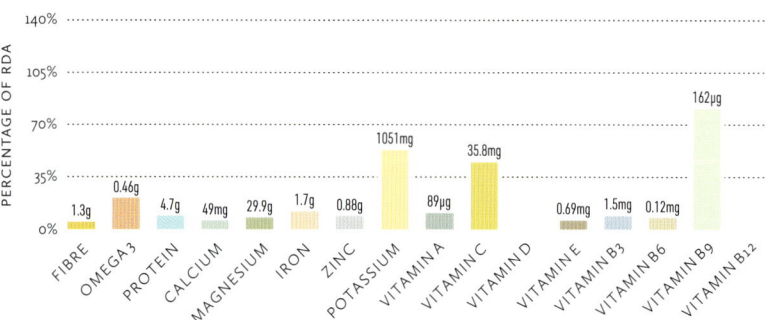

PER 250G PORTION

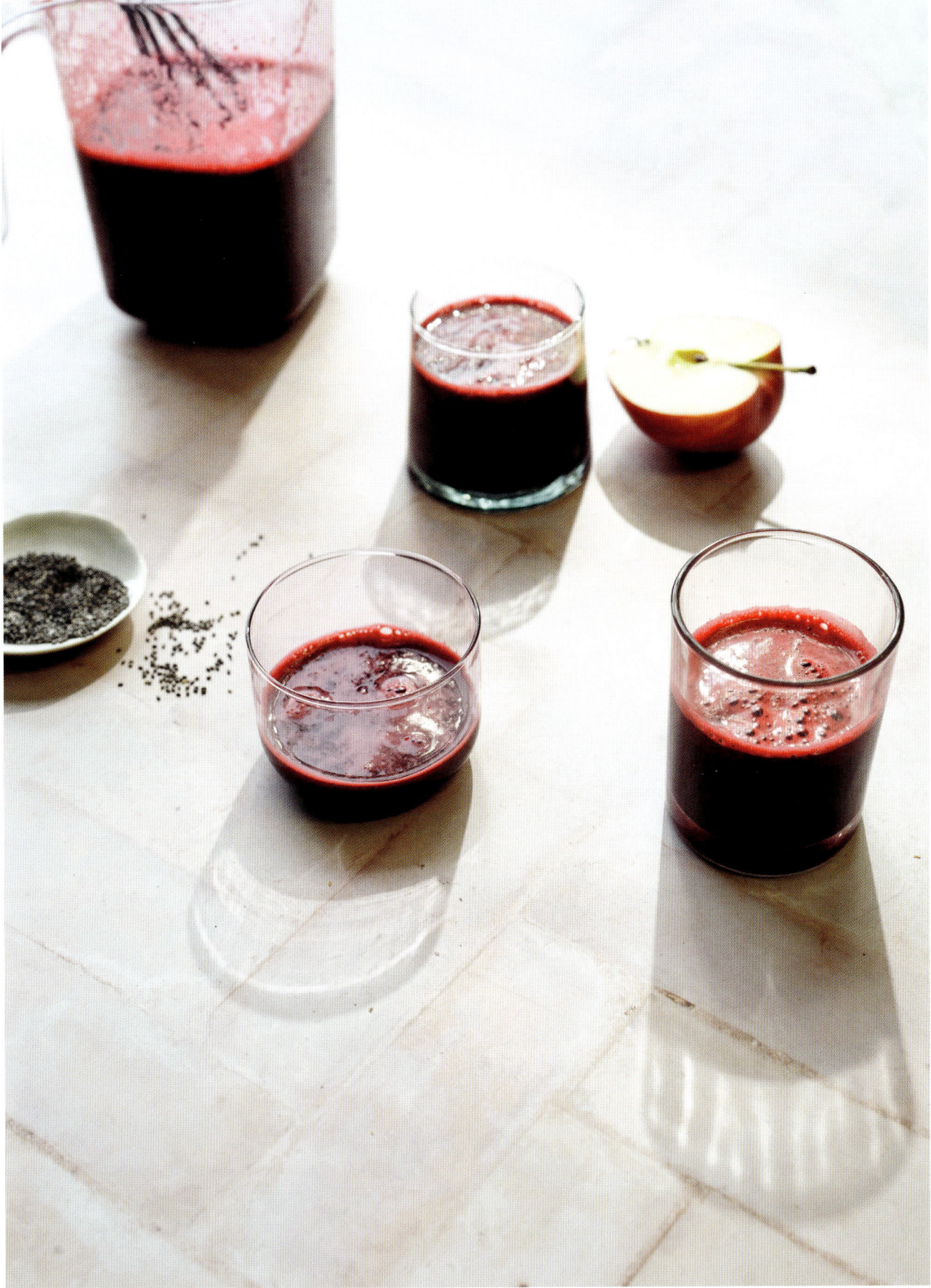

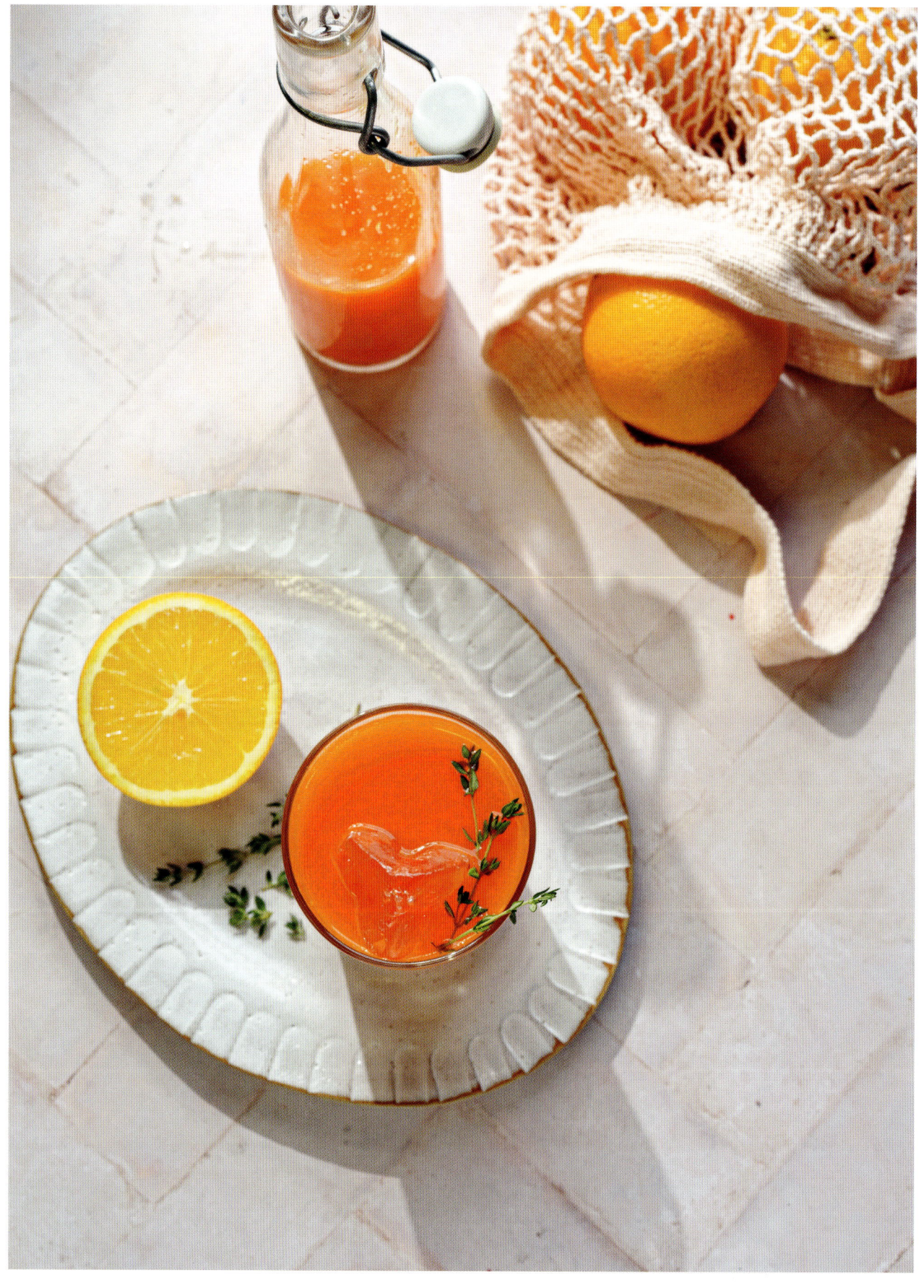

Carrot, Red Pepper, Orange and Ginger Juice

8 carrots, roughly chopped

2 red peppers, roughly chopped

1 thumb-sized piece of fresh ginger, roughly chopped

2 oranges

a drop of hemp seed oil or flaxseed oil (optional)

MAKES: 500ML

Rich in beta-carotene and vitamin C, this is a refreshing summertime juice that tastes really good. The addition of hemp seed oil improves the uptake of these nutrients.

1. Juice the carrots, red peppers and ginger.
2. Juice the oranges separately, then combine with the carrot and red pepper juice.
3. Pour the juice into bottles and store in the fridge.
4. Add a drop of flaxseed oil or hemp oil to improve absorption of vitamin-A-rich nutrients.

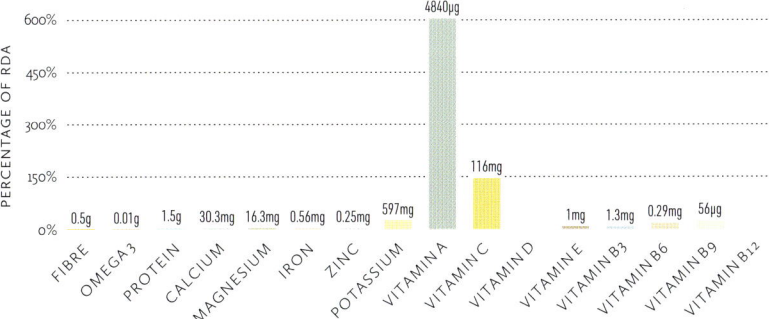

Life-Giving Green Juice

1 head of broccoli
½ fennel bulb
1 apple
30g fresh root ginger
1 large courgette
90g baby spinach leaves
60g kale leaves
bunch of fresh mint
2 limes
1 ripe avocado
broccoli microgreens (optional)

MAKES: 1 LITRE

A hybrid of juice and smoothie, this is a fantastic way to get a concentrated dose of green phytonutrients into your system. It also tastes amazing. You will feel like a new woman!

1. Rinse and roughly chop the ginger, mint and all the fruit and veg, except the avocado.
2. Feed these through the mouth of the juicer one by one, starting with the harder ingredients – that is, broccoli, fennel, apple and ginger, followed by the courgette, then the leaves and fresh lime.
3. When you're ready to serve, put 250ml of green juice in a blender, add a quarter of the avocado and blitz on high until smooth.
4. Top with the broccoli microgreens (if using) and enjoy.
5. Store the remainder of the juice in 250ml food-grade plastic bottles in the fridge or freezer. If freezing, don't fill to the top to allow for expansion. The next time you want some juice, defrost one portion by placing the frozen bottle in a bowl of warm water for 15 minutes. Once defrosted, put the juice in the blender with a quarter of avocado.

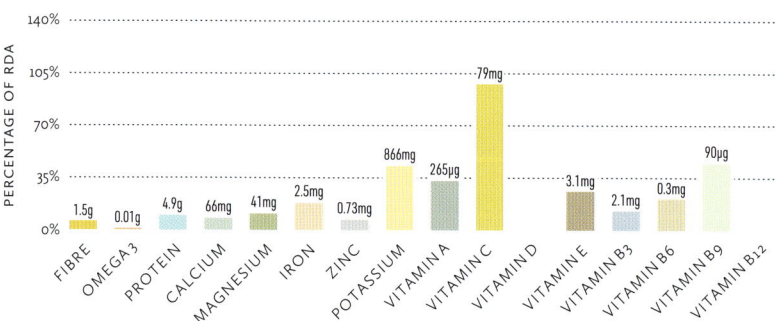

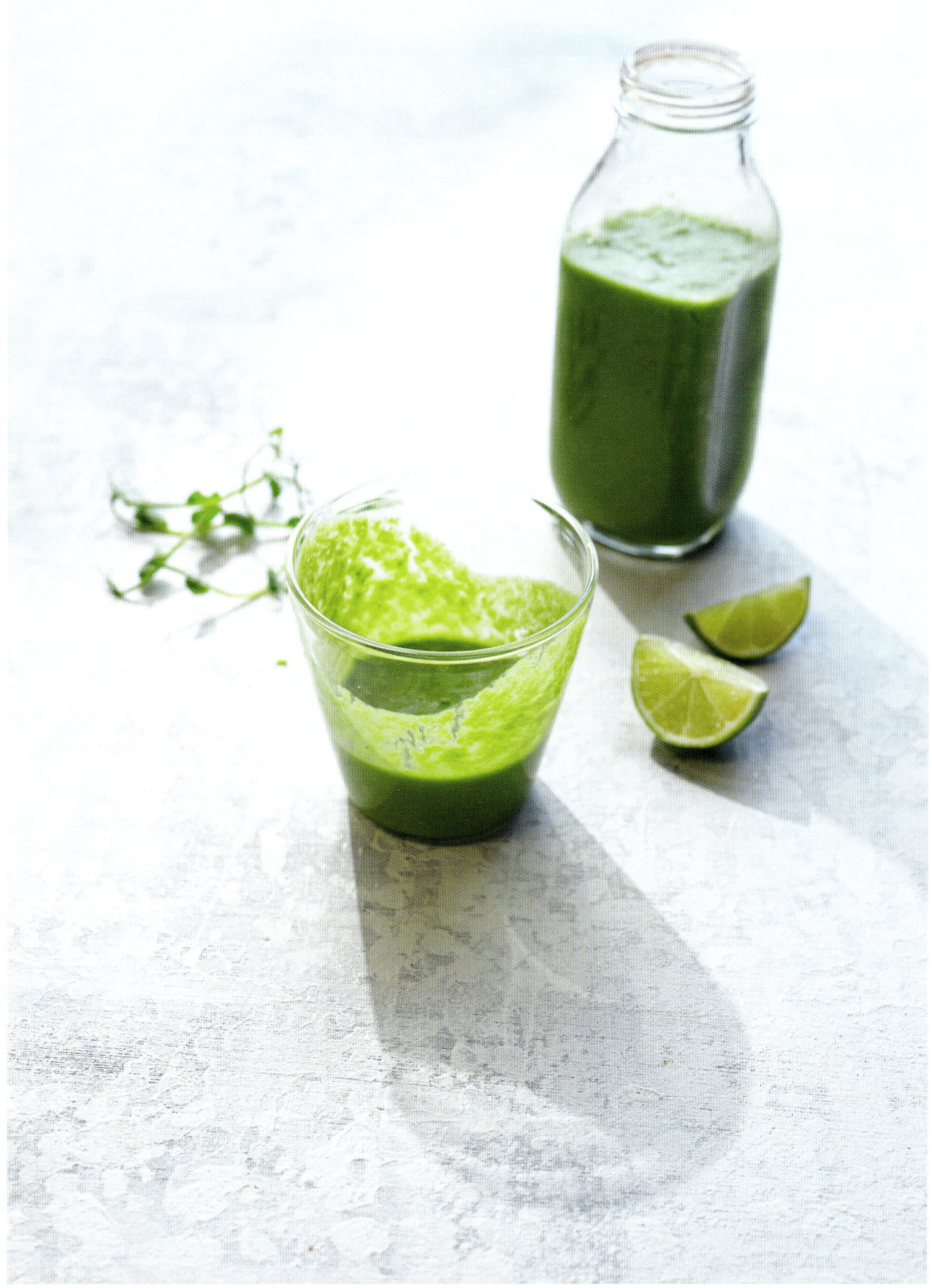

Sweet Potato Toast

1 medium-sized sweet potato, skin on

olive oil

pink Himalayan salt, to taste

TOPPING IDEAS

Vegetarian: smashed avocado, poached egg and roasted red pepper with pan-fried mushrooms

Pescatarian: smashed avocado, poached egg, smoked salmon and balsamic dressing

Sweet: almond butter, sliced banana, maple syrup and granola

MAKES: 4–5 SLICES

These tasty slices work well with both sweet and savoury toppings. I make them as part of my weekly meal prep, and then I top them as per the suggestions below, or I chop them up and add them to salads.

1. Preheat the oven to 180°C.
2. Cut the sweet potato lengthways to get 1–2cm-thick slices.
3. Place on a baking sheet, brush with olive oil and add a sprinkling of Himalayan salt.
4. Roast for 30 minutes, until golden and toasted.

PER 50G PORTION

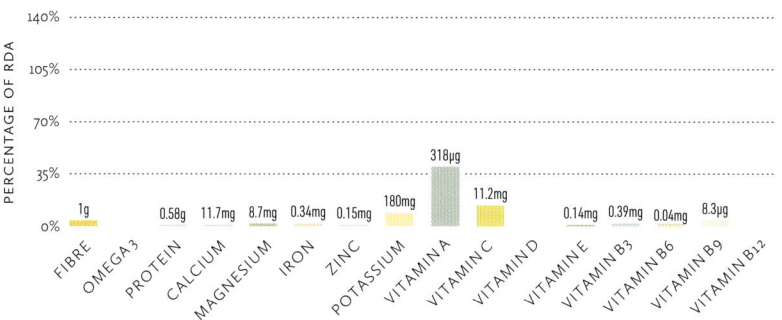

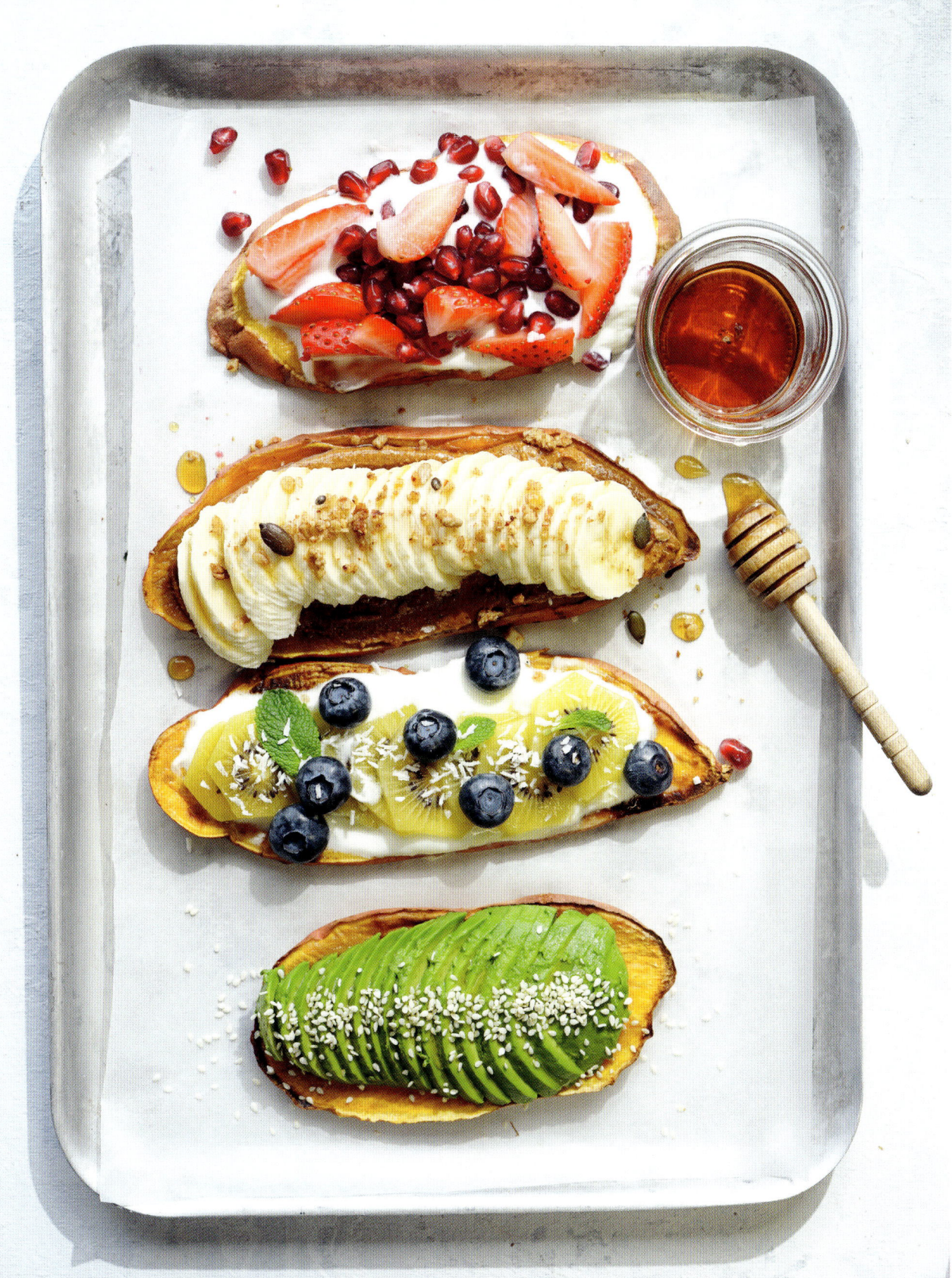

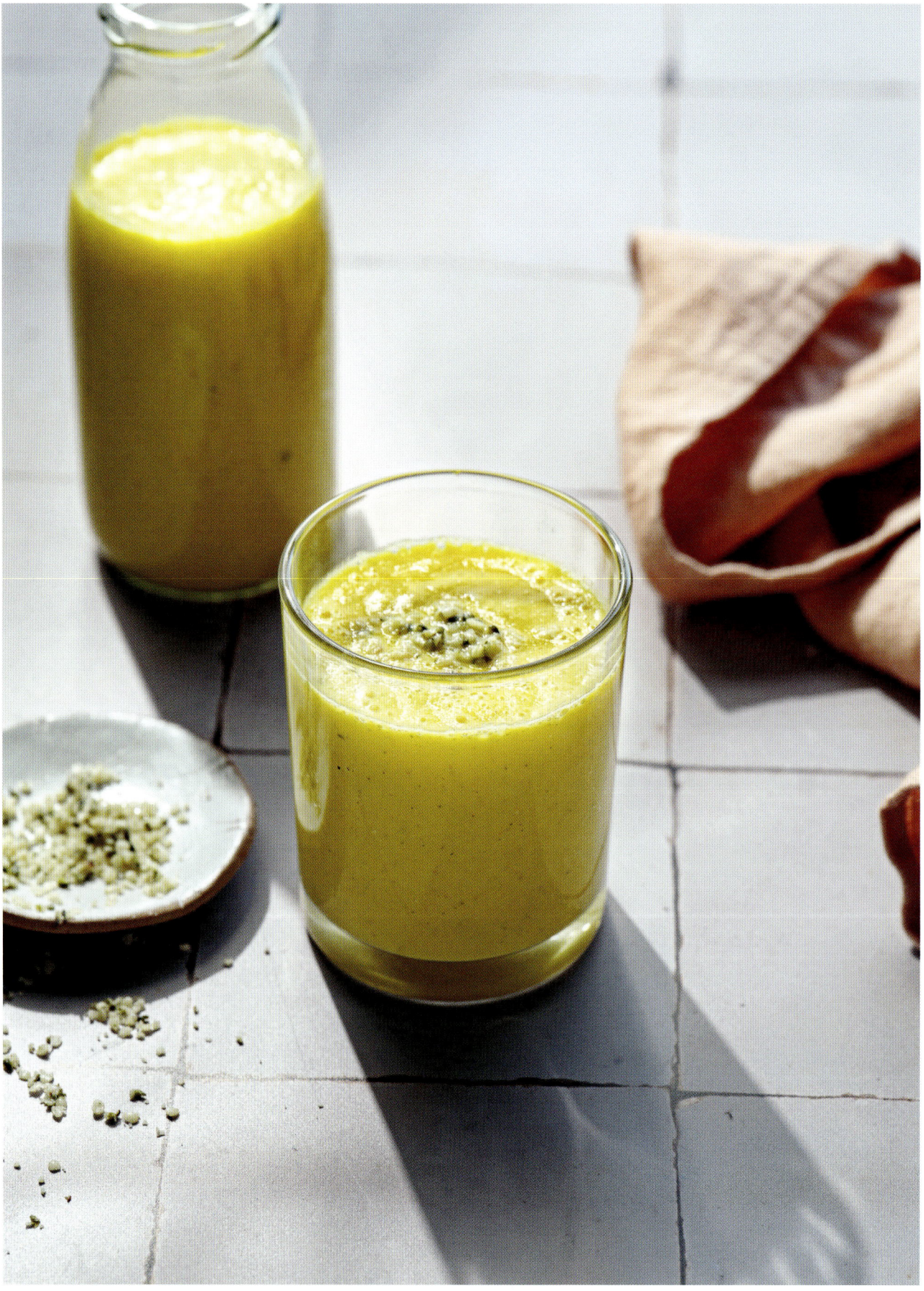

Mango, Turmeric and Hemp Seed Smoothie

1 organic red apple, cored and chopped

2 oranges, segmented

1 mango, peeled and chopped

1 thumb-sized piece of ginger root, peeled

1 thumb-sized piece of turmeric root, peeled, or 1 tsp ground organic turmeric

1 tbsp hemp seeds or cold-milled hemp seeds

1 tsp maca powder

100–150ml coconut water or filtered water

MAKES: 2 PORTIONS

With a distinct hint of turmeric and ginger, this sweet-tasting anti-inflammatory smoothie is a great hormone balancer that is rich in omega-3 and plant protein. To make this into a smoothie bowl, simply add less liquid to give a thicker mixture.

1. Place all the ingredients in a blender and blitz on high until completely smooth.
2. Drink straight away, accompanied by a breakfast cookie (see p110).

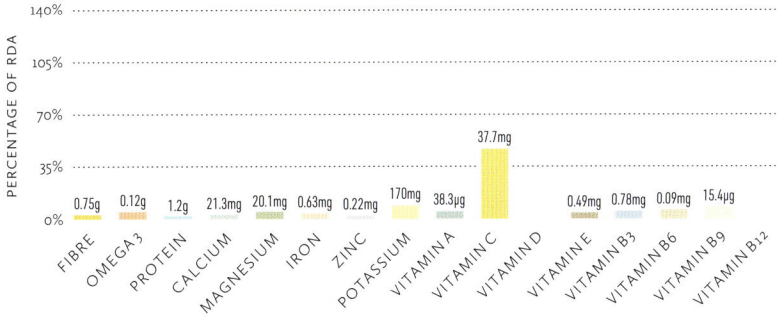

PART FOUR: RECIPES – ANTIOXIDANTS

The Lit-from-Within Chicken Salad

with poached chicken and tender stem broccoli in miso, ginger, chilli dressing

75g butternut squash, peeled and cubed

2 tbsp olive oil

½ tsp garlic powder

½ tsp pink Himalayan salt

1 nest of wholemeal noodles or buckwheat noodles (gluten-free option)

60g tender stem broccoli, cut in half lengthways

3–4 cashews

1 tsp sesame seeds

1 chicken breast, poached or roasted

1 big handful of fresh baby spinach leaves

handful of mangetout, cut into thin strips

¼ red pepper, cut into thin strips

1 spring onion, finely sliced

½ orange, peeled and segmented, or 1 mandarin orange, peeled

DRESSING

100ml walnut oil or olive oil

2 tbsp rice vinegar

1 tbsp fresh lime juice

1 tbsp miso paste

1 tsp grated ginger

1 tsp grated garlic (1 small clove)

¼ finely chopped red chilli

1 tbsp organic maple syrup

SERVES: 1

This Thai-inspired salad, bursting with antioxidants, vitamin C and beta-carotene, is a good source of folic acid too. There are a lot of elements to it, so the secret is to prep ahead.

1. Preheat the oven to 180°C.
2. Drizzle the cubed butternut squash with olive oil, sprinkle with a little garlic powder and salt, then roast for 25–30 minutes until tender.
3. Cook the noodles according to the pack instructions, drain and set aside.
4. Position a colander over a pot of boiling water and place your tender stem broccoli into it, with the lid on, for a couple of minutes. Set aside.
5. Whisk together the dressing ingredients. This will make approximately four servings of dressing, so store the extra in an airtight glass container in the fridge.
6. Toast the cashews and, as they are browning, add the sesame seeds to the dry pan. These will only take a minute to brown.
7. Lastly, shred the chicken breast with your hands or a fork.
8. To assemble the salad, put the noodles and spinach leaves in a mixing bowl, along with half the dressing. Mix well and divide between two salad bowls.
9. Add all the other ingredients on top, finishing with the toasted nuts and the rest of the dressing.

PER 435G PORTION

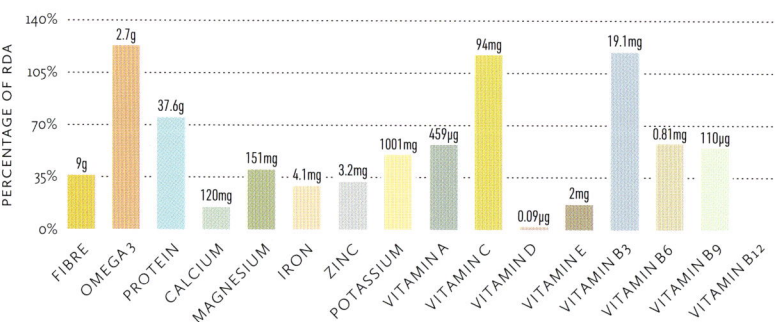

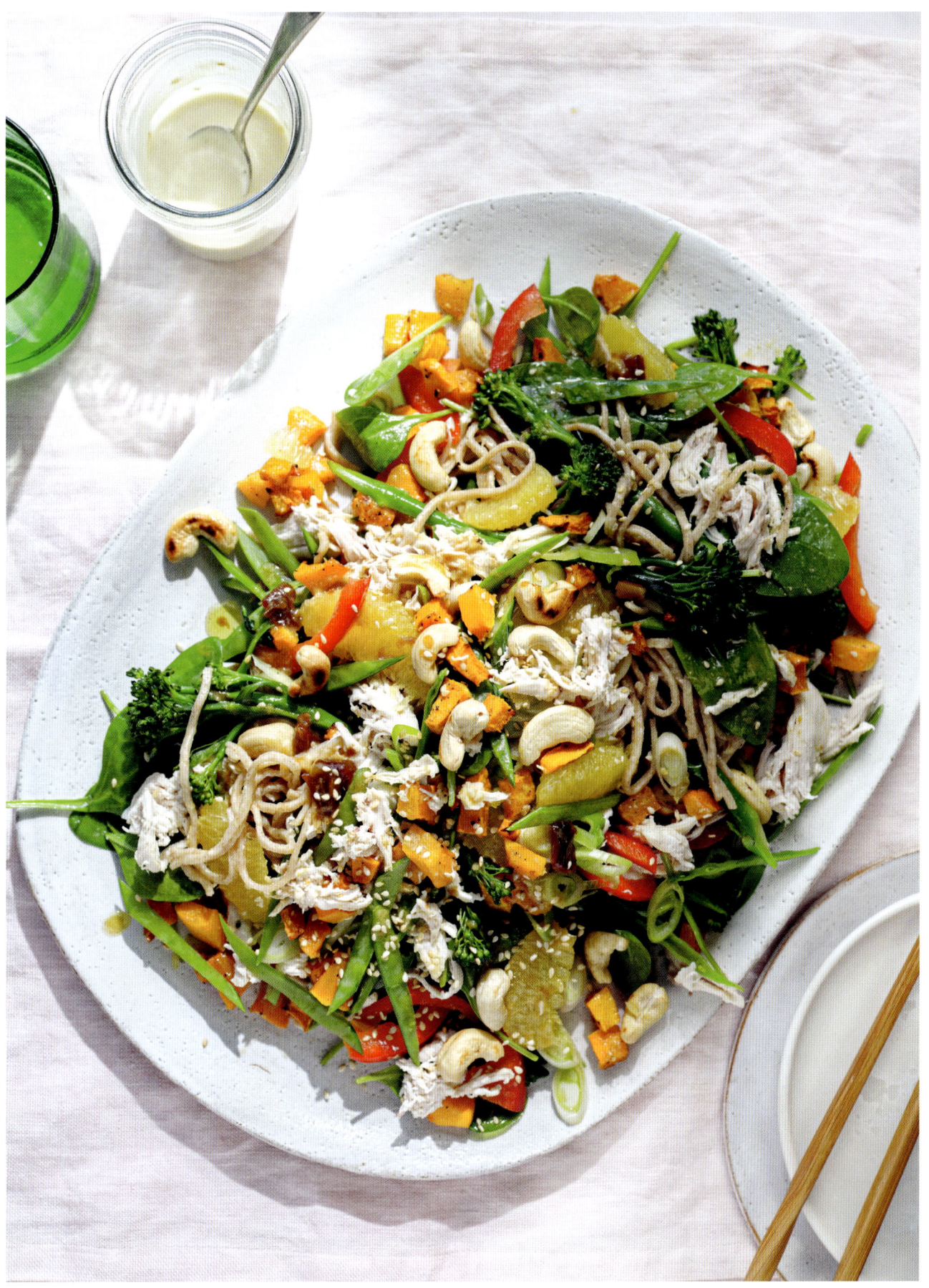

Tomato, Chilli and Fennel Soup

1 tbsp olive oil

1 red onion, peeled and chopped

1 clove of garlic, peeled and chopped

leaves of 3 thyme sprigs, roughly chopped

2 fennel bulbs, sliced

1 tbsp tomato purée

400g tinned tomatoes

500ml filtered water

¼ tsp chilli flakes

salt and pepper, to taste

1 tbsp maple syrup

SERVES: 4

Fennel adds another layer of flavour to this wholesome and warming tomato soup. It tastes great topped with a dollop of yoghurt and fennel seeds.

1. Put a drizzle of olive oil in a pan, and sweat the onions and garlic together, with the lid on, until soft.
2. Add the thyme, fennel and tomato purée and cook for 10–15 minutes.
3. Add the tinned tomatoes, water and chilli flakes (if using), bring to the boil and simmer for 40 minutes, until everything is soft.
4. Add a splash of water if the soup becomes too thick.
5. Once ready, season with salt, pepper and maple syrup, then blend until smooth.
6. Serve – I like to top this with chilli flakes, roasted cherry tomatoes and a few leaves of basil. You can also add a cooling dollop of live probiotic yoghurt.

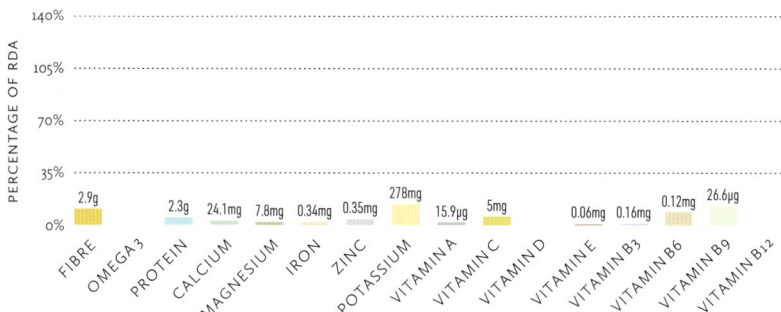

PER 300G PORTION

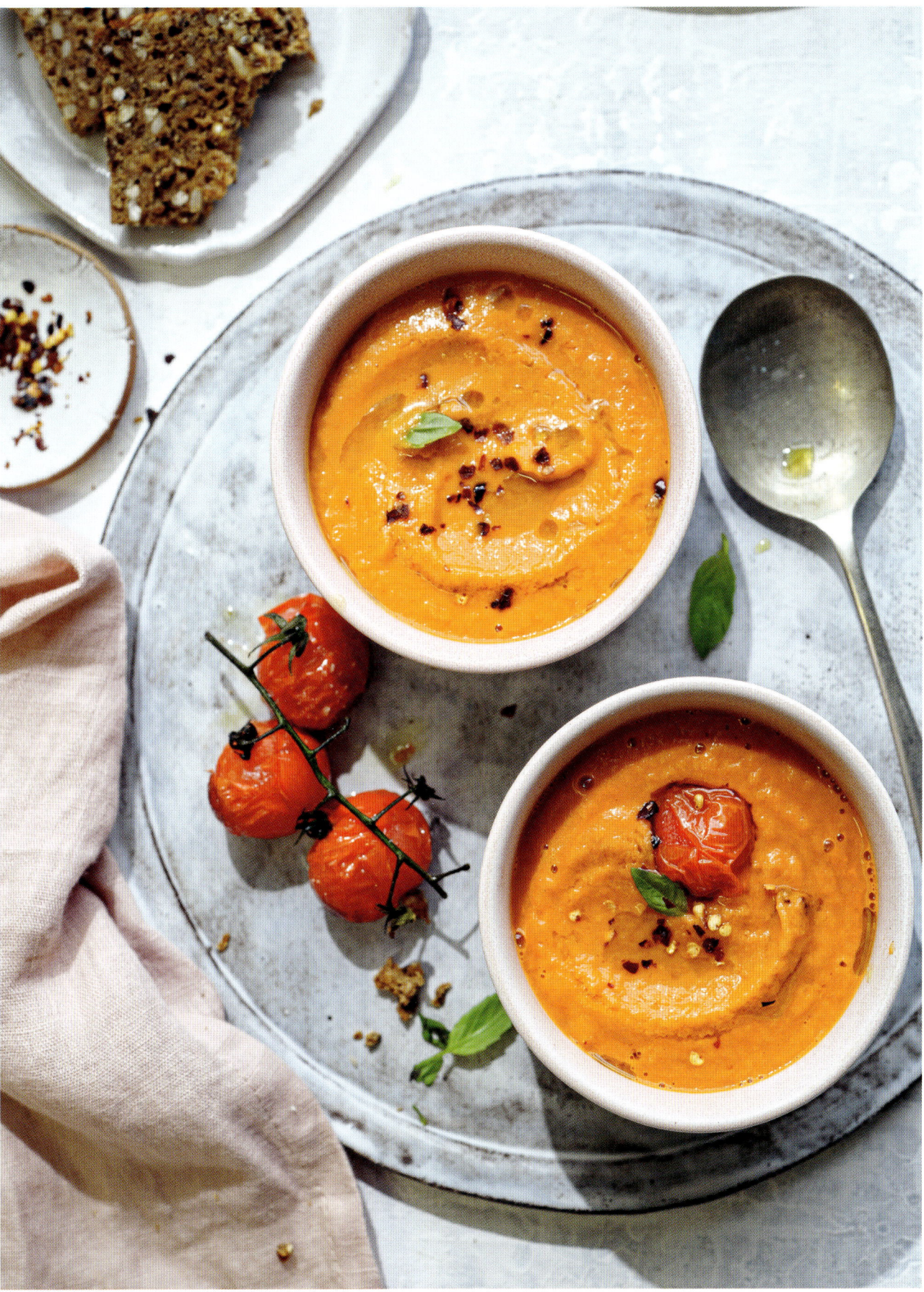

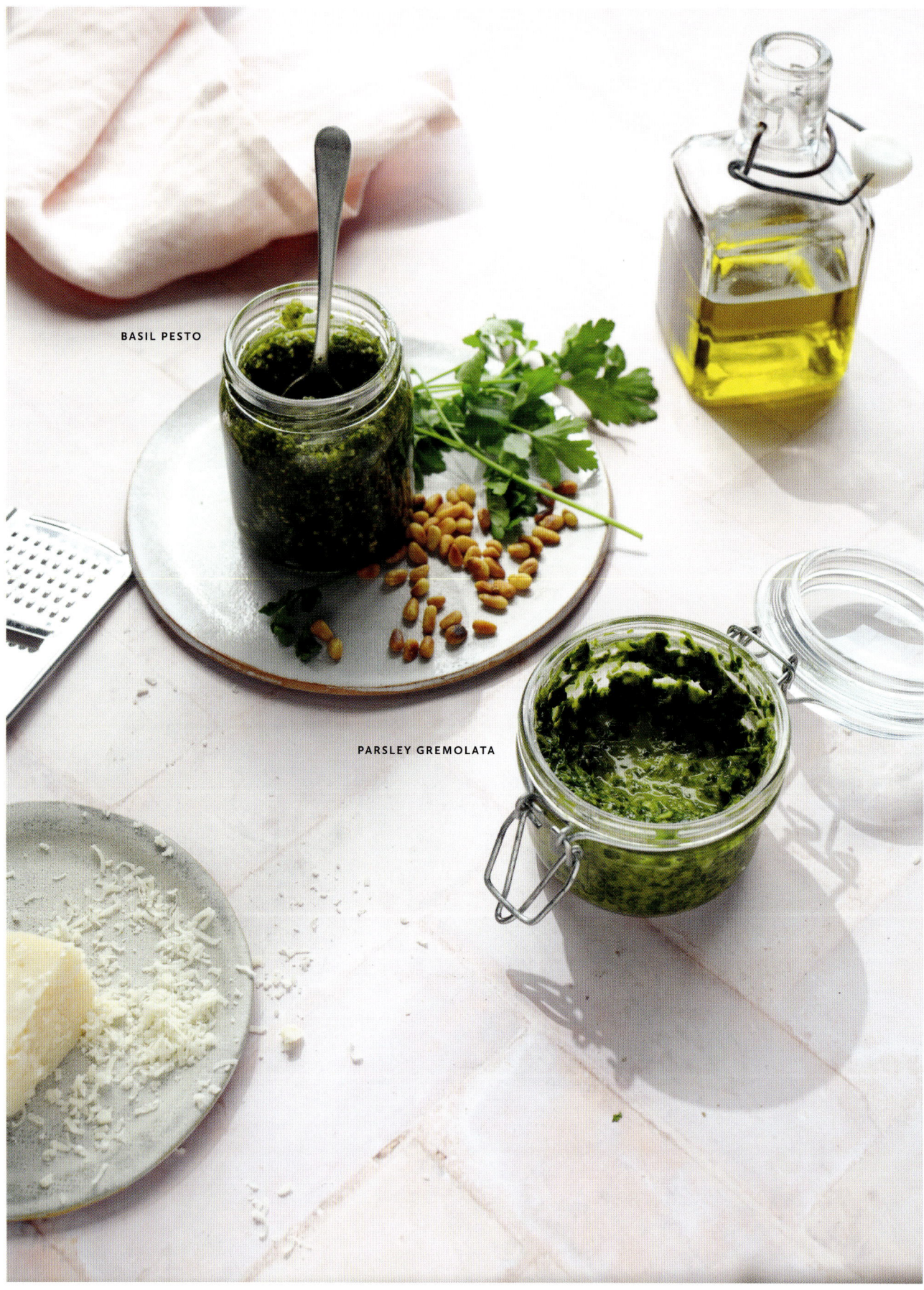

Parsley Gremolata

1 large bunch of fresh flat-leaf parsley (about 35g)

2 cloves of garlic, minced

zest and juice of 1 lemon

5–6 tbsp olive oil

pink Himalayan salt, to taste

MAKES: 10+ PORTIONS

This versatile and tasty condiment can be used as a marinade or as a topping for soups and stews. It keeps well in the fridge and can also be frozen. It really is very handy!

1. Blitz all the ingredients together in a high-speed blender. The resulting texture should be rustic and bitty, not baby-food-smooth.
2. Taste and adjust the seasoning, if necessary, by adding more lemon, garlic or salt.
3. Store in an airtight jar in the fridge for up to 2 weeks, though it is better to use sooner rather than later for optimum nutrition benefits.

PER 14G PORTION

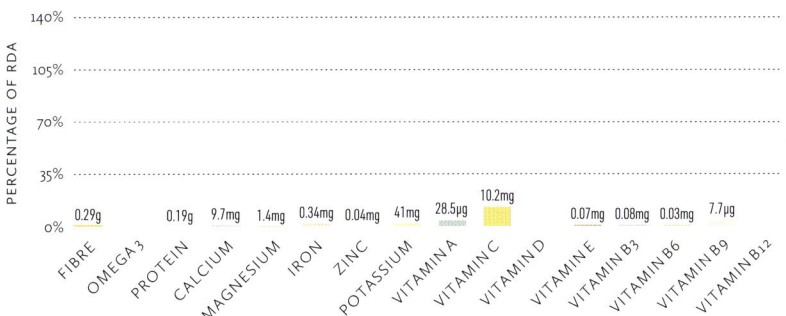

Basil Pesto

100g fresh basil leaves, stalks removed

100ml olive oil

1 clove of garlic

50g pine nuts, toasted

50g cashew nuts, toasted

45g Parmesan cheese or 2 tbsp nutritional yeast

1 tsp pink Himalayan salt

MAKES: 360G

A versatile store cupboard staple, this rustic, chunky pesto packed with nuts is ideal with eggs, pasta, salads and more. You can choose to make it vegan by replacing Parmesan cheese with nutritional yeast flakes.

1. Place all the ingredients in a food processor, and pulse until everything is broken down and well combined. The resulting mixture should be quite rustic in texture.
2. Taste and adjust the seasoning, if necessary, or add more olive oil. Store in an airtight, clip-top jar in the fridge, where it will keep for about a week.

PER 50G PORTION

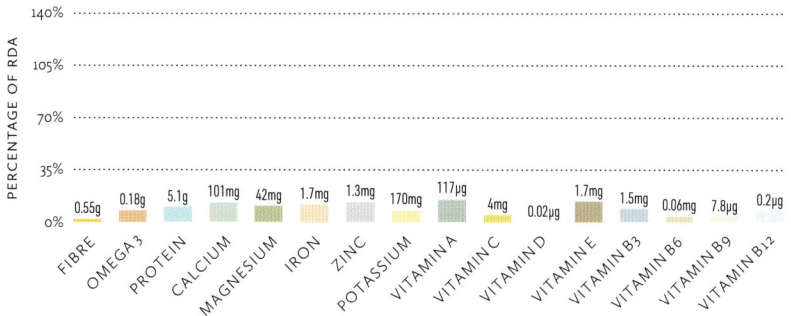

Roasted Mediterranean Vegetables

1 small sweet potato, peeled and roughly chopped

2 red onions, roughly chopped

2 cloves of garlic, minced

1 red pepper, roughly chopped

1 yellow pepper, roughly chopped

1 aubergine, roughly chopped

250g mushrooms (any kind), roughly chopped

1 tbsp extra virgin olive oil

1 tbsp tamari (gluten-free soy sauce)

drizzle of maple syrup

MAKES: 4 PORTIONS

Roasted Med veg – I usually make a big batch of these vegetables and keep them in an airtight glass container in the fridge for up to five days. Then I use them throughout the week in other meals – for example, pasta sauces, salads, wraps and omelettes.

1. Preheat the oven to 180°C, and line a baking sheet with greaseproof paper or a Teflon sheet.
2. Put all the chopped veg in a bowl, and add the olive oil, tamari and maple syrup. Mix well.
3. Lay all the veg out flat on the baking sheet, and roast in the oven for 30–40 minutes, mixing halfway through, until soft and browned.
4. Once the veggies are ready, remove them from the oven and allow them to cool.

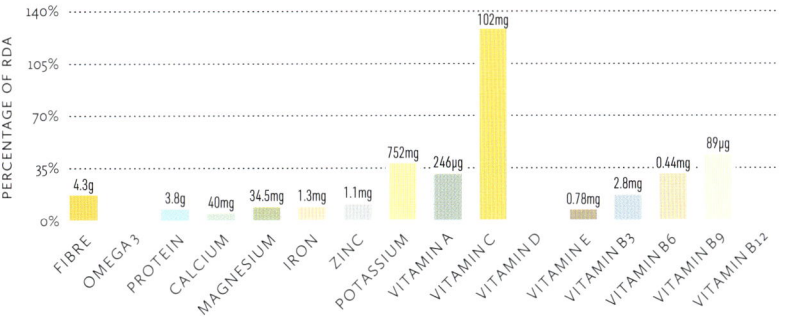

PART FOUR: RECIPES – ANTIOXIDANTS

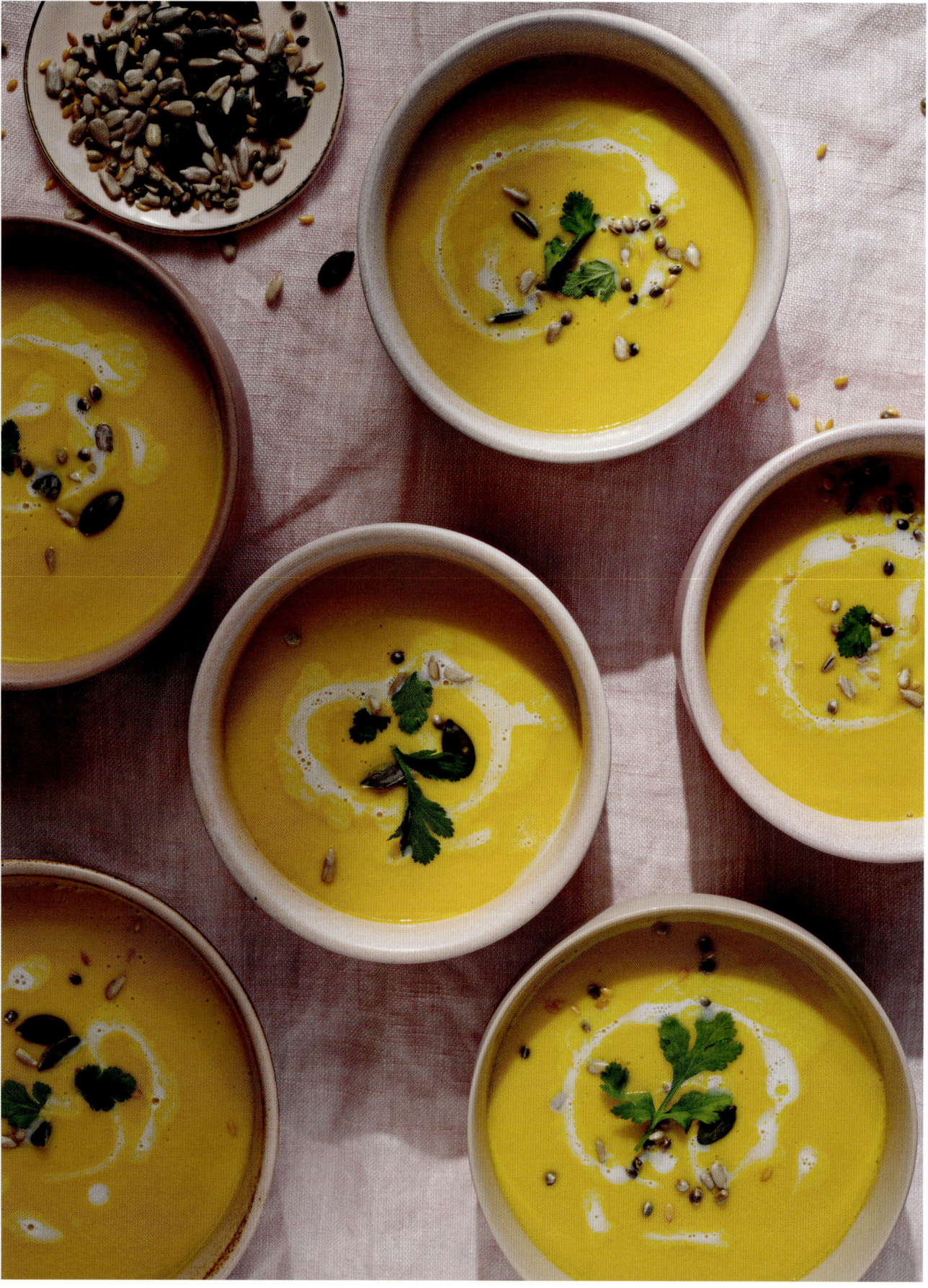

Carrot, Ginger and Celery Soup

2 tbsp olive oil

500g organic carrots, chopped

3 celery sticks, chopped

1 medium white onion, chopped

1 thumb-sized piece of ginger, quartered and peeled

2 cloves of garlic, chopped

600ml vegetable broth

200ml half-fat coconut milk

¼ bunch of flat-leaf parsley

salt and pepper, to taste

SERVES: 5+

Delicious and nutritious, this soup is also quick to make. If you want to elevate the flavour, serve it with a dollop of parsley gremolata on top.

1. Put a drizzle of olive oil in a large stockpot, and add the carrots, celery and onion.
2. Allow to sweat gently with the lid on until softened.
3. Add in the ginger and garlic, stirring gently.
4. Add in the vegetable broth and cook on a low heat for 30 minutes, until the vegetables are tender.
5. Add the coconut milk and parsley, and adjust the seasoning if necessary.
6. Remove from the heat and blend until smooth.
7. Serve – I like to top with some freshly chopped herbs, mixed seeds and a drizzle of coconut milk or natural yoghurt. For even more flavour, add a teaspoon of parsley gremolata (see p195).

PER 300G PORTION

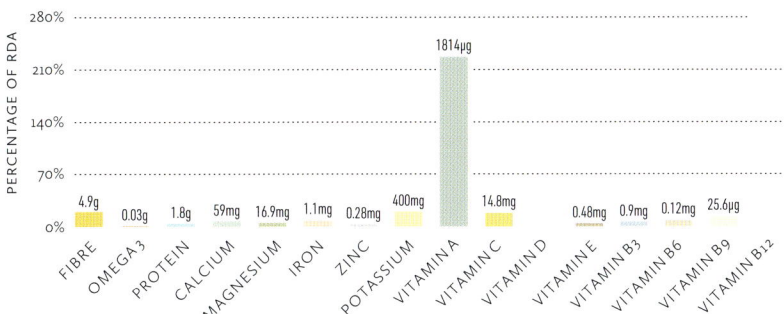

The Glow Bowl

extra-large handful of baby spinach leaves

extra-large handful of kale leaves

small bunch of fresh mint

¼ cucumber

½ avocado

zest and juice of 2 limes

1 piece of ginger, peeled

100ml organic soya milk or oat milk

225g frozen mango (or 1 fresh mango) or 1 whole papaya, seeds removed; or a mix of both

½ tsp spirulina powder

1 scoop of plant-based vanilla protein powder

TOPPINGS

any berries

1 kiwi

1 tbsp goji berries

1 tsp desiccated coconut

MAKES: 3 BOWLS

This smoothie bowl is a powerhouse of superfood ingredients. It is ideal as a satisfying breakfast or as a substantial snack if you've missed a meal.

1. Place all the ingredients in a blender, and blitz on high until all are broken down and smooth.
2. This tastes best straight away; however, it will keep in the fridge in an airtight glass container for up to 3 days. Consume within 24 hours for optimum nutrient benefit. It also freezes well.

Tip: Frozen mango (or papaya) adds a nice chilled creaminess to the smoothie bowl. However, if you don't have any frozen, just proceed with room-temperature fruit.

PER 256G PORTION

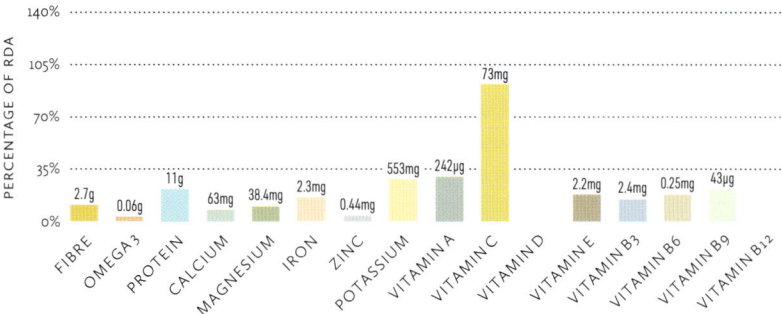

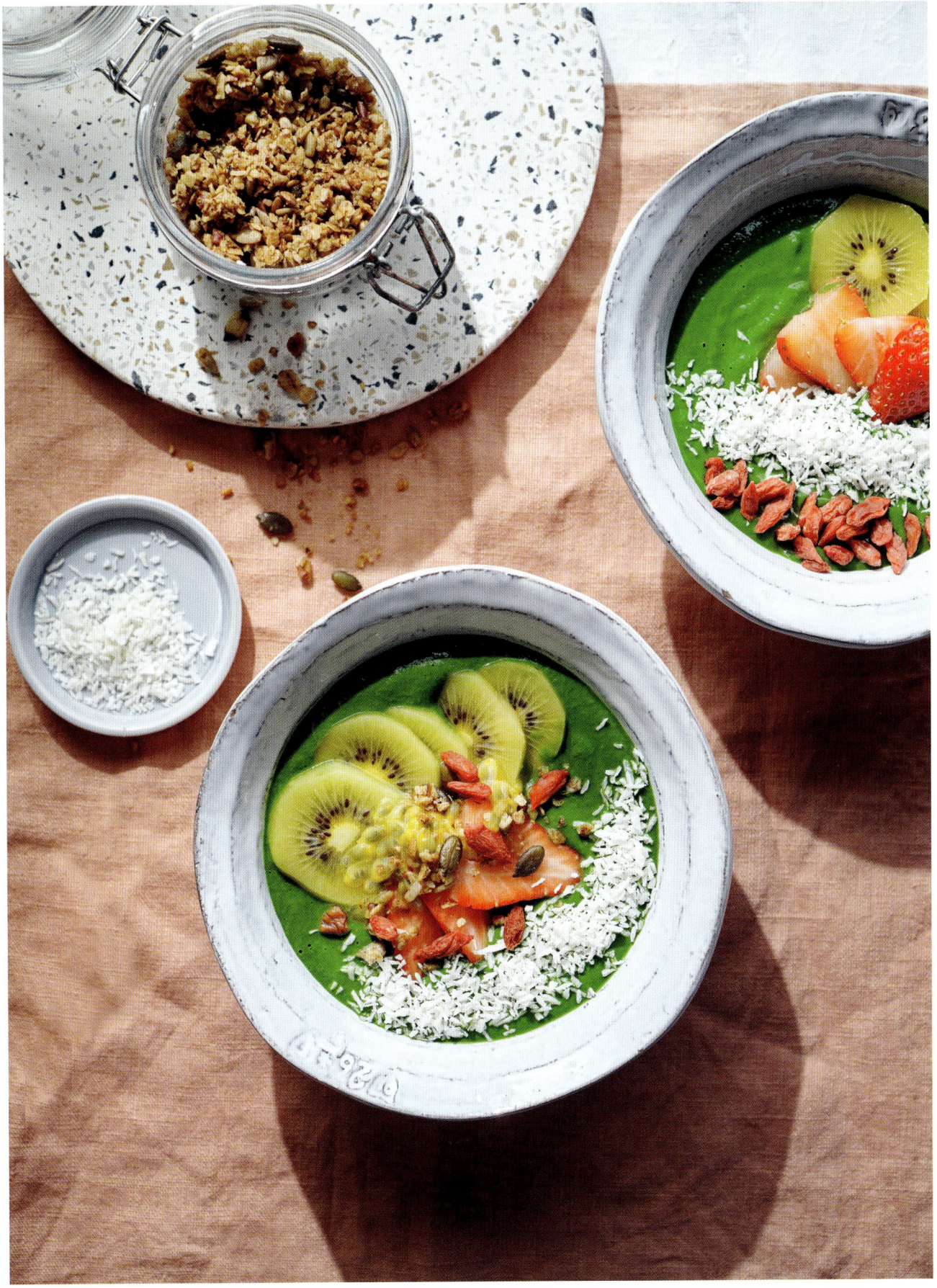

The Fountain-of-Youth Smoothie Bowl

2 heaped tbsp açai powder
1 banana, chopped
150g watermelon
50g frozen blueberries
2 tbsp goji berries

TOPPINGS
berries of choice
cacao nibs
pomegranate seeds
chopped walnuts
desiccated coconut

MAKES: 2 BOWLS

This is a vibrant, dark-purple, antioxidant-packed smoothie bowl. Try it out with different toppings to enhance its nutrient benefits.

1. Place all the ingredients in a blender, and blitz on high until they are broken down and smooth.
2. Spoon into a bowl and serve with your toppings of choice.

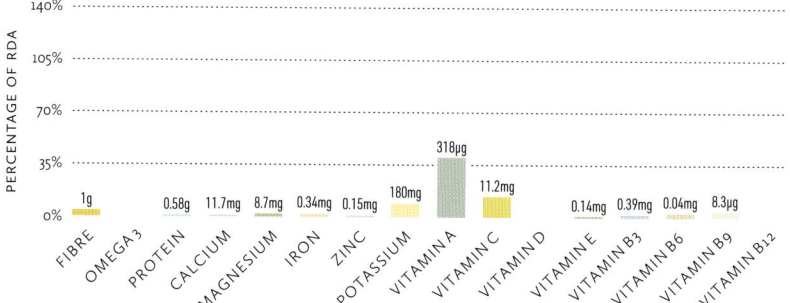

PER 160G PORTION

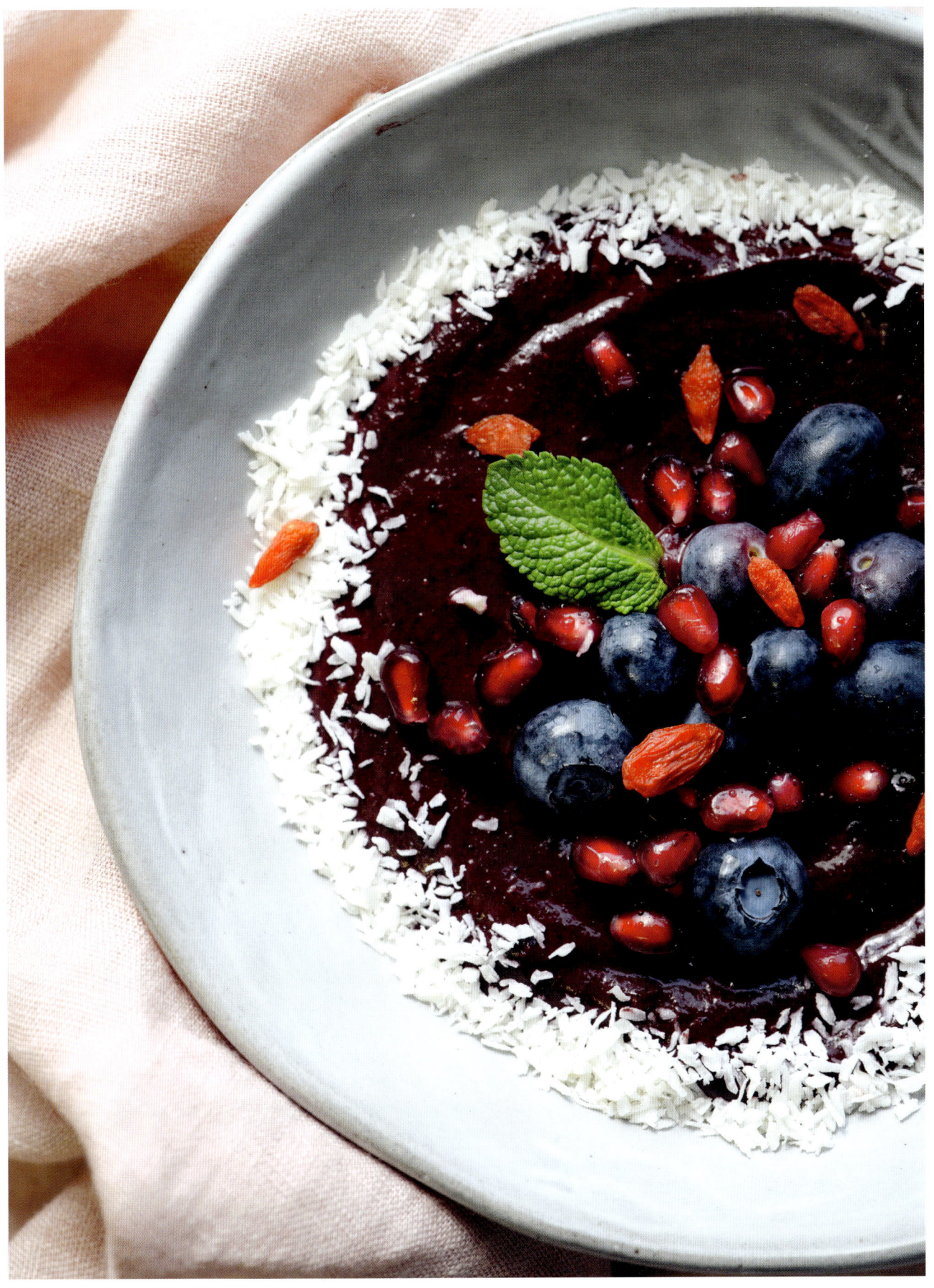

Sweet Potato Gnocchi

with roasted red pepper and tomato sauce

GNOCCHI

2 small to medium-sized sweet potatoes

1 egg

1 tsp salt

200g strong white (or type 00) flour

SAUCE

2 red peppers

2 tbsp olive oil

2 red onions, finely chopped

3 cloves of garlic, minced

800g tinned chopped tomatoes

1 tbsp maple syrup

1 tsp pink Himalayan salt

TOPPINGS

Parmesan cheese, grated

4 tbsp toasted pine nuts

basil pesto (optional, see p196)

MAKES: 4+ PORTIONS

A nice twist on the Italian classic, using beta-carotene-rich sweet potatoes. The red pepper and tomato sauce can be made in bulk and used in other dishes, such as roasted Med veg lasagne (see p207).

1. Preheat the oven to 180°C.
2. Pierce the sweet potatoes with a fork, place them on a baking tray and roast them for 45–60 minutes, or until completely soft. Remove from the oven and allow to cool.
3. While the potatoes are in the oven, make the roasted red pepper and tomato sauce. Start by placing the peppers on a roasting tray in the oven at 180°C for 35–40 minutes. Once browned and roasted, remove, place in a bowl and cover. (This will make it easier to remove the skins.)
4. Add the olive oil, onions and garlic to a large casserole pan with a lid. Place on a low heat and allow to soften. Once the onions are translucent, add the tinned tomatoes and cook for 10 minutes.
5. When the peppers are cool enough to handle, remove the skins. Chop the flesh and add it to the pan. Cook gently for a further 5–10 minutes, then put the sauce in a blender along with the maple syrup and Himalayan salt and blitz until smooth.
6. When the sweet potatoes are cool, slice them open down the middle and scoop out the flesh. Put this in a bowl and mash until perfectly smooth. Add the egg and mix well. Season with salt.
7. Add the flour to the sweet potato mix a little at a time and combine well. The mix will get stiffer as you add the flour, resembling a dough mix. Try not to add too much flour, as this will affect how light and fluffy the gnocchi are once cooked.
8. Knead the dough for a few minutes, then wrap it in cling film and leave for 20–30 minutes to rest.
9. Once rested, cut the dough lengthways into 4 columns. Flour your work surface and roll each section into a log. >

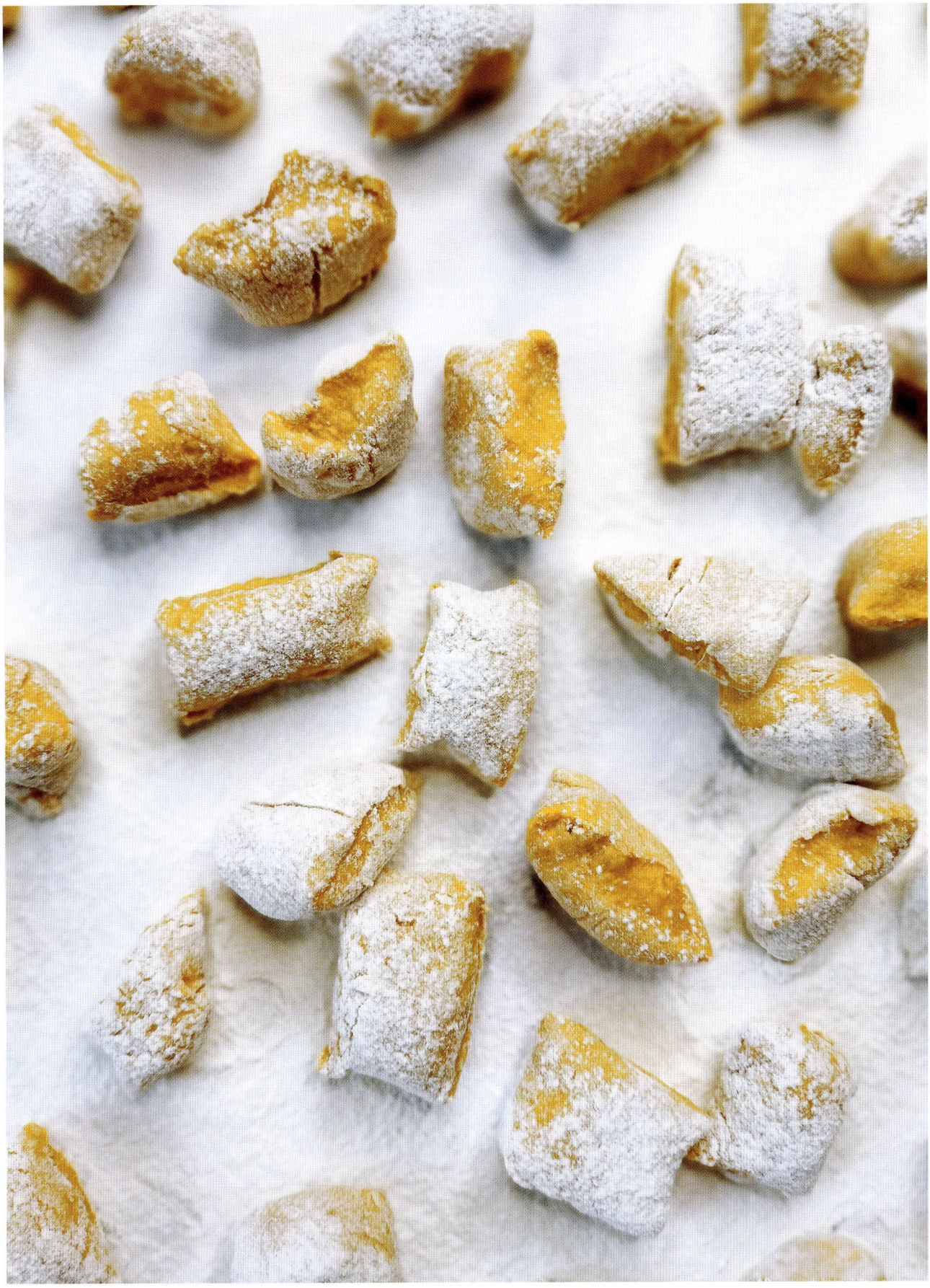

10. Using a pastry cutter or knife, cut each log up into bite-sized pieces. Continue until all the dough is cut up like this. You can now choose to cook it straight away or store it in the freezer.
11. If you are going to eat straight away, bring a pot of water to the boil.
12. Add the gnocchi to the boiling water in batches and allow to cook for a few minutes. They will start to rise and float when they are cooked. Using a slotted spoon, remove from the pan, shake off any excess water and add directly into the warm sauce in a separate pan.
13. Mix well, then plate up immediately. Top with grated Parmesan, toasted pine nuts and a teaspoon of pesto.

PER 315G PORTION

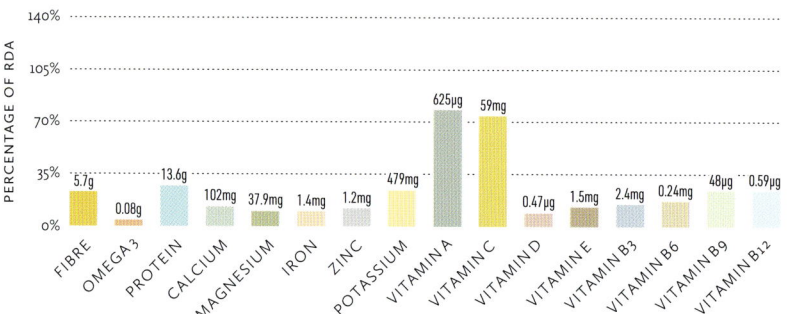

Roasted Med Veg Lasagne

with aubergine, spinach, mushroom and ricotta cheese

SAUCE

2 red peppers

2 tbsp olive oil

2 red onions, finely chopped

3 cloves of garlic, minced

800g tinned chopped tomatoes

1 tbsp maple syrup

1 tsp pink Himalayan salt

LASAGNE LAYERS

2 aubergines, finely sliced lengthways

55ml olive oil

2 punnets of mushrooms (any kind), finely sliced

2 bags of baby spinach leaves

1 small clove of garlic, minced

2 x 250g packets of fresh lasagne sheets

2 x 250g tubs of ricotta cheese

90g Parmesan cheese, grated

1½ tsp pink Himalayan salt

MAKES: 8 PORTIONS

This is a good, tasty option to feed a crowd. It has many elements (some of which you can prepare in advance), but it's well worth the effort. It is made with fresh lasagne sheets, roasted aubergine slices and ricotta cheese (instead of béchamel), with a sweet red pepper and tomato sauce.

1. Preheat the oven to 180°C, and line a roasting tray and three baking sheets.
2. Follow steps 3–5 of my sweet potato gnocchi recipe (see p204) to make the roasted red pepper and tomato sauce, and set aside.
3. Place the aubergine slices on the baking sheets, brush with a little olive oil and sprinkle with a grind of salt. Roast for 20+ minutes, keeping an eye on them so they don't burn.
4. While the aubergine slices are roasting, put the mushrooms in a frying pan with 1 tablespoon of olive oil and a little salt, and cook on a medium heat. When ready, move to a bowl and set aside.
5. Pan-fry the spinach with the minced garlic and 1 teaspoon of olive oil. Pour off any excess liquid.
6. Now it's time to assemble everything in a large ovenproof lasagne dish. Brush some olive oil all over the base and sides.
7. Add a couple of spoons of the roasted red pepper and tomato sauce to the base, followed by a layer of fresh lasagne sheets to cover the base and sides. (This will overlap up the side of the dish, which is fine.)
8. Add a few spoons of ricotta cheese, spreading it around the base.
9. Add a layer of roasted aubergine slices, followed by some spinach and some mushrooms.
10. Grate some Parmesan over the top, then repeat each ingredient until you have completed three layers in total.
11. Finish with a layer of fresh pasta topped with tomato sauce and grated Parmesan.
12. Place in the oven for 30–40 minutes, or until golden brown. >

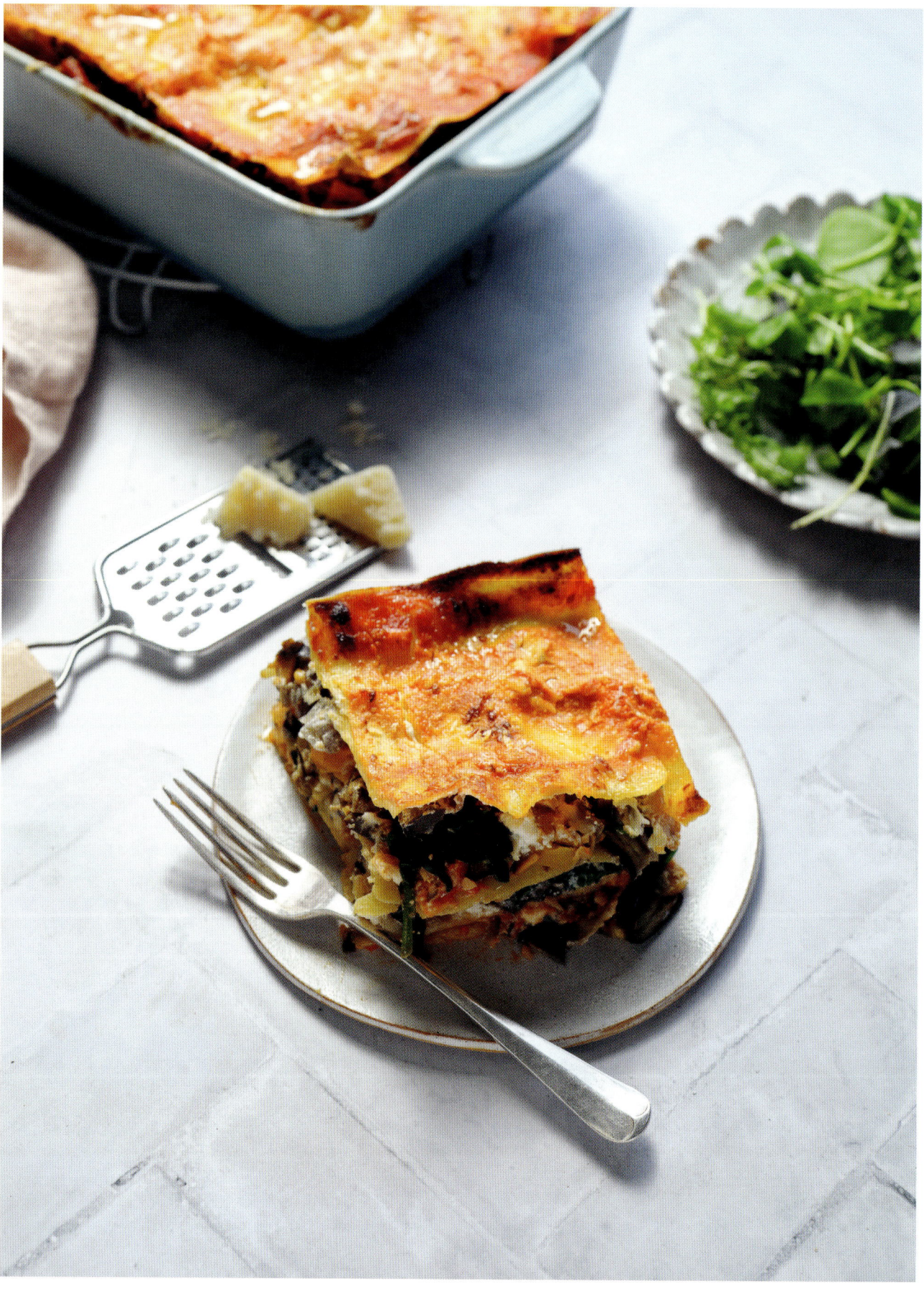

13 Serve directly to the table with plenty of grated Parmesan cheese (or see my tip if you're planning to serve later). Enjoy!

Tip: If you're making your lasagne in advance and storing in the fridge, bring it back to room temperature before roasting in the oven.

PER 575G PORTION

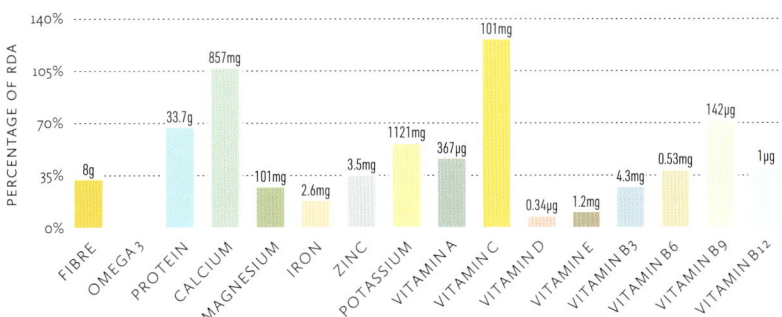

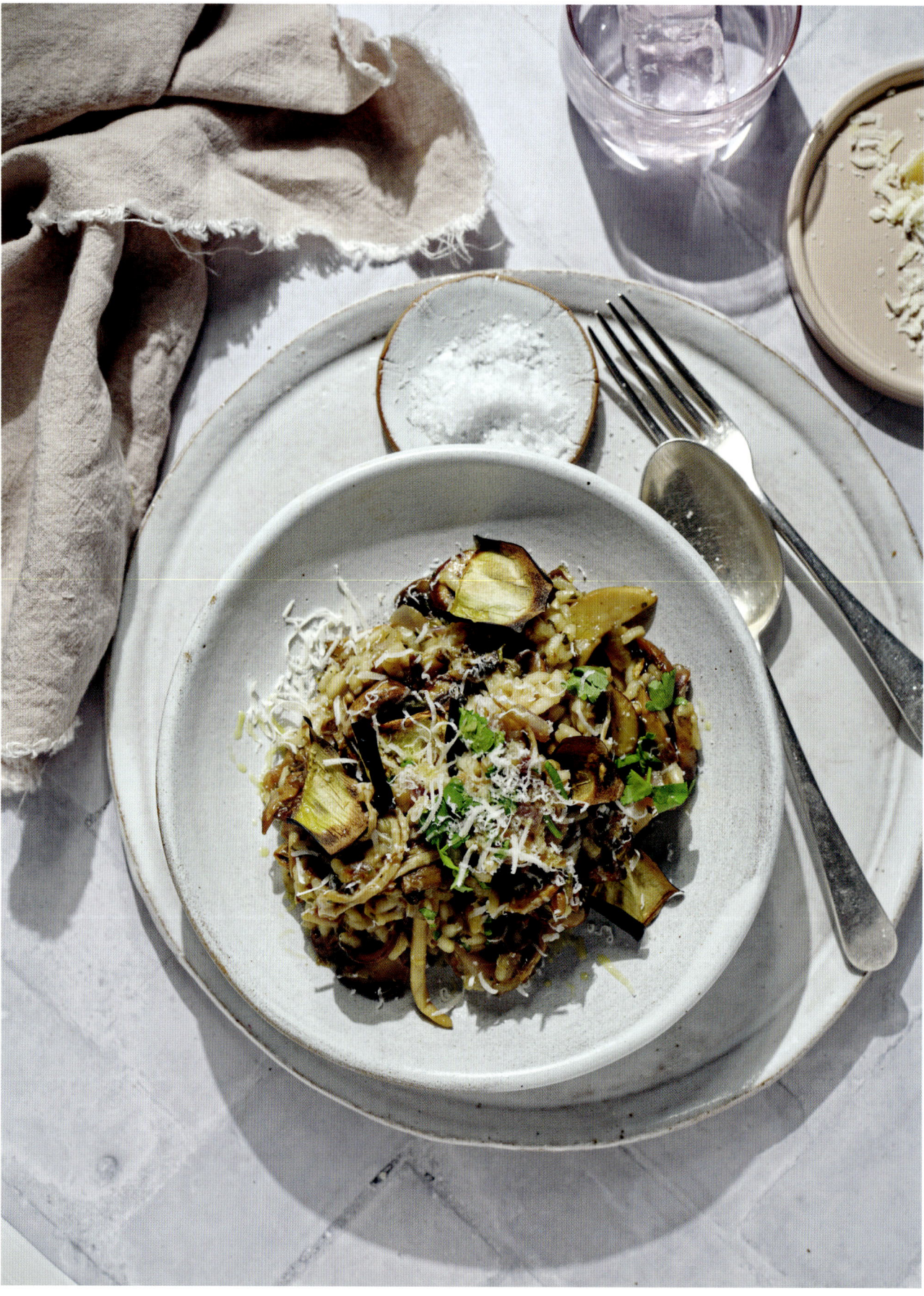

Porcini Mushroom Risotto

with roasted aubergine crisps

1 whole aubergine, finely sliced into ½cm rounds, then cut into quarters

8 tbsp olive oil

675g fresh mixed mushrooms, including 100g shitake mushrooms

100g dried porcini mushrooms

3 cloves of garlic, minced

handful of freshly chopped parsley or 1 tsp parsley gremolata (see p195)

1 red onion, finely chopped

300g risotto rice

1 litre veg stock

75ml white wine or prosecco

freshly grated Parmesan cheese

1 tsp butter (optional)

pink Himalayan salt and pepper, to taste

SERVES: 4

One of my favourite go-to risottos, this crowd-pleasing recipe is full of immune-boosting mushrooms with a real depth of flavour. It's great for an occasion meal with family or friends, served either with my kale salad (p276) or rocket, pine nut and Parmesan salad (p268).

1. Preheat the oven to 200°C.
2. Arrange the aubergine quarter slices on a lined baking sheet, brush with 1 tablespoon of olive oil and season with salt.
3. Roast until golden brown; this should be about 15 minutes, depending on the thickness of your aubergine slices. Remove from the oven and keep warm until the risotto is ready to serve.
4. Gently heat 4 tablespoons of olive oil in a large heavy-based saucepan.
5. Add all the fresh mushrooms and allow to cook gently for 10–15 minutes.
6. Meanwhile, rehydrate the porcini mushrooms by covering them in hot water for 10 minutes or so.
7. When the fresh mushrooms are ready, remove them from the pan and put in a bowl (keep warm). Wipe the pan clean with some kitchen paper and add another tablespoon of olive oil.
8. Drain the porcini mushrooms, retaining the soaking liquid. Finely chop the porcini and add to the pan along with the minced garlic. Allow to cook gently on a low heat. When the garlic begins to colour, add in half the porcini soaking liquid. Simmer gently until reduced.
9. Add the fresh mushroom mix, and stir to combine. Season with salt and pepper, then remove from the heat, and add the parsley or gremolata. Mix well and keep warm in a bowl.
10. Put the saucepan back on the heat with a tablespoon of olive oil and gently sweat the onion until translucent.
11. Add the risotto rice and stir until it becomes coated with the onions and oil. Add the other half of the porcini liquid and 2 ladles of hot veg stock. Stir to combine until the liquid has been absorbed. This will take a few minutes. Repeat the process: keep adding a ladle or 2 of veg stock to the rice until

all of the liquid has been absorbed and the rice is soft but still al dente (with a bite).

12 Finally, add the white wine or prosecco, stir and allow it to be absorbed before adding the mushroom mix. Combine well and add the finishing touches: a handful of grated Parmesan and the butter (if using).

13 To serve, plate up a heaped ladle of risotto mix into a shallow, warmed bowl, top with the roasted aubergine crisps, grated Parmesan cheese and a drizzle of olive oil.

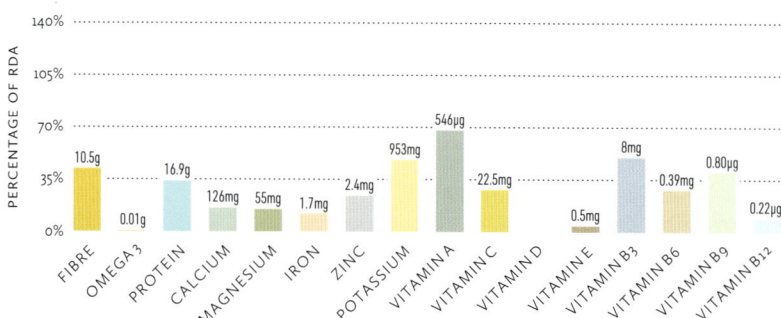

PER 600G PORTION

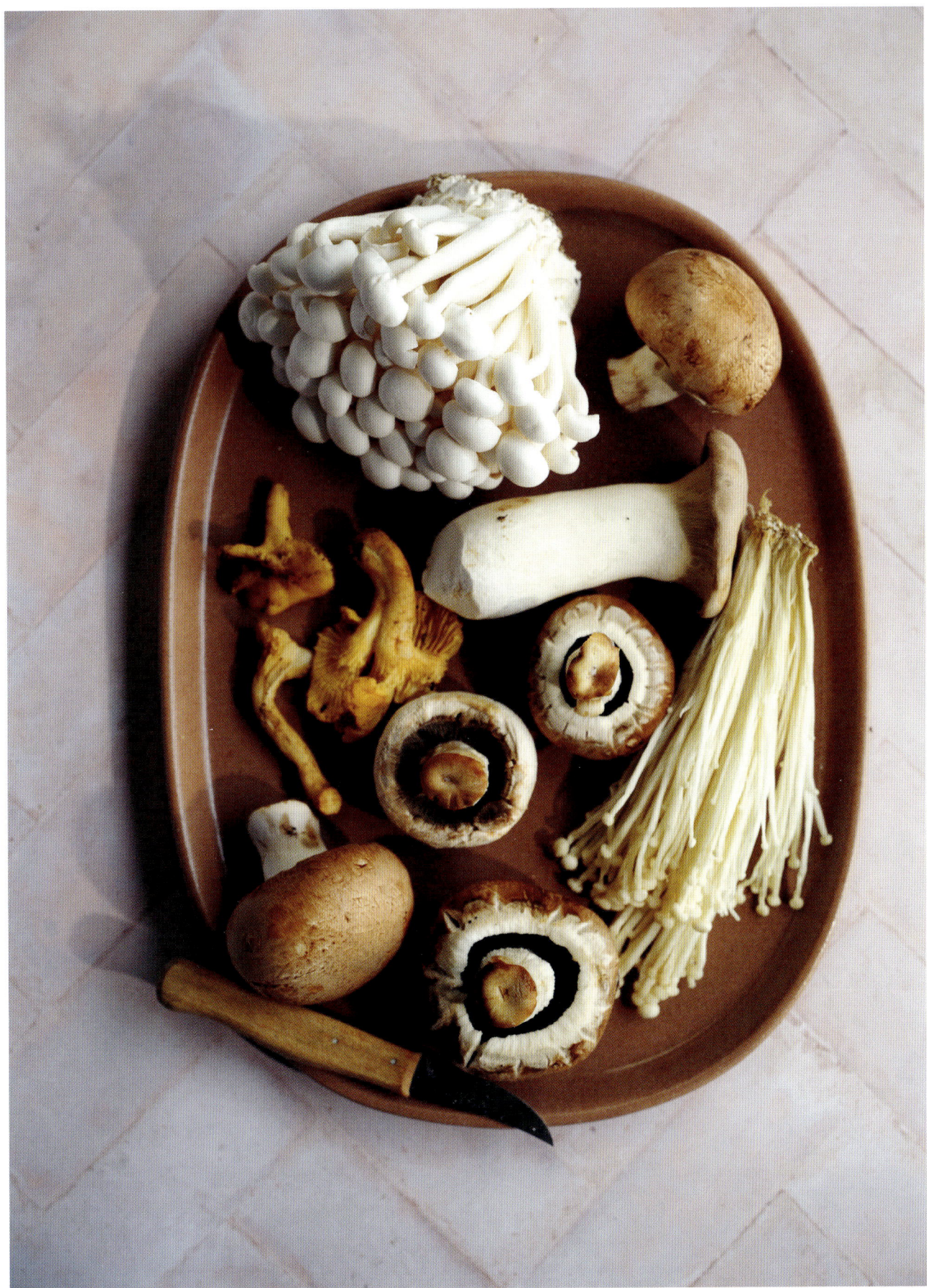

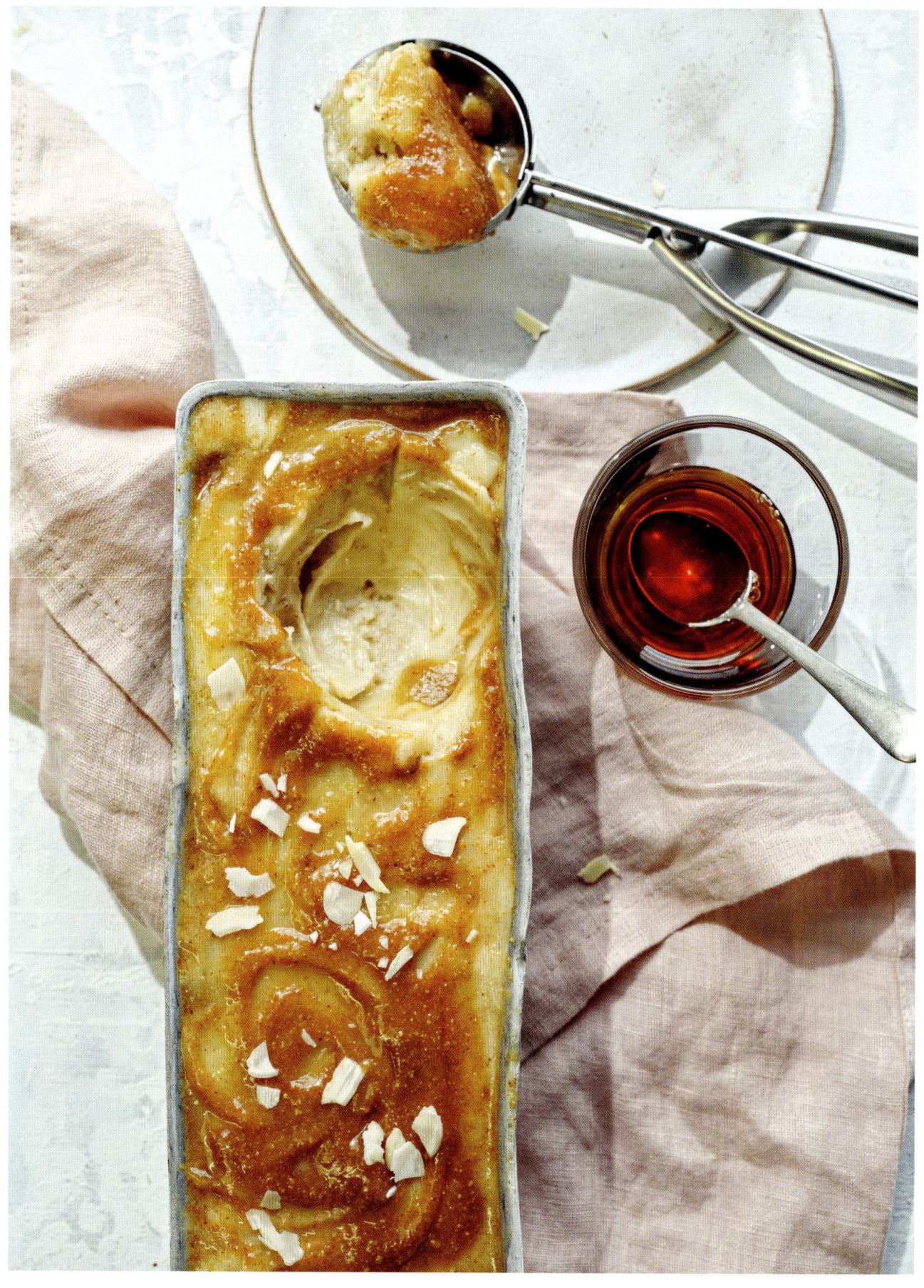

Banana Nice-Cream

with maple nut butter swirl

10 frozen bananas, chopped up into chunks

splash of oat milk

1 tbsp good-quality vanilla bean paste or vanilla essence

200g almond butter (see p170)

100ml maple syrup

SERVES: 4+

Who knew you could transform bananas into ice-cream – or nice-cream, as I prefer to call it! This dairy-free and saturated-fat-free ice cream is creamy and easy to make. It is a real treat drizzled with a little extra maple syrup and sprinkled with chopped nuts.

1. Put the bananas in a high-speed blender along with the oat milk, and blitz on high, using a tamper to keep the mixture moving in the blender until broken down and well combined. The mixture should resemble creamy soft-serve ice cream. Add the vanilla bean paste and mix by hand.
2. Remove from the blending jug and place in a bowl in the freezer while you prepare the flavouring.
3. Put the almond butter and maple syrup in a separate bowl and mix with a fork. The mixture should be runny in texture.
4. Line a loaf tin with parchment paper. Remove the nice-cream from the freezer and put half the mixture into the loaf tin.
5. Add a spoon or two of maple almond butter on top and swirl it around. Add the remaining nice-cream, and finish with the remaining maple butter swirled across the top.
6. Cover with cling film and freeze for 2–3 hours. You can then serve it with an ice-cream scoop.

Tip: Use well-ripened bananas for a sweeter ice cream.

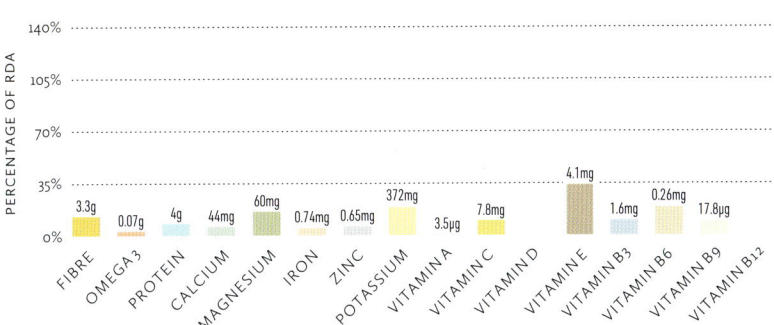

6. Protein

One of my key recommendations for women going through menopause is to increase the number of plant proteins in their diet. As well as aiding your digestion, a diet rich in plant protein sources can reduce your risk of cancer and heart disease and improve your bone health – and, of course, it can help to reduce the carbon footprint of what you're eating as well.

This section includes both animal and plant protein recipes; of the latter, the lentil Bolognese is a midweek staple in our house. It's quick and easy to prepare and a worthy substitute for the original Italian version!

Roasted Med Veg Frittata

6 large organic eggs

1 tbsp olive oil

1 tbsp feta cheese, crumbled

300g roasted Med veg (see p197)

1 tsp Himalayan salt and pepper

SERVES: 4

This is a tasty brunch option for family and friends that uses more of my batch-friendly Med veg. I like to serve the frittata with pesto and rocket leaves, or you can cut it up into wedges and store it in the fridge as a handy snack for when hunger strikes …

1. Preheat the oven to 180°C.
2. Break the eggs in a large mixing bowl, and season with salt and pepper.
3. Wet a large sheet of parchment paper, scrunch it up and use it to line a medium-sized, ovenproof frying pan or skillet. Push the paper into the edges of the pan.
4. Add the olive oil to the paper and swirl it around with a pastry brush.
5. Pour the egg mix into the pan.
6. Add the feta cheese, followed by the roasted Med veg.
7. Mix the egg around so that most of the vegetables are covered.
8. Place the pan, uncovered, in the oven for 15–20 minutes, until the mixture feels firm to touch.
9. Once the frittata is cooked, remove it from the oven and allow it to cool slightly. Enjoy now, or it can be cut into wedges and stored in the fridge as a handy grab-and-go snack.

PER 186G PORTION

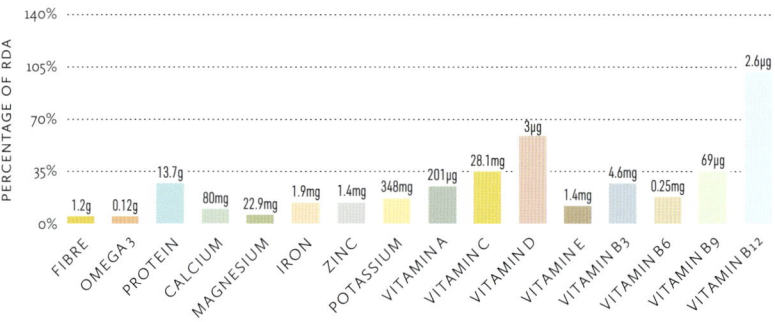

Courgette Rolls

with edamame bean hummus, Moroccan quinoa and asparagus

bunch of asparagus

150g Moroccan quinoa (see p226)

125g edamame bean hummus (see p91)

1 tsp pink Himalayan salt

1 tbsp finely chopped coriander, plus extra leaves for filling

½ courgette (halved lengthways), cut into ribbons with a peeler

2 tbsp sesame seeds, toasted

¼ red pepper, finely sliced (julienne)

1 small red onion, finely sliced

MAKES: 6+ PORTIONS

These are really tasty and easy to put together using up leftovers from the edamame bean hummus and the Moroccan quinoa. They look fabulous, too – the perfect way to impress your friends and family at a party.

1. Preheat the oven to 180°C.
2. Chop off more than half the stems of the asparagus, leaving you with just the tips (about 4cm in length). Place these on a roasting tray in the oven for about 10 minutes, or until tender. Remove and set aside.
3. Combine the quinoa, hummus, salt and chopped coriander in a bowl, and mix well.
4. Using a palette knife, spread this mix on to each courgette slice. Don't overload it, or it will spill out when rolling.
5. Sprinkle with toasted sesame seeds.
6. Place 2 red pepper sticks at the bottom of a courgette slice; top with 2 asparagus spears and 2 rounds of red onion. All these elements should hang over on one side, so they are visible.
7. Top with a coriander leaf and start rolling. Carefully roll to the top of the slice.
8. Place on a board and sprinkle with more sesame seeds to finish. Repeat for the rest of the slices. Any leftovers will keep for up to a day in the fridge in an airtight glass container.

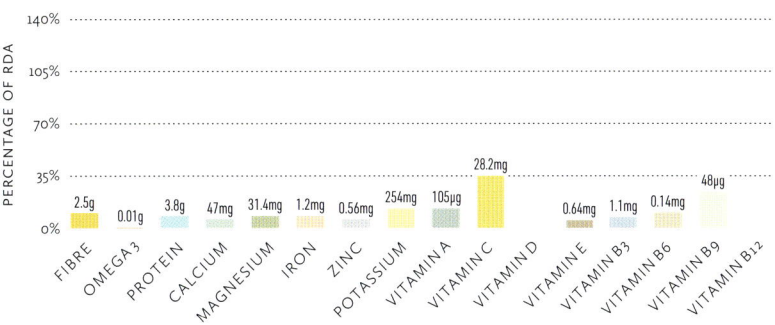

PER 100G PORTION

Shakshuka

baked Moroccan eggs

1 tbsp olive oil

2 kale leaves, washed and de-stemmed

½ onion, finely chopped

½ red pepper, finely chopped

½ small chilli, finely chopped

½ courgette, finely chopped

1 clove of garlic, finely chopped

1 tsp pink Himalayan salt and pepper

400g tinned tomatoes

2 sun-dried tomatoes in oil

1 tbsp maple syrup

4 large organic eggs

handful of coriander, finely chopped

spring onions, finely sliced

SERVES: 2

A really tasty brunch or supper recipe, this is ideal served with porridge bread (see p102) or my four-seed rye sourdough bread (see p256).

1. Preheat the oven to 180°C.
2. Add your olive oil to a heavy-based, ovenproof saucepan with a lid and heat gently. Put the kale leaves, onion, red pepper, chilli, courgette and garlic in and cook on a low heat.
3. Season with salt, pepper and a drizzle of olive oil, and allow to cook gently for a few minutes with the lid on until the onions are translucent.
4. Put the tinned tomatoes and sun-dried tomatoes in a blender with the maple syrup. Blitz on high until smooth, then add to the saucepan and stir. Cook for another 5 minutes.
5. Once the salsa is cooked and the veg are tender, make four wells in the sauce with the back of a spoon.
6. Add a drizzle of olive oil to each well, then crack an egg into each one. Put the lid on the pan and transfer to the hot oven for up to 5 minutes, or until the egg whites are firm.
7. Sprinkle with coriander and spring onions and serve to the table directly from the pan. I like to dish this up with slices of avocado or my favourite home-baked bread.

PER 482G PORTION

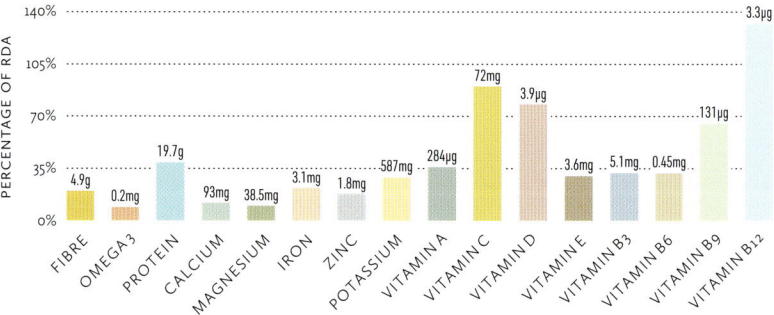

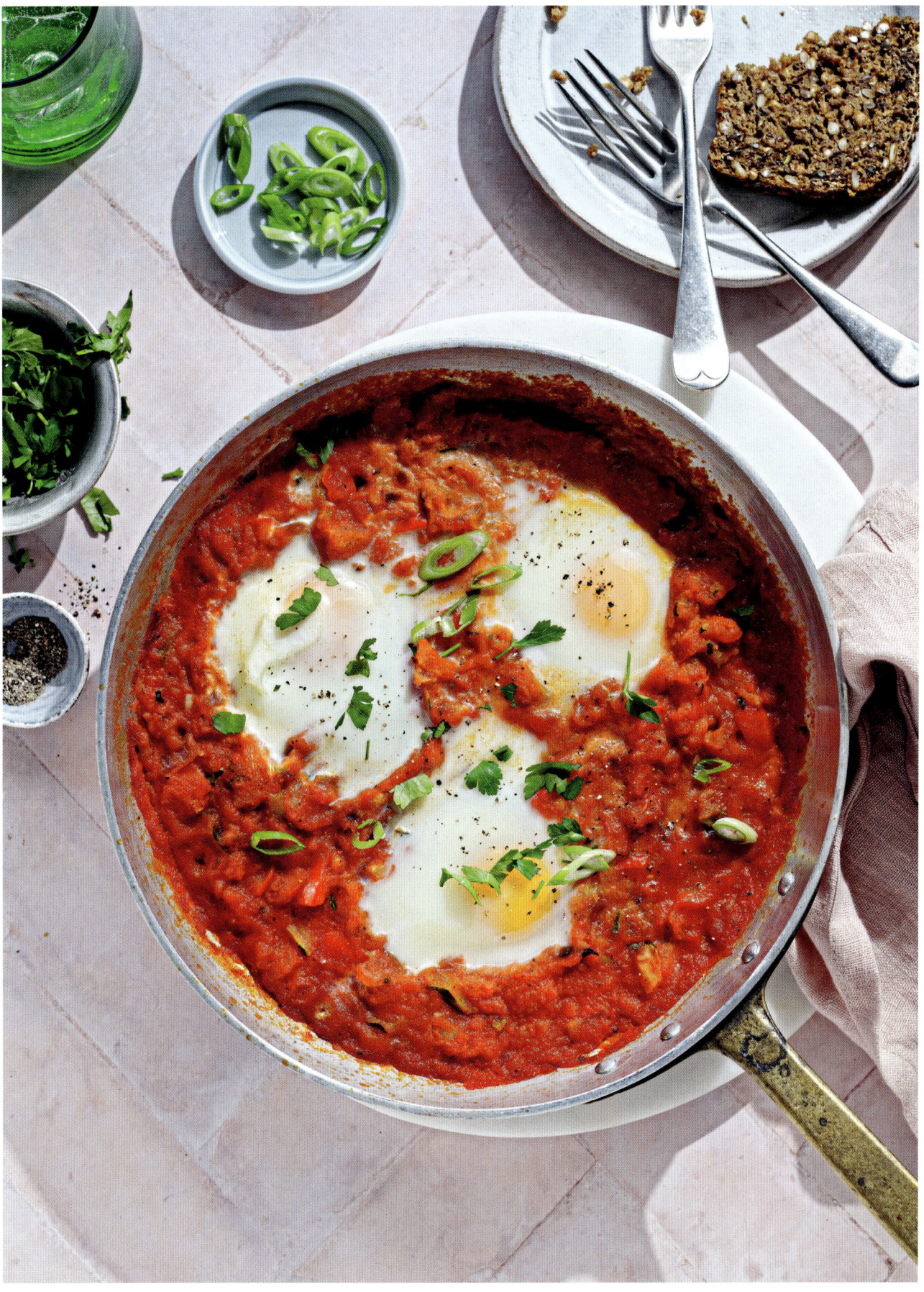

Courgette Tortillas

2 large courgettes

1 tsp pink Himalayan salt

1 egg

2 tbsp nutritional yeast

FILLING OPTIONS

tofu scramble (see p80)

smoked salmon, avocado, broccoli sprouts and red onion

wholegrain rice, beetroot ketchup (see p121), spring onions, tomato, prawns and broccoli sprouts

MAKES: 6 PORTIONS

Made with just three ingredients, these gluten-free tortillas taste great with a variety of fillings – see my suggestions below, or let your imagination (and taste) guide you.

1. Preheat the oven to 230°C, and line two oven trays with parchment paper.
2. Grate the courgettes and place in a large sieve or colander over a bowl to drain the liquid.
3. Add the salt and mix well (this will help to drain the liquid even further in the next step).
4. Squeeze the courgettes with your hands to get as much water out as possible. Leave for 5 minutes to drain.
5. Transfer to a bowl and add the egg and nutritional yeast. Mix well.
6. Take around 3 tbsp of the mixture and place on the lined tray, then spread this out as thinly as possible with your hands to approximately a 15cm round. Repeat with the remaining mix to make up to 6 tortillas.
7. Roast the tortillas in the oven for 10–15 minutes, or until browned.
8. Remove from the oven and carefully peel the tortillas off the paper. Allow to cool on a wire rack before adding your filling of choice – don't overfill the tortillas, as they are soft and fragile. The tortillas can be stored in the fridge in an airtight container for a couple of days.

PER 58G PORTION

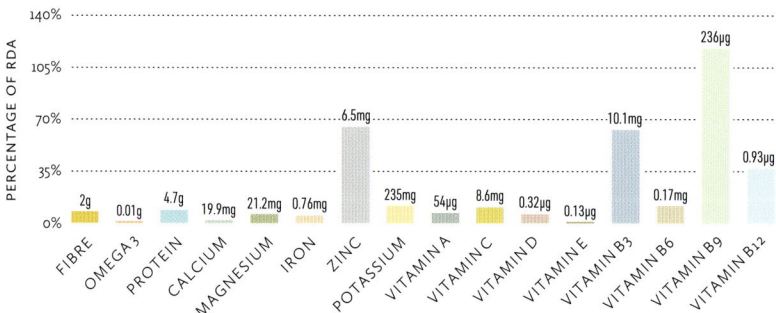

Falafel Wrap

with avocado and beetroot ketchup

1 kale quinoa wrap (see p163)

1 tbsp beetroot ketchup (see p121)

1 tsp sesame seeds, toasted

¼ red onion, finely sliced

¼ avocado, sliced

2 x 30g falafels (see p99), cut in half

1 tbsp cashew cream (see p113)

handful of broccoli sprouts (microgreens)

MAKES: 1 WRAP

Using a home-made kale quinoa wrap increases the protein and fibre content of this tasty and filling recipe, which further improves its nutrient density; however, if you don't have any, just use a large cos or iceberg lettuce leaf.

1. On a kale quinoa wrap, spread the beetroot ketchup and sprinkle the sesame seeds.
2. Add the onions and avocado, and top with the falafel halves. Drizzle the cashew cream on top of the falafels, and finish with a good bunch of broccoli sprouts.

Tip: To make a burrito-style wrap, keep the filling in the centre of the wrap; fold in the sides, squash down the filling slightly, then wrap and roll. The wrap is a little fragile, but if it splits, just cut it in half and eat with both hands!

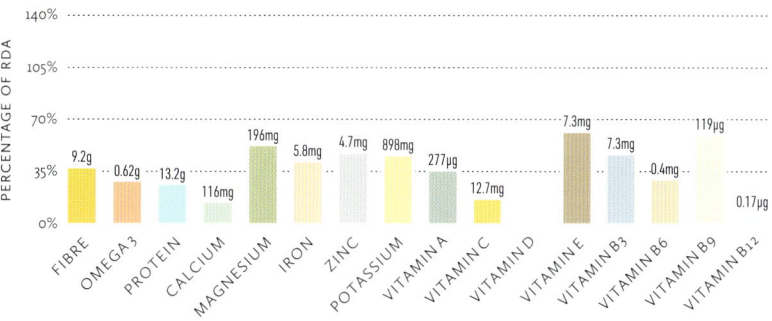

PER 230G PORTION

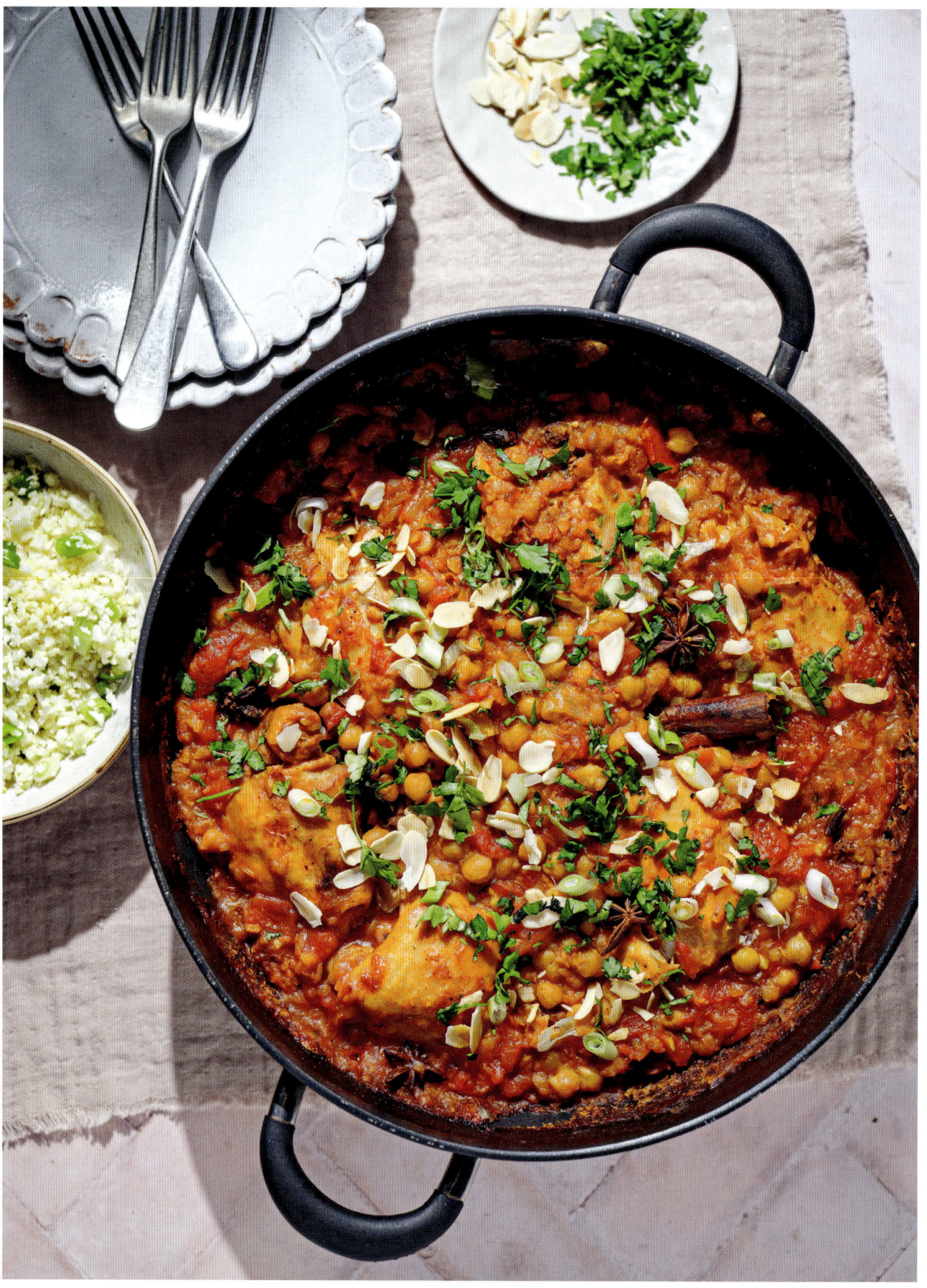

Moroccan Spiced Chicken Tagine

MARINADE

1 tsp ground ginger

1 tsp cinnamon

1 tsp smoked paprika

black pepper

grated zest of 1 lemon

50ml olive oil

TAGINE

800g chicken thighs, skinless and boneless

2tbsp olive oil

3 red onions, finely chopped

4 cloves of garlic, minced

800ml chicken stock

1 cinnamon stick

400g tinned peeled chopped tomatoes

60g raisins

400g tinned chickpeas, drained

1 tsp ras el hanout

3–4 star anise

2 tbsp honey

1 tsp harissa paste

1 cup dried red lentils

pink Himalayan salt and ground black pepper, to taste

TO SERVE

Moroccan quinoa (see p226) or wholegrain brown basmati rice

large handful of coriander leaves, chopped

handful of flaked almonds, toasted

SERVES: 4+

This recipe requires overnight marination of the chicken thighs to tenderise them and maximise their flavour. It's the perfect family dinner: bursting with taste and quick and easy to prepare.

1. Combine all the marinade ingredients in a large glass food storage container and mix well.
2. Add the chicken thighs to the container and coat them well with the marinade. Cover and refrigerate overnight.
3. The next day, preheat the oven to 180°C.
4. Put the olive oil, onion and garlic in a heavy-based, ovenproof saucepan, and cook with the lid on, on a medium heat, until soft and translucent.
5. Add the chicken stock and stir to loosen any sediment from the bottom.
6. Add the chicken pieces to the pan, along with the cinnamon stick. Season with salt and pepper.
7. Add the tinned tomatoes, raisins, chickpeas, ras el hanout, star anise, honey, harissa paste and red lentils. Cook for 1.5 hours in the oven with the lid on, until the chicken is tender and the sauce has thickened.
8. Serve with Moroccan quinoa or wholegrain brown basmati rice, topped with coriander and toasted flaked almonds.

PER 600G PORTION

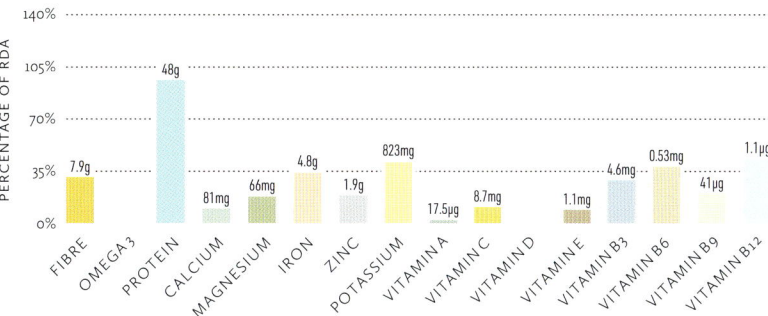

Moroccan Quinoa

with toasted pistachios

| 1 tbsp olive oil |
| 1 tsp ground cumin |
| ½ tsp ground cinnamon |
| 1 tsp paprika |
| 1 red onion, finely diced |
| 1 stick of celery, finely diced |
| 500ml vegetable stock |
| 180g quinoa |
| 35g raisins (optional) |
| 35g roasted unsalted pistachios, shelled, or flaked almonds, toasted |
| 20g fresh coriander, chopped |
| handful of pomegranate seeds |

MAKES: 8 PORTIONS

This tasty quinoa recipe is very versatile – it can be used as part of a salad bowl, as a wrap filling or to accompany hot dishes like turmeric roasted chicken breast (see p243) and Moroccan spiced chicken tagine (see p225). Quinoa is both gluten-free and a good source of protein.

1 Put the olive oil in a heavy-based saucepan, add the spices and let them sizzle.
2 Add the onion and celery, toss everything together and cook with the lid on until softened.
3 Add the stock and the quinoa, mix well and put the lid back on the saucepan.
4 Allow to cook gently until all the liquid has been absorbed (10–12 minutes). The quinoa will sprout little tails when ready. It should be soft to taste, while still retaining a little bite.
5 If including raisins, remove your pan from the heat, add the raisins and stir. Put the lid back on and allow to steam for 5–10 minutes so the raisins swell. (If you aren't adding raisins, you can skip this step.)
6 Chop the roasted pistachios roughly and add to the quinoa, along with some fresh coriander and a handful of pomegranate seeds for decoration.

Tip: You can store your quinoa in the fridge in an airtight container for up to 5 days. If doing so, add your fresh herbs and roasted pistachios just before serving.

PER 125G PORTION

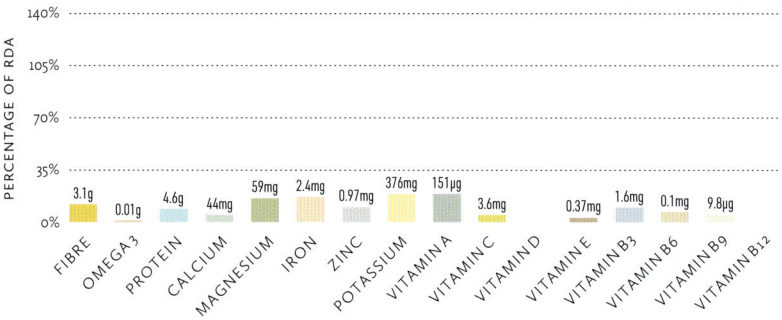

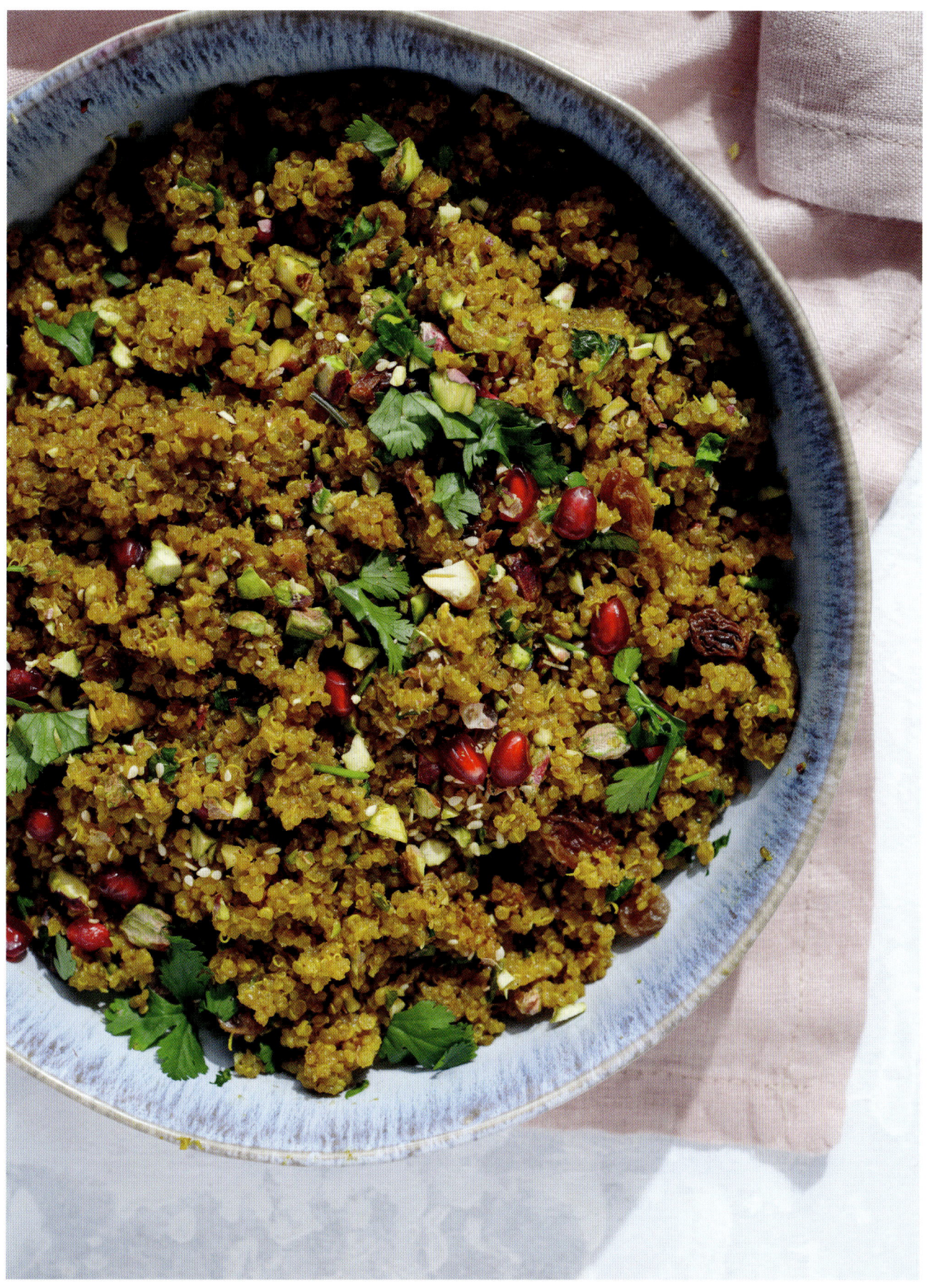

Lentil and Mushroom Burgers

with quinoa crust

1 onion
2 cloves of garlic
handful of spinach leaves
4 tbsp olive oil
150g pumpkin seeds
250g mushrooms of choice
2–3 tbsp ground almonds
400g lentils, cooked
2 tbsp tomato purée
2 sun-dried tomatoes
1 tsp smoked paprika
pinch of pink Himalayan salt
1 tbsp nutritional yeast
100g quinoa
nut oil (sesame, walnut or avocado)

MAKES: 10 BURGERS

These burgers are delicious and well worth making ahead of time – they freeze well and are a versatile addition to lots of meals. In terms of nutrition, these are high in plant protein, fibre and minerals, and offer a great-tasting, minimally processed vegan burger.

1. Blitz the onion, garlic and spinach in a food processor. Gently pan-fry this mixture in 2 tablespoons of olive oil until the onions are soft. Move to a large mixing bowl.
2. Blitz the pumpkin seeds in the food processor until they resemble breadcrumbs, then add to the bowl.
3. Blitz the mushrooms in the food processor, then gently fry in your remaining olive oil until golden. Add to the mixing bowl, along with the ground almonds. This will help to bind the mixture.
4. Blitz the cooked lentils, tomato purée, sun-dried tomatoes, paprika and salt in the food processor until it resembles a paste. Stir it into the mixing bowl along with the nutritional yeast.
5. Using your hands, shape the mixture into 10 burgers.
6. Place the burgers on some silicone paper and allow them to firm up in the fridge for 2–3 hours.
7. Preheat the oven to 180°C.
8. Blitz the quinoa to a coarse flour in a blender. Empty the contents onto a plate and dip each burger into the mix to coat.
9. Add some nut oil to the pan and gently brown each burger. Place on a lined baking tray and put in the oven for 10 minutes to warm through.
10. Serve per your preference – I like to dish these up on a roasted whole mushroom, or in a large iceberg lettuce leaf with beetroot ketchup (see p121) and avocado.

Tip: Make your burgers ahead of time and chill them in the fridge (this will prevent them from falling apart when cooking). They will keep in an airtight container in the fridge for up to 5 days, and can also be frozen.

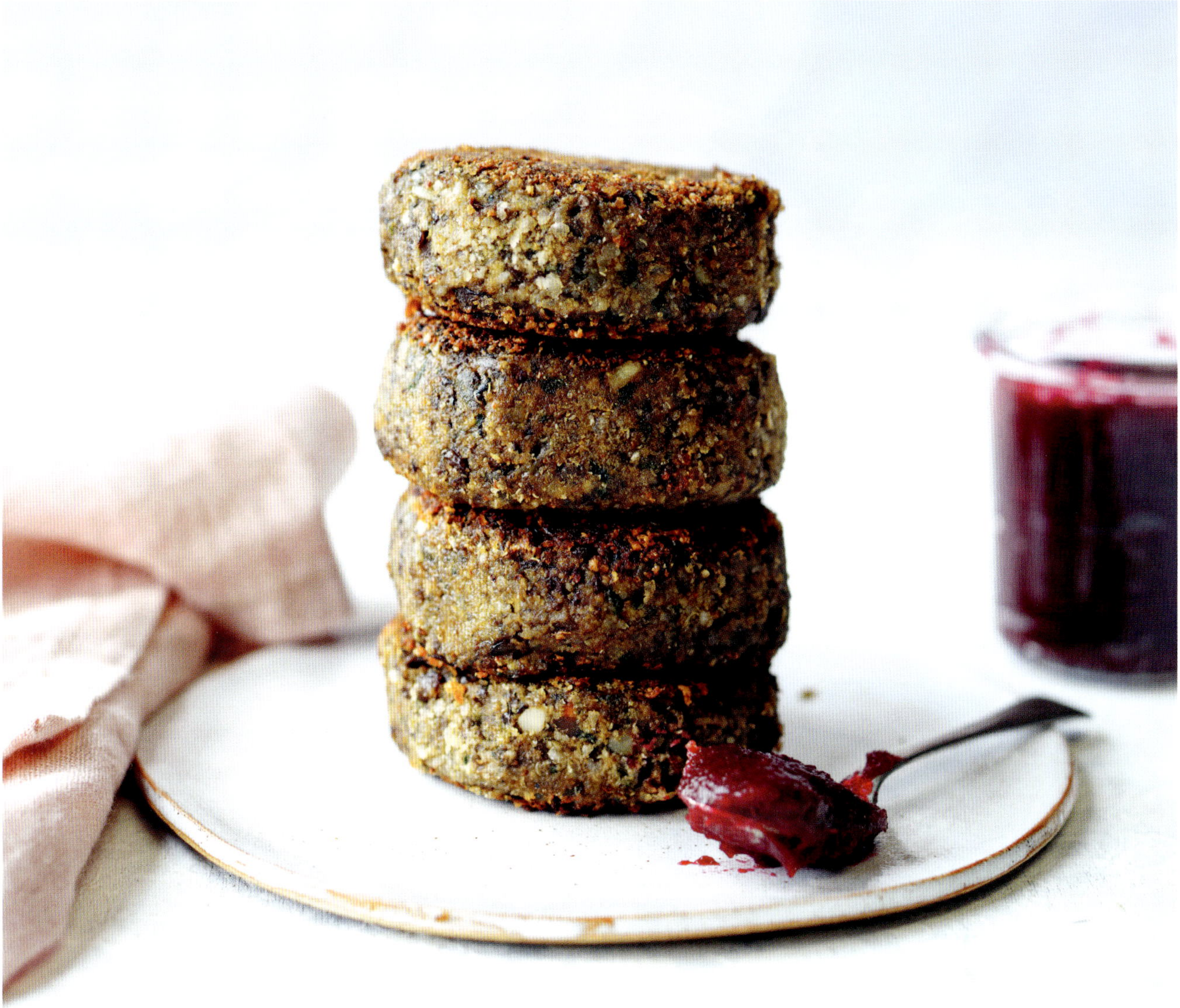

PER 125G PORTION

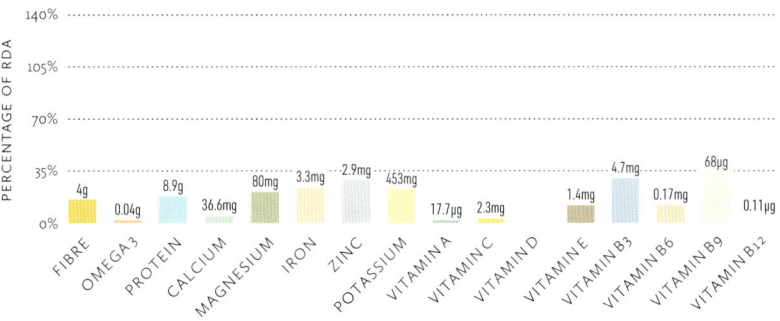

PART FOUR: RECIPES – PROTEIN

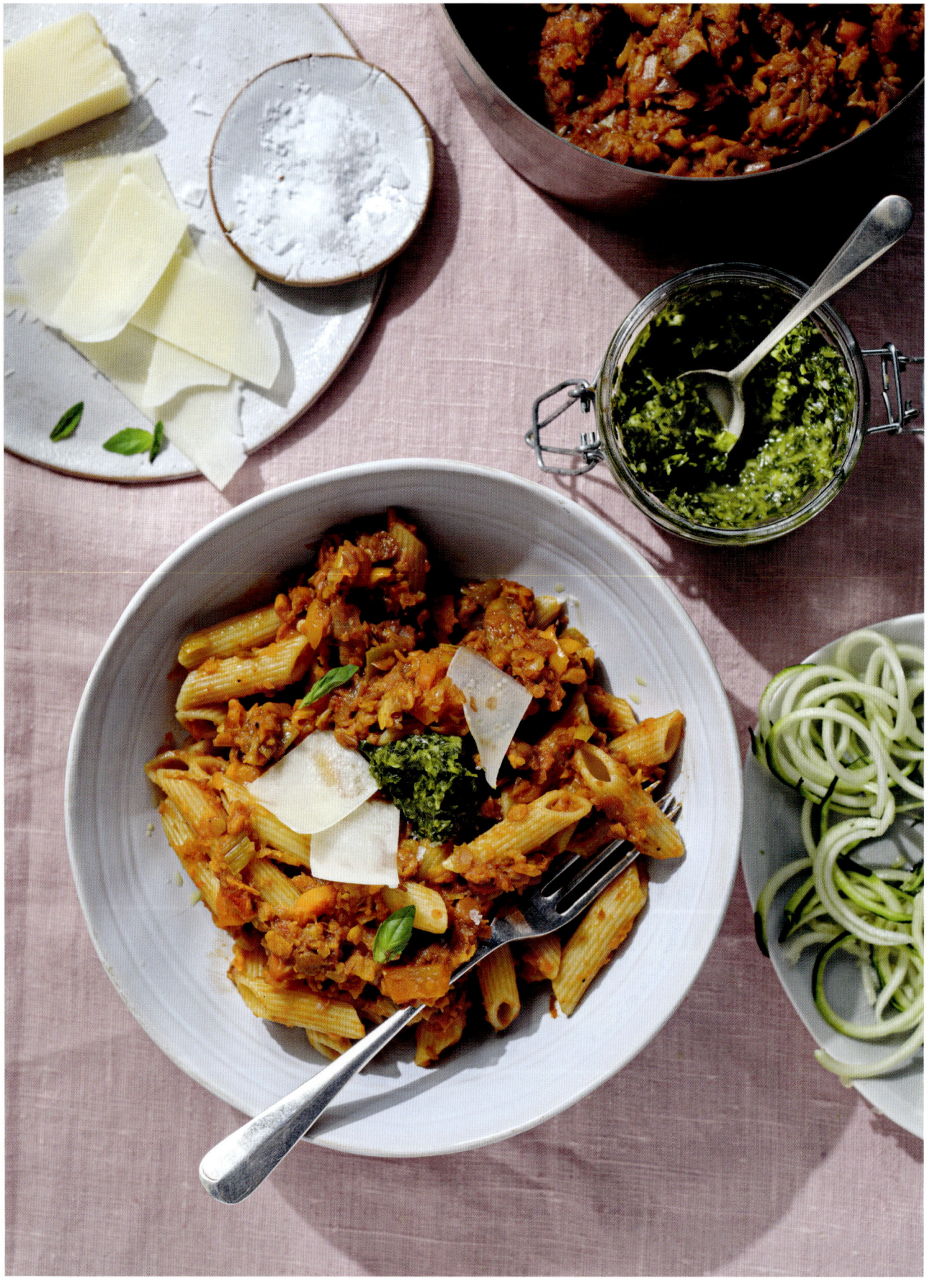

Lentil Bolognese

1 tbsp olive oil
1 carrot, finely grated
1 stick of celery, finely sliced
1 leek, finely sliced
1 small sweet potato, grated
800g tinned organic chopped tomatoes
1 glass of red wine
1 tsp veg stock powder
100g mushrooms, sliced
1 small green or yellow pepper, finely chopped
2 large bay leaves
190g dried red lentils
230g cooked brown lentils
1 tsp honey
1 tbsp sun-dried tomato paste
pink Himalayan salt and pepper, to taste
1 red onion, finely diced
4 cloves of garlic

TO SERVE

100g wholewheat penne pasta or 1 medium-sized courgette (per person), spiralised
fresh basil
Parmesan shavings (optional)
parsley gremolata (see p195)

MAKES: 8 PORTIONS

This is a worthy substitute for the original recipe: a tasty, easy, make-ahead, plant-based meal with all the classic Italian flavours.

1. Sweat the onions and 3 cloves of garlic in the olive oil on a very low heat until the onions are translucent.
2. Add the carrot, celery, leek and sweet potato to the pan, and cook gently until soft.
3. Season with salt and pepper.
4. Add the tinned tomatoes, red wine and stock powder.
5. Add the mushrooms, green pepper, bay leaves and both types of lentils, and simmer gently for 1 hour.
6. Allow to cool, then season again with a freshly grated garlic clove.
7. Adjust the seasoning as necessary, with a pinch of salt, some honey or sun-dried tomato paste.
8. Serve with either wholewheat penne or spiralised courgetti, plus fresh basil.

PER 350G PORTION (INCL. 100G PASTA)

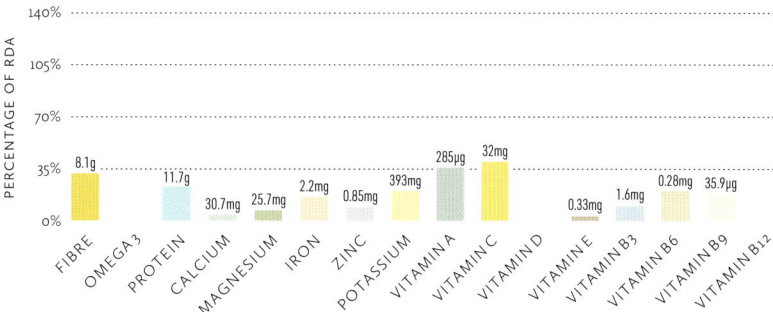

Mushroom and Lentil Shepherd's Pie
with roasted root veg mash

2 tbsp olive oil

5 large portobello mushrooms, finely chopped

150g fresh shitake mushrooms, finely chopped

2 onions, finely chopped

2 celery stalks, finely chopped

2 leeks, finely sliced

6 cloves of garlic, minced

3 small carrots, finely chopped

2 tbsp sun-dried tomato paste

300ml vegan red wine

2 tbsp Worcestershire sauce

1 bay leaf

1 sprig of fresh rosemary

350ml vegetable stock

250g pre-cooked brown lentils

100g frozen peas

salt and pepper, to taste

1 tbsp maple syrup

handful of fresh chopped parsley

ROASTED ROOT VEG MASH

2 medium sweet potatoes, chopped small

½ butternut squash, chopped small

½ celeriac root, chopped small

2 tbsp olive oil

½ tsp grated nutmeg

1–2 tbsp plant milk (optional)

pink Himalayan salt and black pepper, to taste

SERVES: 8

This is healthy comfort food to feed a crowd! You could also top it with olive oil mash to satisfy the kids. Shitake mushrooms have medicinal properties that benefit our immune system, so it's worth getting them fresh from your greengrocer, but any mushrooms will do.

1. Put one tablespoon of olive oil in a large casserole dish or saucepan, and heat gently. Add the mushrooms and allow them to brown gently. Remove the mushrooms from the pan with a slotted spoon and set aside.
2. Add another tablespoon of olive oil to the pan, and add the onions, celery, leeks and 4 cloves of garlic.
3. Cover with the lid and cook for a few minutes until translucent.
4. Add the carrots. (These will take the longest to cook, so make sure they're chopped small.)
5. Add a tablespoon of sun-dried tomato paste, the red wine, Worcestershire sauce, cooked mushrooms, bay leaf and rosemary sprig to the pan, along with the veg stock and the cooked lentils.
6. Cook over a low heat with the lid off for about 1 hour, until the carrots are soft. Add the frozen peas towards the end, with 5 minutes to go.
7. Set aside and allow to cool. If possible, make it in advance and store in the fridge overnight – this will allow the flavours to develop and intensify.
8. For the root veg mash, preheat the oven to 200°C.
9. Place all the veg in a mixing bowl with one tablespoon of olive oil and the seasoning, then move them to a large lined roasting tray and roast until tender – about 45 minutes. When soft, remove from the oven and put in a mixing bowl. Blitz with a stick mixer, adding the rest of the olive oil, plant milk (if using), nutmeg, salt and pepper. Season to taste. >

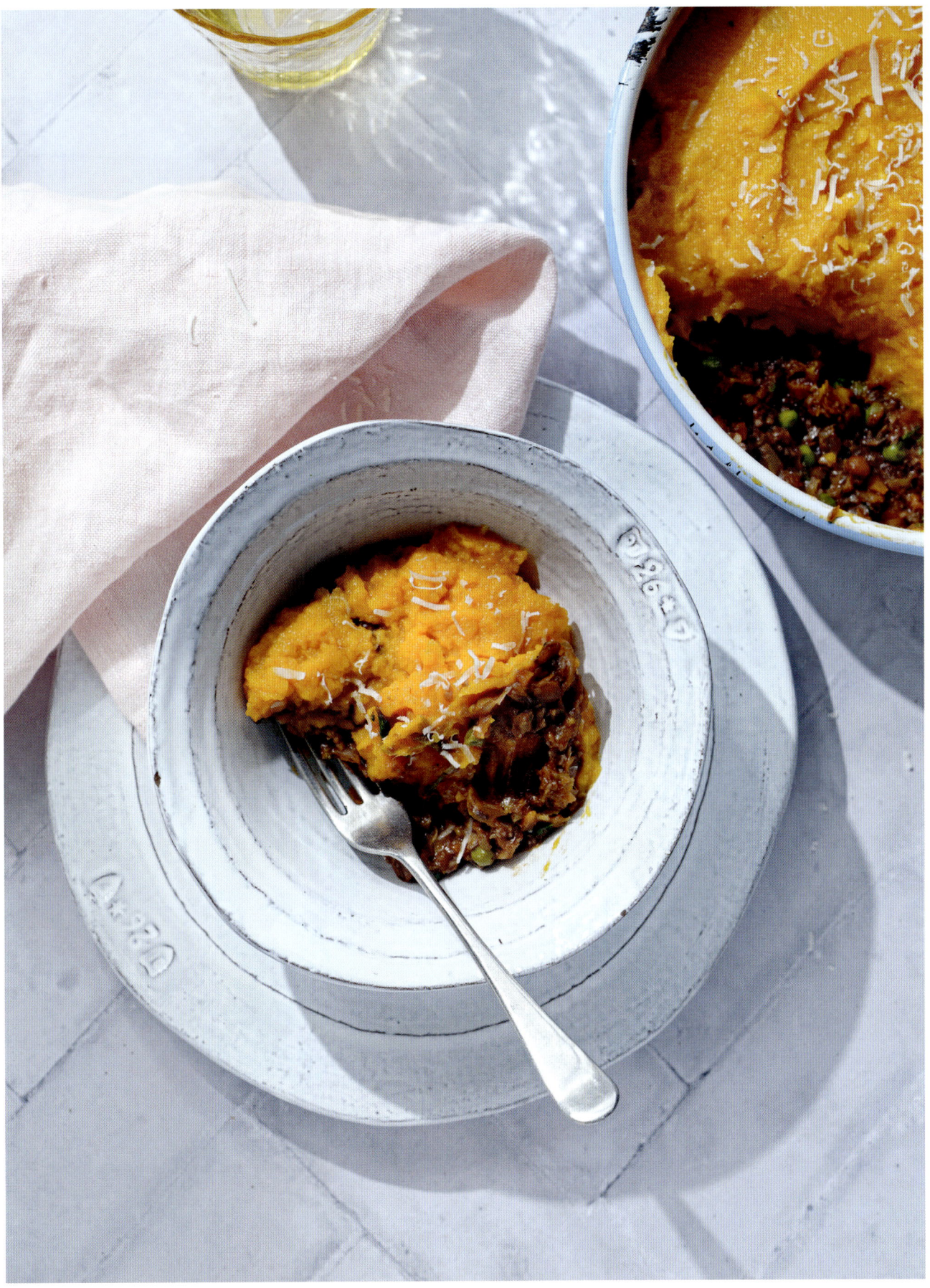

10. Time to assemble the shepherd's pie. If you have chilled the mushroom/lentil mix, reheat slightly in a pot and check the seasoning – I like to add salt and pepper, maple syrup, another tablespoon of tomato paste, the rest of your minced garlic and some fresh parsley at this point. Then spoon your mixture into either individual pie dishes or one large dish to the halfway mark. Top with the roasted root veg mash, forming decorative peaks with a fork. At this stage, you could also add a layer of olive oil mashed potatoes.
11. Roast in the oven at 200°C for around 20 minutes, until warmed through and crispy on top, and then place directly on the table to serve sharing-style. If you like, you can finish it off with a drizzle of olive oil, chopped herbs and vegan Parmesan.

Tip: Use a food processor to prep the veg quicker. This recipe can be made in stages ahead of time to save time. It also freezes well.

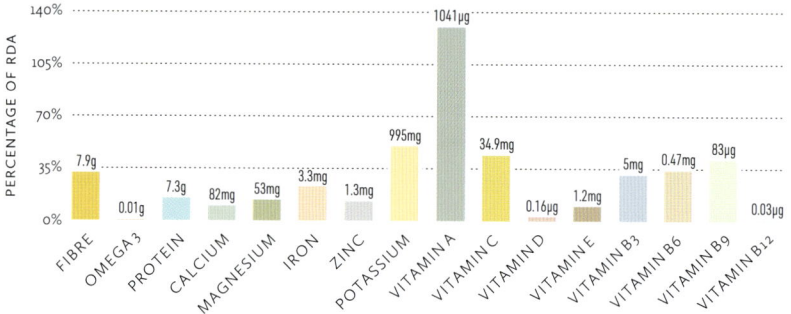

PER 400G PORTION

Chicken Bone Broth

1 tbsp olive oil

2 medium-sized organic carrots, cut into large chunks

1 leek, cut into large chunks

1 medium organic onion, quartered

pink Himalayan salt, to taste

1 organic/free-range carcass of a cooked chicken

1 garlic head, cut in half

2 celery sticks

2 bay leaves

1 tbsp apple cider vinegar (see p255)

2 tsp black/pink peppercorns

MAKES: 1–1.5 LITRES

Bone broth contains essential amino acids which are the raw ingredients for all our hormones, and provides a source of bioavailable nutrients in a very easy-to-digest form. It also contains collagen – which is fantastic for your skin, hair and nails – and glucosamine and chrondroitin sulphates, which support joint health.

1. Heat the olive oil in a stockpot, then add the carrots, leeks and onions. Stir to combine and sprinkle with Himalayan salt.
2. Add your chicken carcass to the stockpot and fill it with water (1–2 litres), making sure to cover the bones. Add the garlic, celery, bay leaves, apple cider vinegar and peppercorns, as well as more water if necessary.
3. Bring to a gentle boil, keeping the lid (slightly skewed) on the pan. Reduce and simmer on a very low heat for at least 8 hours and up to 24 hours. You may need to top it up with water during this process.
4. Once cooking time is complete, discard the bones and vegetables, and strain the broth using a fine mesh sieve. Once cool, it can be refrigerated. The solidified fat that will form on the top can be removed, but be careful not to remove the precious jelly-like substance underneath – this contains all the collagen!

Tip: The longer this cooks, the more savoury and concentrated it will become. This is ideally made in a slow cooker or left in a cool oven or bottom Aga.

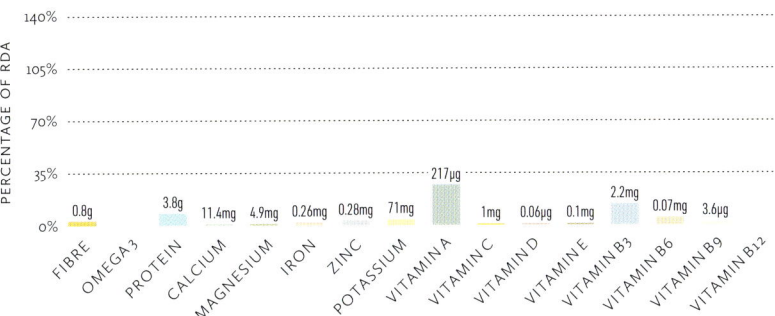

PER 500ML PORTION

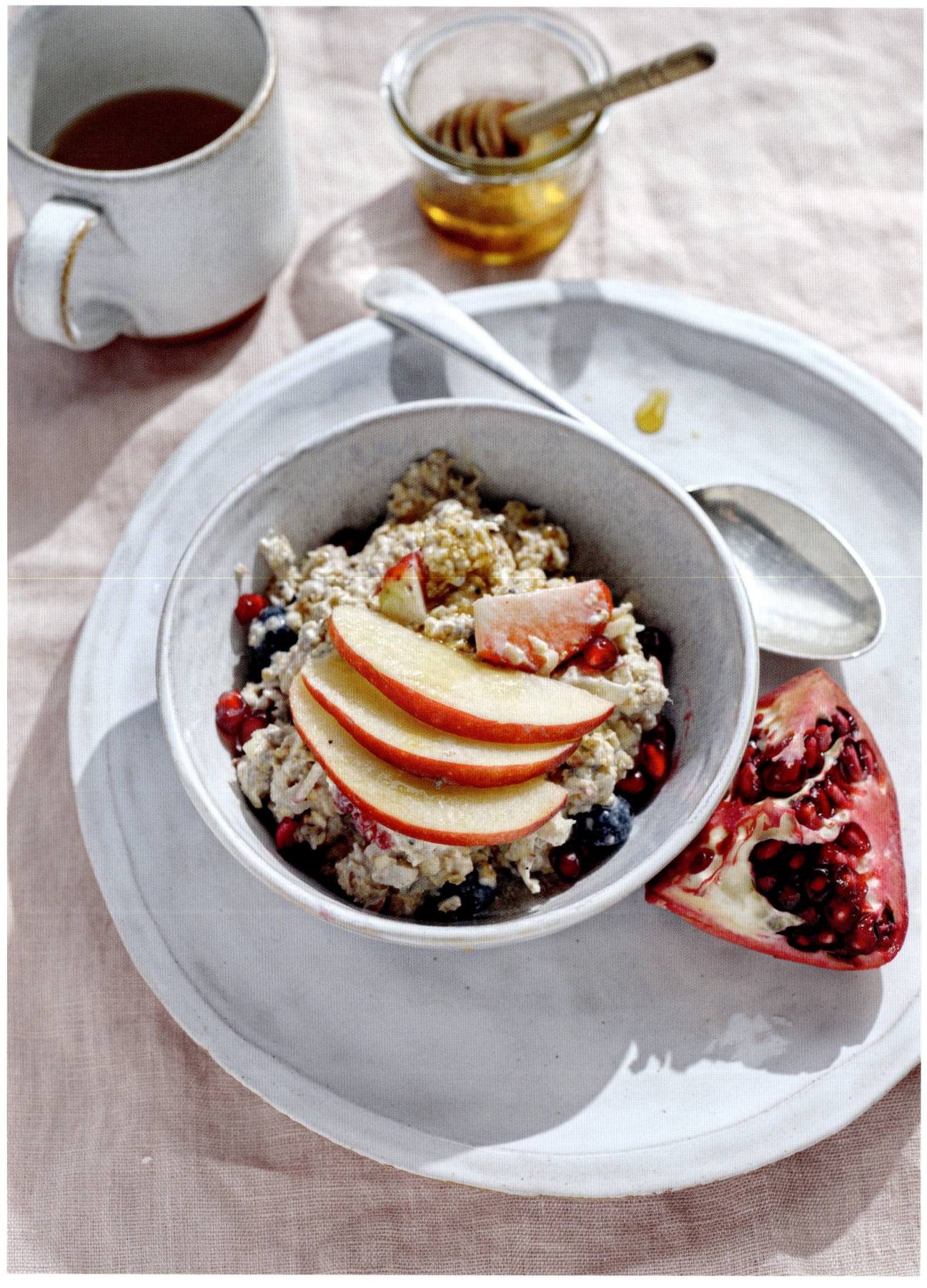

Bircher Muesli

6 tbsp pecan cinnamon granola (see p107)

4 tbsp porridge oats

1 tbsp chia seeds

1 organic apple, grated

75g fresh blueberries

75g fresh berries of choice

150ml live probiotic natural yoghurt

50ml oat milk

TOPPINGS

1 tbsp almond butter per pot

sprinkling of coconut shards

sprinkling of goji berries or fresh red currants

¼ apple, sliced

MAKES: 3 POTS

Perfect for breakfast or a snack, this traditional Austrian recipe is a version of overnight oats, made with live probiotic yoghurt and lots of seeds and berries. It's really tasty and nourishing, as well as rich in plant protein and fibre.

1. Combine all the ingredients in a bowl and mix well.
2. The mixture should be loose and not too dry, so adjust accordingly.
3. Spoon into three small glass jars, seal and refrigerate for a couple of hours or overnight.
4. When ready to consume, top as per the above suggestions. These will keep for up to 4 days in the fridge.

Tip: The chia seeds will absorb a lot of the moisture, so you may need to use a little extra liquid to prevent the muesli from becoming too dry.

PER 210G PORTION

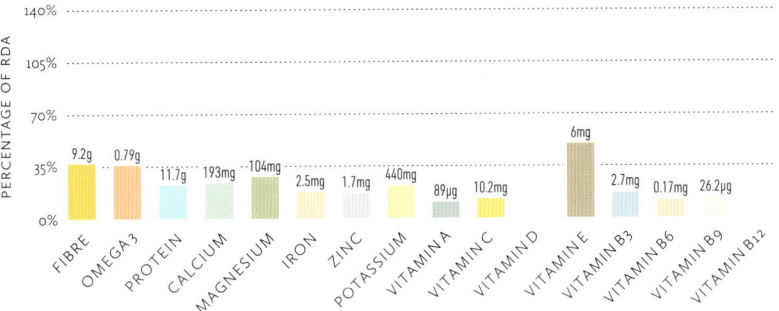

Mocha Chia Protein Overnight Oats

80g porridge oats
1 tbsp whole chia seeds
1 tbsp ground flaxseeds
1 Medjool date, pitted
235ml plant milk (oat, almond or organic soya)
1 tbsp raw cacao powder
½ tbsp almond butter (see p170)
¼ cup strong coffee (americano or espresso)
½ tsp vanilla bean paste or essence
½ scoop vanilla protein powder or cold-milled hemp seeds
pinch of pink Himalayan salt or sea salt

TOPPINGS

sliced banana
almond butter
goji berries
strawberries

MAKES: 2 PORTIONS

These taste so luxurious, you could serve them for dessert! They are also full of plant protein and fibre, which is why they are so filling. Omit the coffee if you want to skip the caffeine hit.

1. Put the dry ingredients (oats, chia seeds and flaxseeds) in a mixing bowl.
2. Place all the other ingredients in a blender, and blitz on high until smooth and well combined.
3. Add the wet mix to the dry mix and stir.
4. When all is well combined, allow to sit and thicken in the fridge for 1–2 hours.
5. To serve, just spoon into the individual jars – ¾ full, to leave space for the toppings!
6. These can be made in advance and will keep in the fridge in an airtight container for several days. When you are ready to eat, simply open the jar, add your toppings of choice and enjoy!

PER 185G PORTION

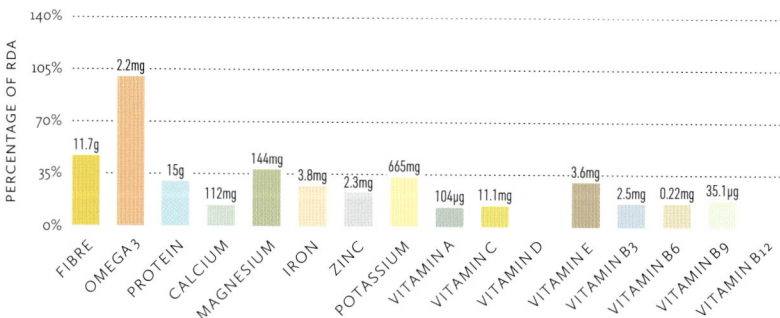

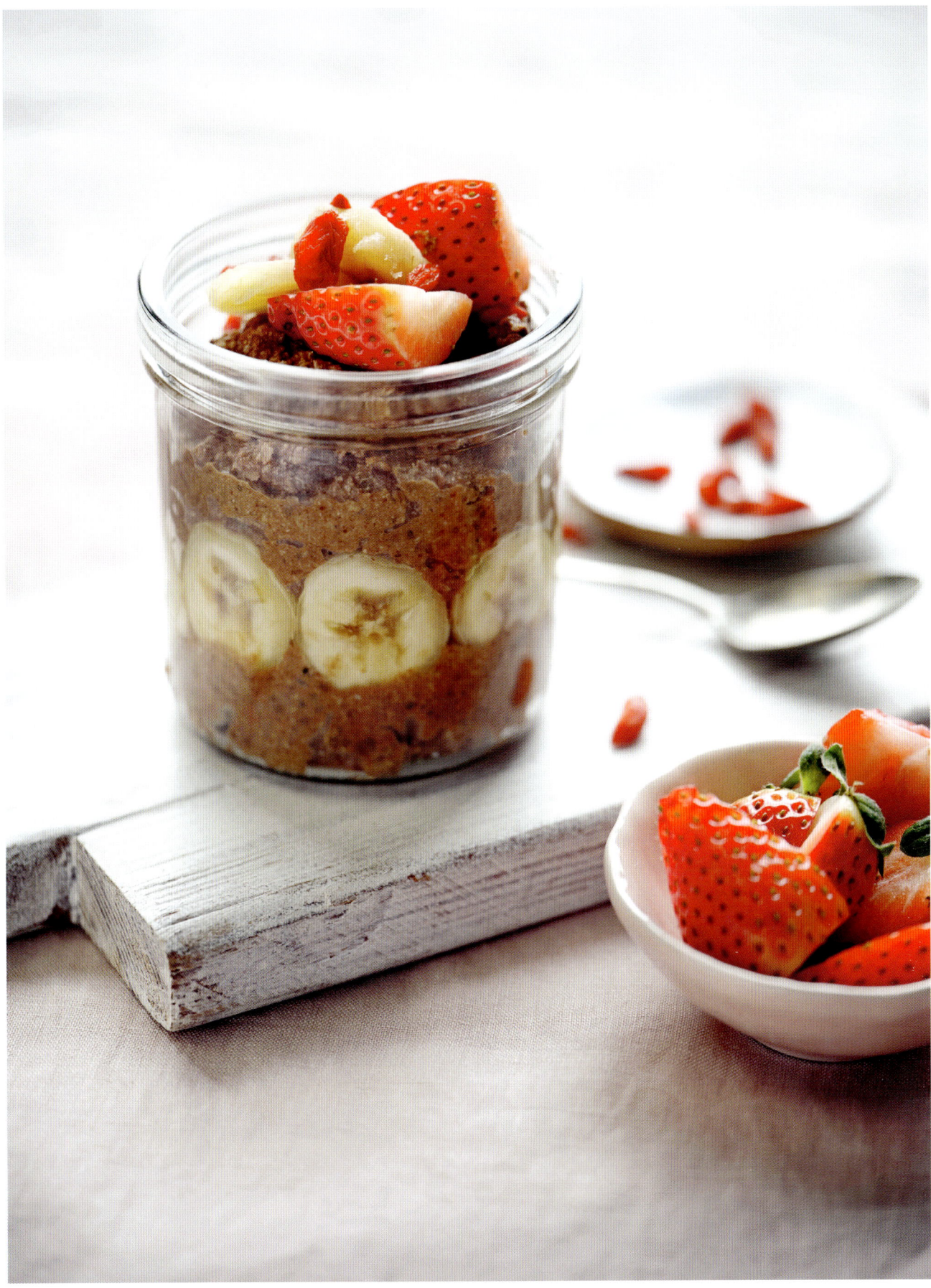

Pear-a-misu

with overnight oats parfait

OATS LAYER

4 tbsp organic porridge oats

1 tbsp organic chia seeds

1 tbsp ground flaxseeds

1 tsp Ceylon cinnamon

1 tbsp maple syrup

120ml organic soya milk

PARFAIT LAYERS

2 small firm pears

8 tbsp live probiotic yoghurt

8 tsp raw cacao powder

8 tbsp rhubarb, pear and apple compote (see p128)

TOPPING

4 tbsp pecan cinnamon granola (see p107)

any leftover pear to decorate

MAKES: 4 PORTIONS

Inspired by the classic Italian dessert, this recipe contains poached pears, live probiotic yoghurt, a fruit compote and raw cacao, with the overnight oats adding plenty of fibre-rich goodness. Try it for a tasty breakfast or a delicious, dessert-like snack.

1. Put all the oats layer ingredients in a bowl and combine well. The resulting mix should be loose and not too dry. The chia seeds will absorb moisture, so use more liquid (if necessary) to avoid it being too dry.
2. Spoon the oaty mixture into four small glass jars, seal and refrigerate until ready to use.
3. Poach the pears by cutting them in half and placing them face down in some water. Simmer gently for up to 10 minutes. Remove and allow to cool, then dice into small pieces, leaving some larger slices for decoration.
4. Add the diced pear to the glass jars and mix through, followed by one layer of natural yoghurt.
5. Sprinkle raw cacao powder on top (using a small sieve), then add 1 tablespoon of compote.
6. Repeat this process with the yoghurt, cocoa powder and compote for a second layer, finishing with a sprinkling of raw cacao and a handful of pecan cinnamon granola.

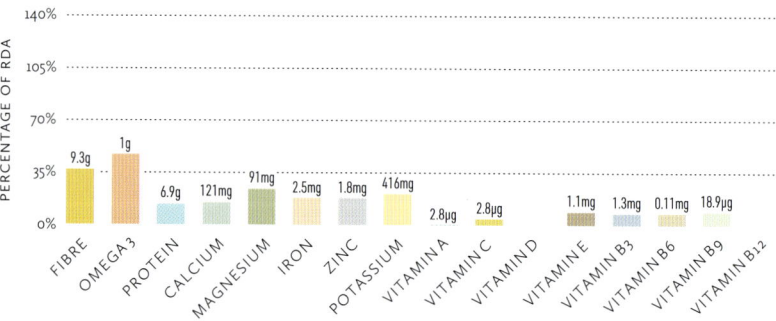

PER 160G PORTION

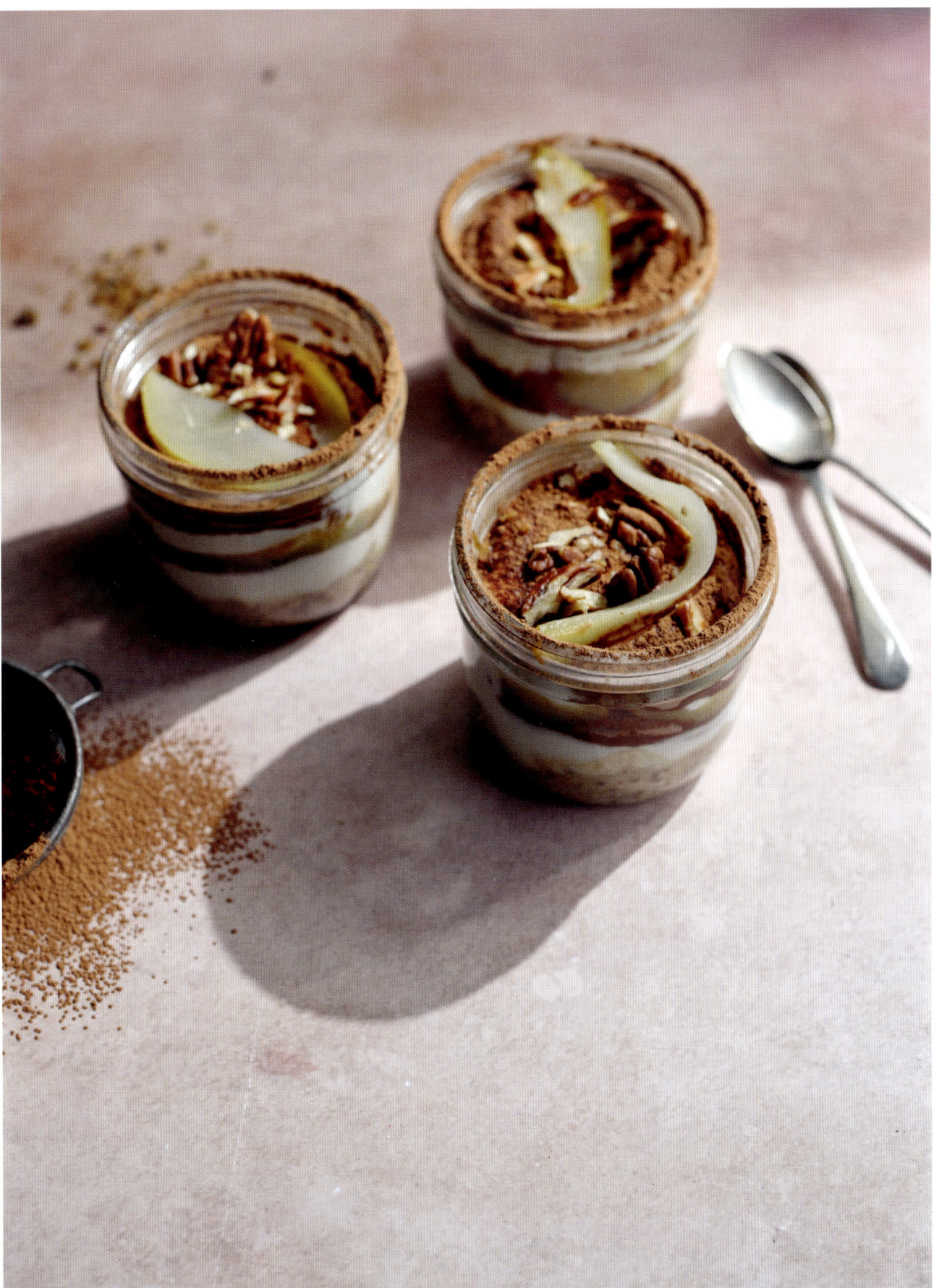

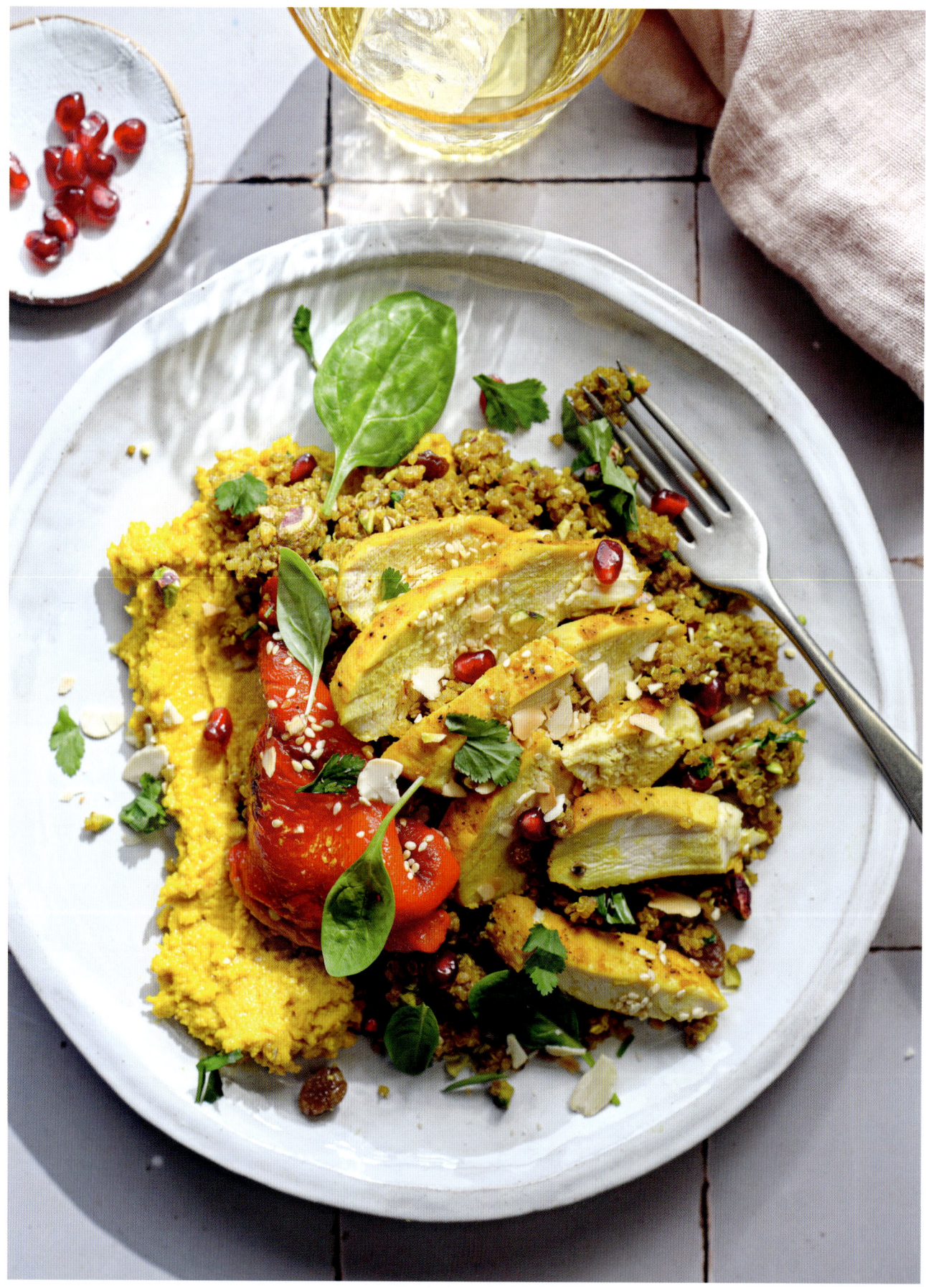

Turmeric Roasted Chicken Breast

with roasted carrot and yellow pepper hummus, whole roasted red pepper and Moroccan quinoa

1 tsp good-quality turmeric powder

3 tbsp olive oil

sea salt and black pepper, to taste

2 free-range chicken breasts, skinless

1 red bell pepper

1 tbsp walnut oil

bunch of green asparagus, stalks removed

100g Moroccan quinoa (see p226)

1 heaped tbsp roasted carrot and yellow pepper hummus (see p117)

fresh coriander, finely chopped

handful of toasted pistachios

SERVES: 2

A great special-occasion meal that is easy to prepare, this is packed with delicious flavours, quality protein and antioxidant-rich ingredients.

1. Preheat the oven to 180°C.
2. Mix the turmeric, 1 tbsp olive oil, salt and black pepper in a bowl to make a marinade.
3. Toss the chicken breasts into the marinade and set aside (the longer, the better).
4. Roast the red pepper in the oven. When brown and soft, remove and place in a covered bowl for about 30 minutes. Peel off the skin and chop into four pieces.
5. Using 1 tbsp of walnut oil, sear the chicken on a hot pan for 3–4 minutes on each side, then finish in the oven until cooked through.
6. At the same time, put the asparagus spears on a baking tray, drizzle with olive oil and sprinkle with sea salt. Roast in the oven alongside the chicken for 15–20 minutes until browned.
7. Slice each chicken breast at an angle into three pieces, and serve on the Moroccan quinoa and hummus, with the asparagus to the side. Sprinkle with some chopped coriander, toasted pistachios and a drizzle of olive oil.

PER 550G PORTION

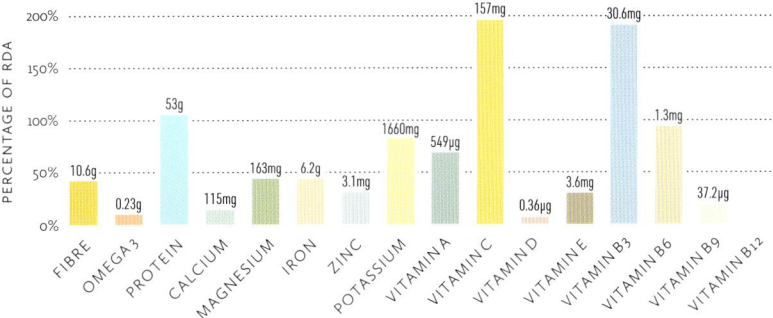

Daily Dahl

with chickpea pancakes

2 tbsp olive oil
1 onion, finely chopped
3 cloves of garlic, finely chopped
1 tbsp fresh ginger, grated
1 tbsp curry powder (madras)
1 tsp turmeric
¼–½ tsp chilli flakes
1 small sweet potato, peeled and diced
2 carrots, peeled and diced
200g dried red lentils, rinsed
1 litre veg stock
3 tomatoes, chopped
pink Himalayan salt and pepper, to taste

CHICKPEA PANCAKES

150g chickpea flour
1 egg
200ml water
1 tbsp sesame oil

TO SERVE (PER PORTION)

small handful of leaves of choice
¼ apple, grated
1 tbsp toasted flaked almonds
1 tbsp chopped fresh coriander
1 tbsp coconut yoghurt (see p253)

SERVES: 4

Packed with anti-inflammatory properties, this dahl is powerful stuff! The chickpea pancakes are a gluten-free, high-protein alternative to naan bread.

1. Heat the oil in a large saucepan, and add the onion and garlic, along with the ginger and spices.
2. Sauté for 10 minutes on a low heat till the onion softens.
3. Add the sweet potatoes and carrots, and sauté for 5 minutes.
4. Add the red lentils and veg stock. Bring to a gentle simmer for about 30 minutes, or until the lentils are cooked. Stir from time to time to make sure nothing is sticking.
5. In the last 5 minutes of cooking, add the tomatoes and stir through.
6. Season with salt and pepper.
7. While the dahl is cooking, make the pancakes. Sieve the flour into a bowl.
8. Add the egg and stir in enough water to make a smooth batter. Whisk it to remove any lumps. (Use less water if making blinis.)
9. Heat some sesame oil in a frying pan – you'll need about ½ tsp for each pancake. Add a spoonful of batter and tilt the pan to spread it out.
10. Cook it until the edges are golden, then flip it and cook the other side. (If making blinis, use a dessertspoon to measure out the batter.) Keep warm.
11. To serve, spoon a little dahl on to the centre of a pancake with some leaves of choice, then roll it up and eat it like a burrito. If you've gone for blinis, just add the dahl alongside them with the toppings listed above.

PER 300G PORTION (INCL. 1 X 50G PANCAKE)

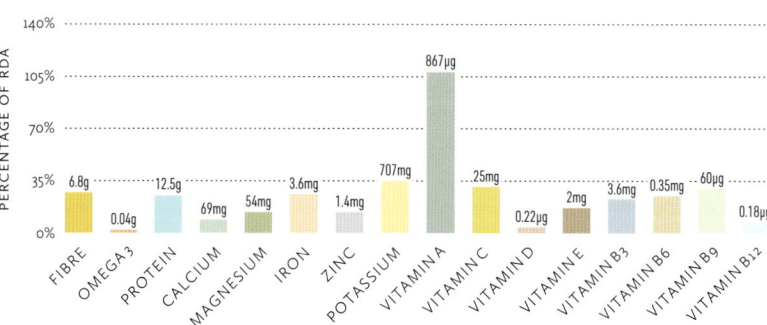

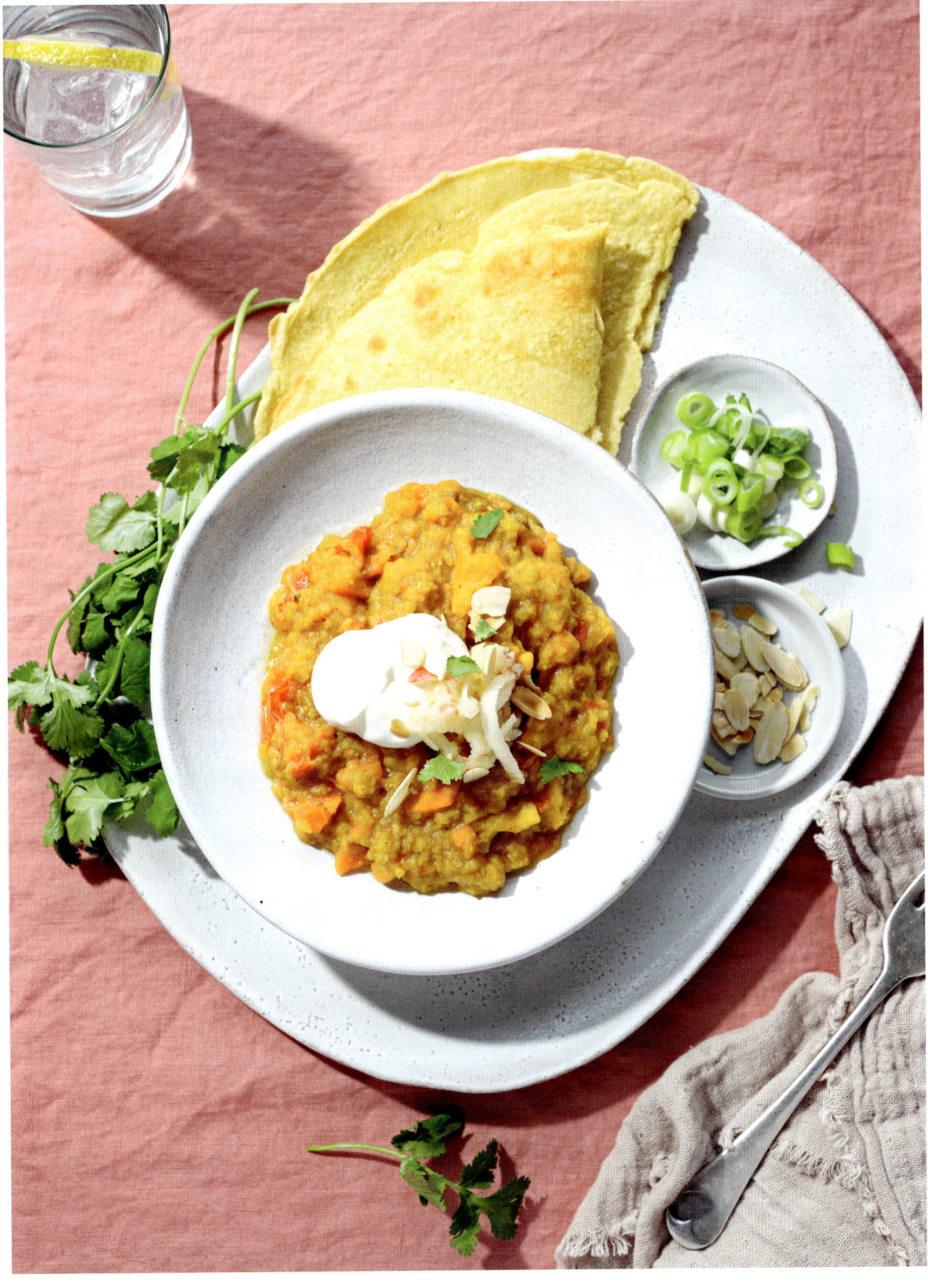

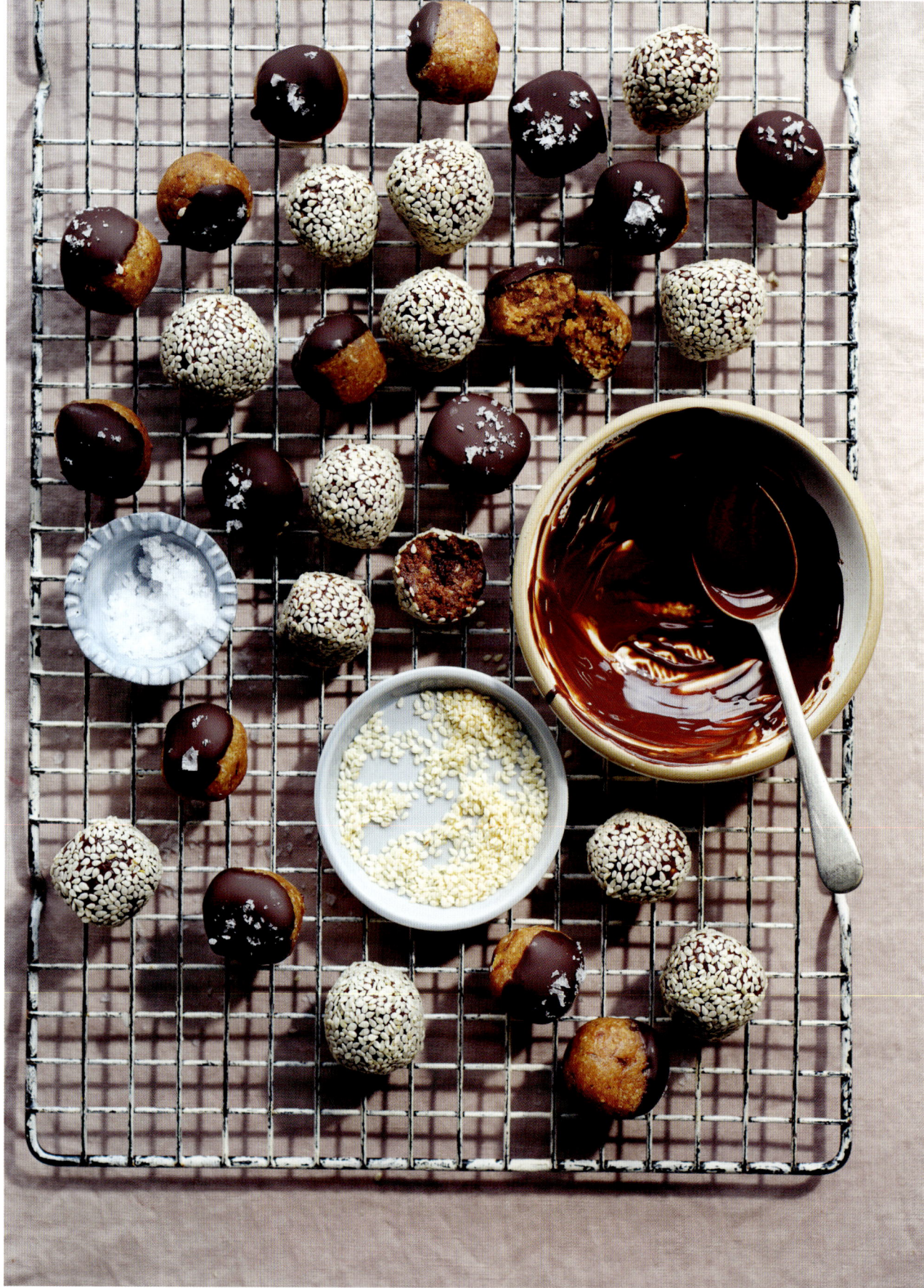

Thrive Protein Balls

50g porridge oats

1 heaped tbsp ground flaxseeds

1 scoop vanilla plant protein powder

3 soft Medjool dates, pitted and chopped small

2 tbsp water

1 tbsp olive oil

4 heaped tbsp almond butter (see p170)

2 tbsp maple syrup

pinch of sea salt (optional)

1 tbsp cacao nibs

TOPPINGS

25g 85% dark chocolate

sprinkling of desiccated coconut

sprinkling of flaked sea salt

MAKES: ABOUT 25 BALLS

Protein- and fibre-rich, with plenty of good fats and antioxidants, these delicious balls are also filling, satisfying any sweet cravings. Store them in an airtight container in the fridge.

1. Blitz the porridge oats in a food processor until you have a smooth flour.
2. Add in the ground flaxseeds and protein powder, and blend again.
3. Add the dates to the food processor, along with the water, olive oil, almond butter and maple syrup, and blitz until all is well combined. Taste and add a little salt if needed.
4. Put the mixture in a bowl, add in the cacao nibs and mix well.
5. Empty the contents of the bowl on to a silicone mat. Fold the edges over the mix one by one and press down until you form a square or rectangle with the mix.
6. Using a pastry cutter, cut the mix into evenly spaced columns lengthways, then across, until you end up with even-sized squares.
7. Lift one square at a time, shape it with your fingers into a ball, then roll it gently in the palm of your hands. The mix will get oily, which is ideal for rolling. Chill in an airtight container in the fridge for 2 hours before decorating.
8. To decorate, melt the dark chocolate in a bain-marie, then dip the protein balls into the chocolate and leave them on a cooling rack.
9. While the chocolate is still wet, sprinkle the balls with desiccated coconut and flaked sea salt (do this quickly and in batches).

PER 18.5G PORTION

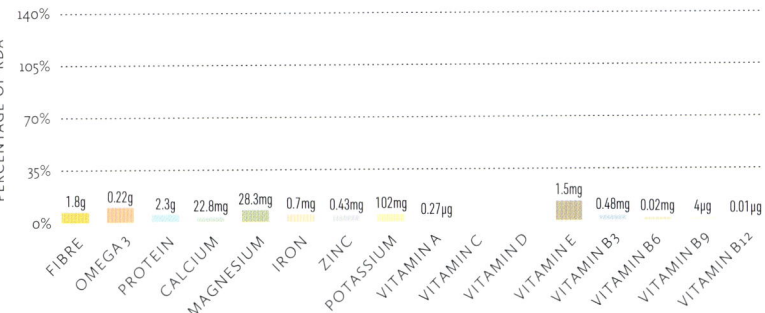

7. Probiotics

Probiotic-rich foods are fermented foods – sauerkraut, miso, kombucha and yoghurt, to give a few examples. They contain strains of friendly bacteria that we want in abundance in our gut. Probiotics help to support our immune system and have been shown to have a positive effect on mood, reducing symptoms of anxiety and depression. They can also help to promote healthy vaginal bacteria, which can reduce vaginal dryness and discomfort.

Some of these recipes are great fun to make: stocking up on apple cider vinegar is so simple and satisfying, and the four-seed rye sourdough is my favourite bread of all time.

Note: Live probiotic strains cannot be analysed using the available software. The nutrient density of the ingredients contained in these section's recipes may also be further enhanced as a result of the fermentation process. The nutrient profile, where provided, is as a guide only.

Sauerkraut with Fennel and Apple

1.4kg green cabbage, trimmed of the outer leaves (set these aside for sealing)

1 fennel bulb, stalks and fronds removed

1 white onion, peeled

2 apples, cored

1 tbsp pink Himalayan salt

1 tsp fennel seeds

MAKES: 15+ PORTIONS

Your gut health is central to your overall well-being. Fermented foods like sauerkraut support digestive health by contributing probiotic-rich nutrients. You can serve this as part of a meze plate or use it for a sauerkraut salad – my favourite recipe mixes a portion of sauerkraut with orange segments, the juice of another orange and a tasty balsamic dressing.

1. First, sterilise a large (2-litre) jar. You can do this using either of the following methods:
Method 1: Preheat the oven to 180°C. Remove the rubber ring from the jar's lid and soak it in hot water for about 10 minutes, before drying thoroughly. Fill the jar with boiling water, empty it and place it in the oven for 10 minutes to dry. Remove carefully and put to one side to cool.
Method 2: Put the jar through the dishwasher on a normal cycle.
As a final protective step for either method, splash a little white wine vinegar into the jar, swirl it around and discard. Use a paper kitchen towel to wipe out the inside, and the jar is now ready to use.
2. Thinly slice the cabbage, ideally in a food processor for speed and size consistency. If slicing by hand, cut the cabbage into manageable quarters first, then slice as finely as you can using a sharp knife.
3. Repeat with the fennel, onion and apples, until everything is a similar size.
4. Transfer to a large mixing bowl and add the salt and fennel seeds.
5. Using your hands, mix and massage the vegetables intensely for about 10 minutes, until tender and juicy. They should release a lot of juice. Don't rush this part – it's an important step! Set the vegetable juice aside for later.
6. When sufficient juice has been released, transfer the mix to your sterilised jar. Pack it down with your hand and fill the jar to almost the top – about ¾ full, which allows space for gases to release. >

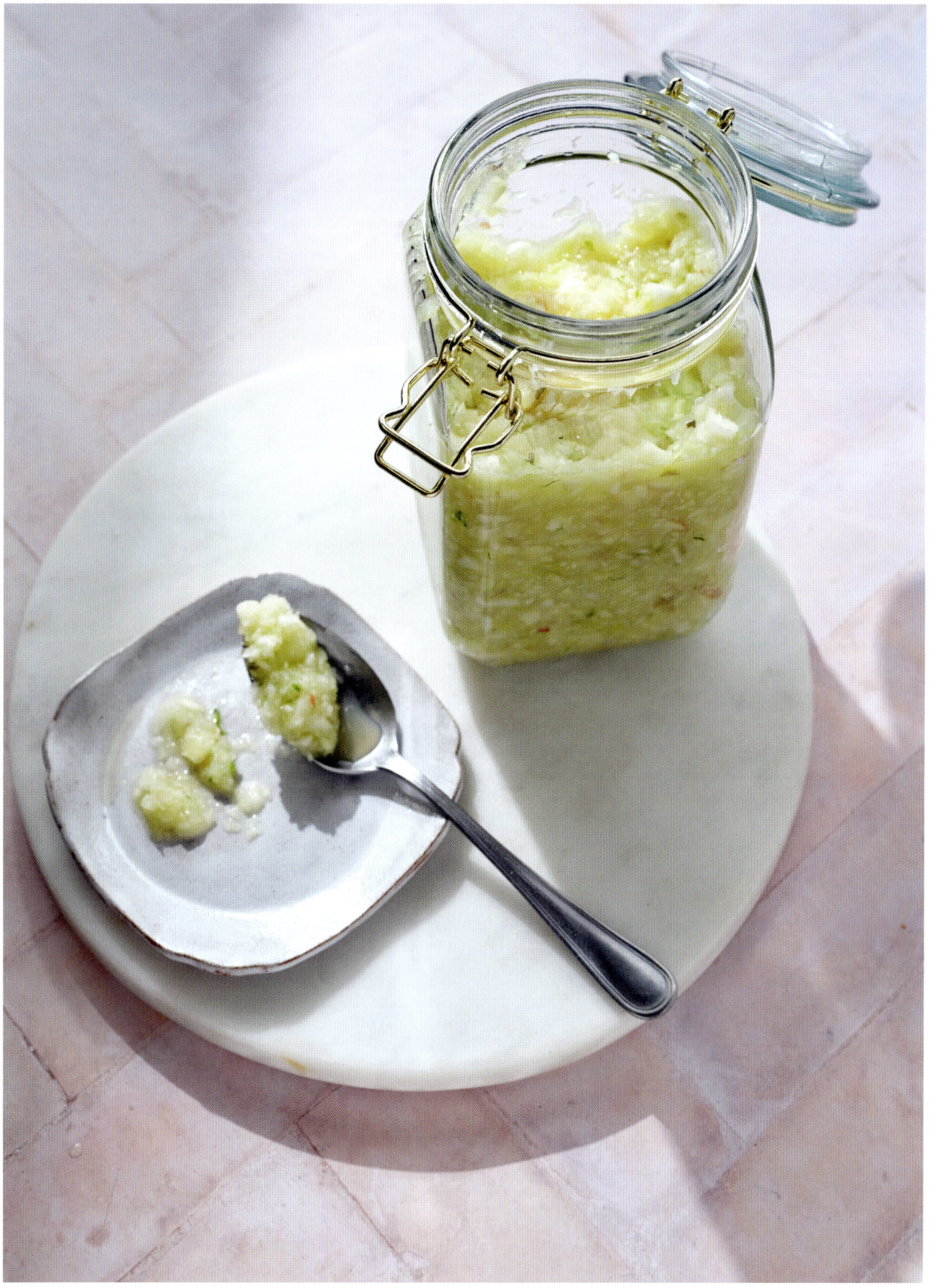

7. Pour the vegetable juice from step 5 in on top so that the cabbage is immersed. Top with the large outer leaves you set aside earlier – this helps to keep the veg mix immersed under the liquid. You can even place a weight on top.
8. Seal the jar and store at room temperature, away from direct sunlight, for 2–4 weeks.
9. During this time, especially in the beginning, you will need to open the lid to allow the gases to escape. Do this twice a day for the first week, then once a day. This process is called burping.
10. When ready, the sauerkraut should be soft (not mushy) and have a fresh, spicy, acidic flavour. You can now remove the cabbage leaves and store the sauerkraut in the fridge – it will keep for a few months with enough liquid to keep it moist.

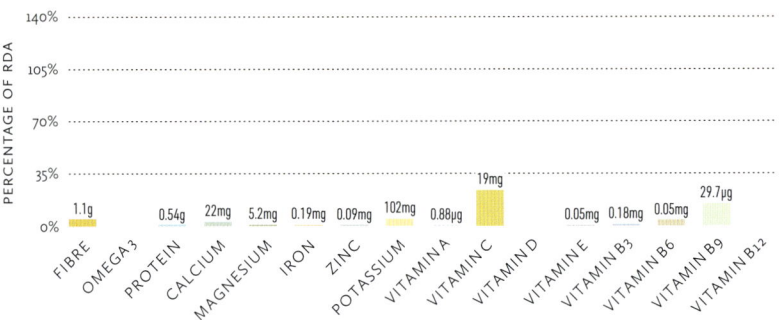

Coconut Yoghurt

400ml full-fat coconut milk

¾ tbsp agar flakes

2 capsules of probiotics

fruit or fruit purée of choice (optional)

MAKES: 250ML

This is a good non-dairy alternative to yoghurt. It has no additives, and it doesn't even require a yoghurt maker!

1. Pour the coconut milk into a saucepan and add ¾ of a tablespoon of agar flakes.
2. Stir gently on a constant heat until dissolved – about 10 minutes. Do not rush this important step.
3. Once the flakes are dissolved, put the mixture in a blender and blend on high.
4. Set aside and leave to cool for several hours.
5. Open the probiotic capsules and empty them into the mixture. Use a whisk or blender to mix well.
6. When you are satisfied that all is well combined, pour into a glass or ceramic bowl.
7. Cut a circle into a sheet of greaseproof paper and place this on top of the bowl to prevent a skin forming. (Alternatively, simply place a plate on top of your bowl.)
8. The longer you leave it to ferment, the higher the concentration of beneficial bacteria. I usually place mine beside the Aga for 12–16 hours, or you can put it in a warm airing cupboard for up to 24 hours. Don't be alarmed if it looks like it has curdled or is very runny – just give it a whizz with an electric whisk.
9. Pour the mixture into a clip-top glass jar and place it in the fridge to thicken for a few hours. The longer you leave it, the thicker it will be.
10. After it has thickened, add some chopped fruit or fruit purée.
11. This will keep for up to 10 days in the fridge (plain) or 3–4 days if you include fresh fruit.

PER 100G PORTION

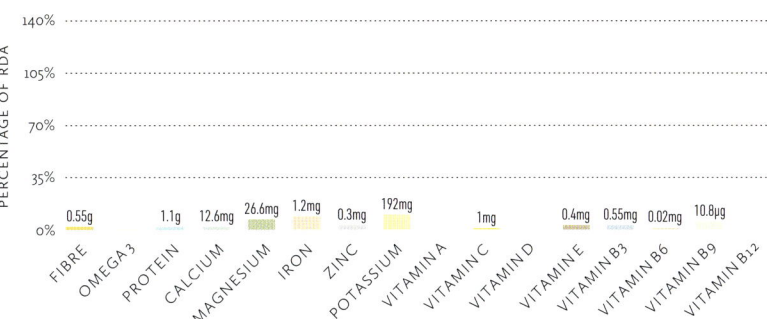

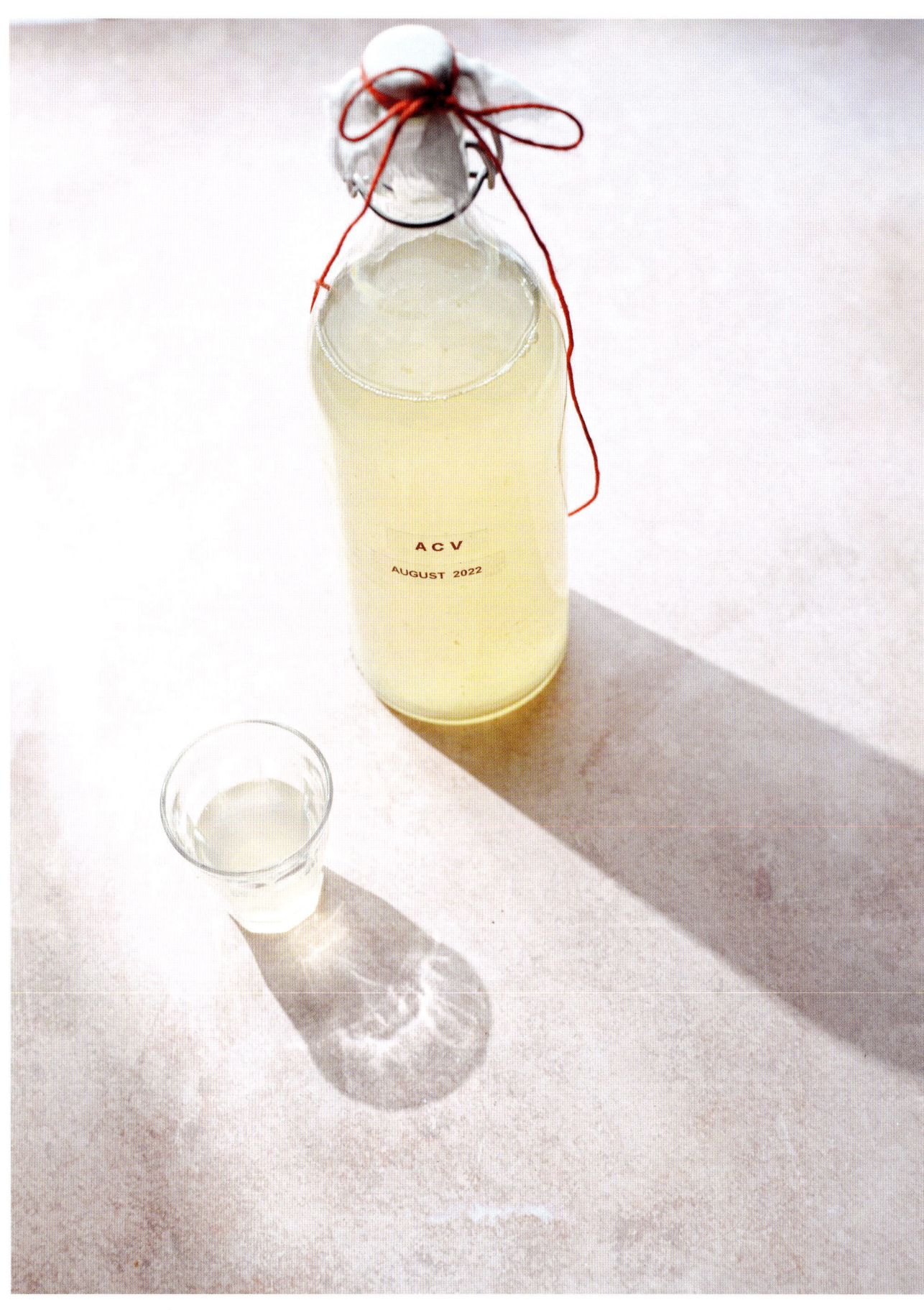

Apple Cider Vinegar

3 large apples of choice, washed and chopped into large chunks

1¼ litres room-temperature filtered water

75g raw organic cane sugar

MAKES: 1 LITRE

You'll have to be patient with this three-ingredient recipe – the fermentation process takes at least one month. But it's worth it in the end, producing a vinegar that's great to use in salad dressings, juice cocktails and invigorating morning drinks.

1. Sterilise a wide-mouthed 2-litre glass jar (see p250).
2. Put the apples in the jar. They should fill at least half the jar.
3. Pour in the water until the jar is around ¾ full, leaving about 5cm at the top.
4. Stir in the raw cane sugar until fully dissolved.
5. Cover the top of the jar with cheesecloth (or a thin clean dishcloth or a coffee filter), and secure with an elastic band.
6. Leave on the counter for about a week, stirring gently once a day. Bubbles will begin to form as the sugar ferments into alcohol. (You will also smell this.)
7. After about a week, the apples will sink to the bottom of the jar. This means it's time to strain them off.
8. Once you have strained the apples, pour the liquid into a fresh glass jar, cover with a fresh piece of cheesecloth and secure with a rubber band.
9. Leave it on the counter for an additional 3–4 weeks to allow the alcohol to transform into acetic acid. A new mother culture may also form on top, just like when you are making kombucha. (This is not a problem.)
10. After a month, taste your vinegar to see if it has the right level of acidity for you. If it still isn't strong enough, leave it for another week. If you accidentally leave it too long and it is too acidic, you can simply dilute it with some filtered water.

Tip: Pour hot water over a tablespoon of this vinegar, the juice of half a lemon and a teaspoon of local honey to make a morning drink that will kick-start your digestion.

Four-Seed Rye Sourdough Bread

100g rye flakes

140g buckwheat

110g flaxseeds

110g sunflower seeds

100g hemp seeds

2 tbsp blackstrap molasses

400g activated sourdough starter (see p69)

800ml filtered water

dried fruit (such as apricots, raisins, figs), chopped (optional)

270g organic strong white flour

270g organic rye flour (wholegrain rye or wholegrain sprouted)

15g pink Himalayan salt

MAKES: 2 LOAVES

Tasty and nutritious, this healthy, filling bread is packed with prebiotic fibre to feed your gut bacteria and benefit your gut microbiome. It's great for sandwiches, or toasted with some almond butter (see p170) and a sliced banana.

1. In a large bowl, mix together the rye flakes, buckwheat, flaxseeds, sunflower and hemp seeds, molasses, sourdough starter, water and dried fruit, if using. Allow this to soak for 8–10 hours (or overnight), stirring well halfway through.
2. Add the strong white flour, rye flour and Himalayan salt to the mix, and leave (covered) for a further 1½–2 hours. The mix will grow and firm up.
3. Preheat the oven to 180°C.
4. Spoon the mixture into two loaf tins lined with siliconised liners to avoid the dough sticking. (You can sprinkle on some toppings at this point if you'd like – I like to use dukkah, oat flakes or sesame seeds.)
5. Bake for 40–45 minutes. To see if it is cooked, insert a knife into the centre; if it comes out clean, it is ready.
6. Leave to cool completely before slicing.
7. This can be cut in half and wrapped in greaseproof paper. It also freezes well.

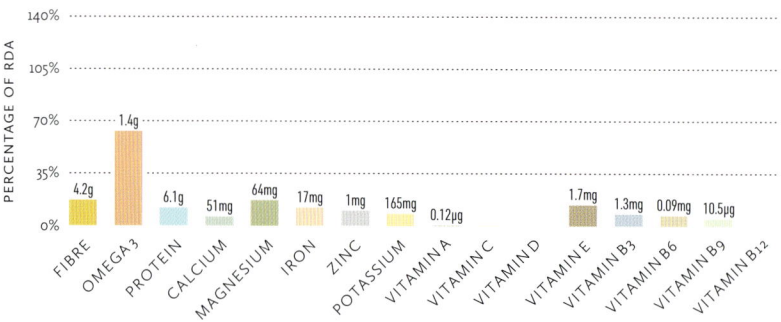

PER 75G PORTION

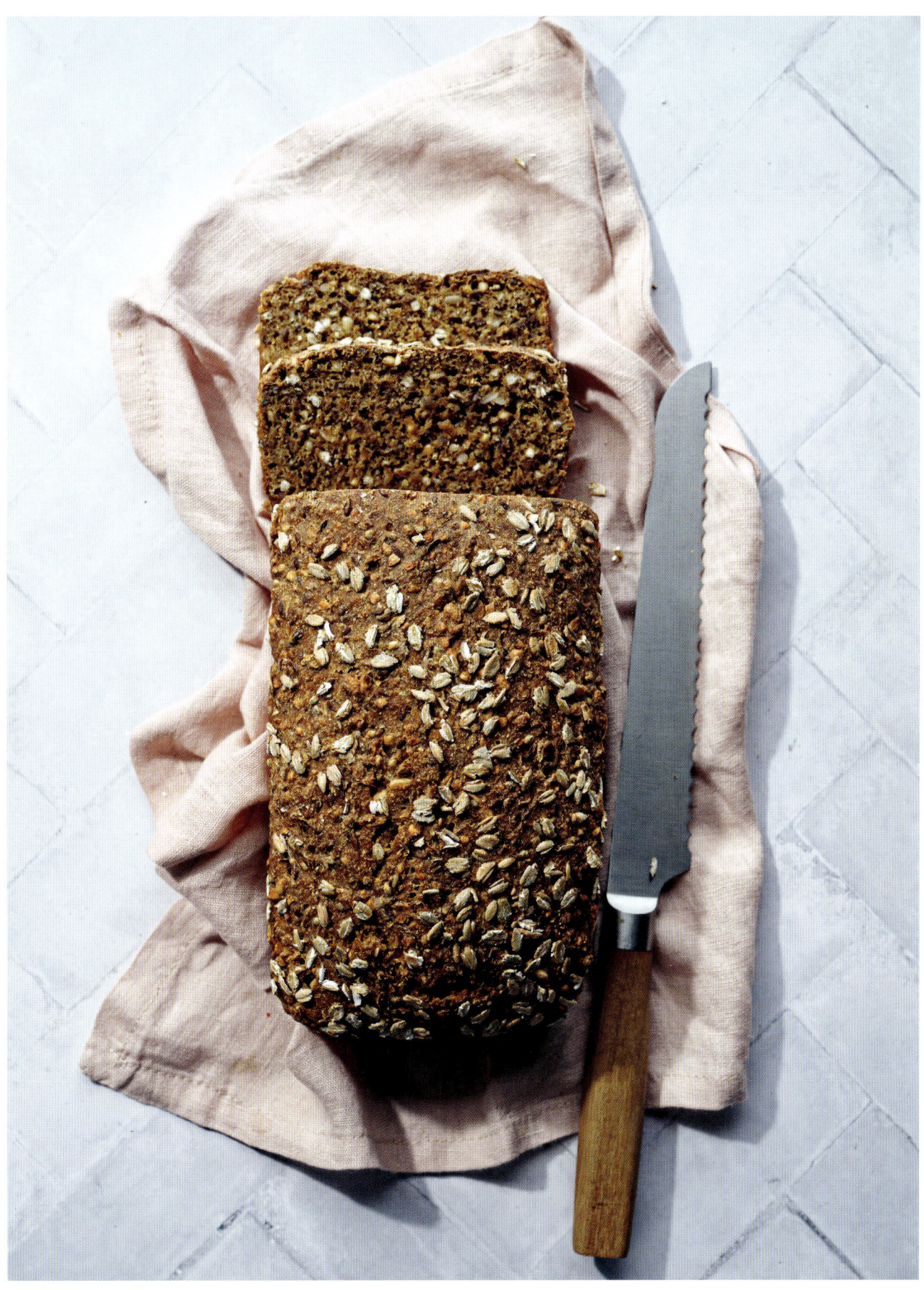

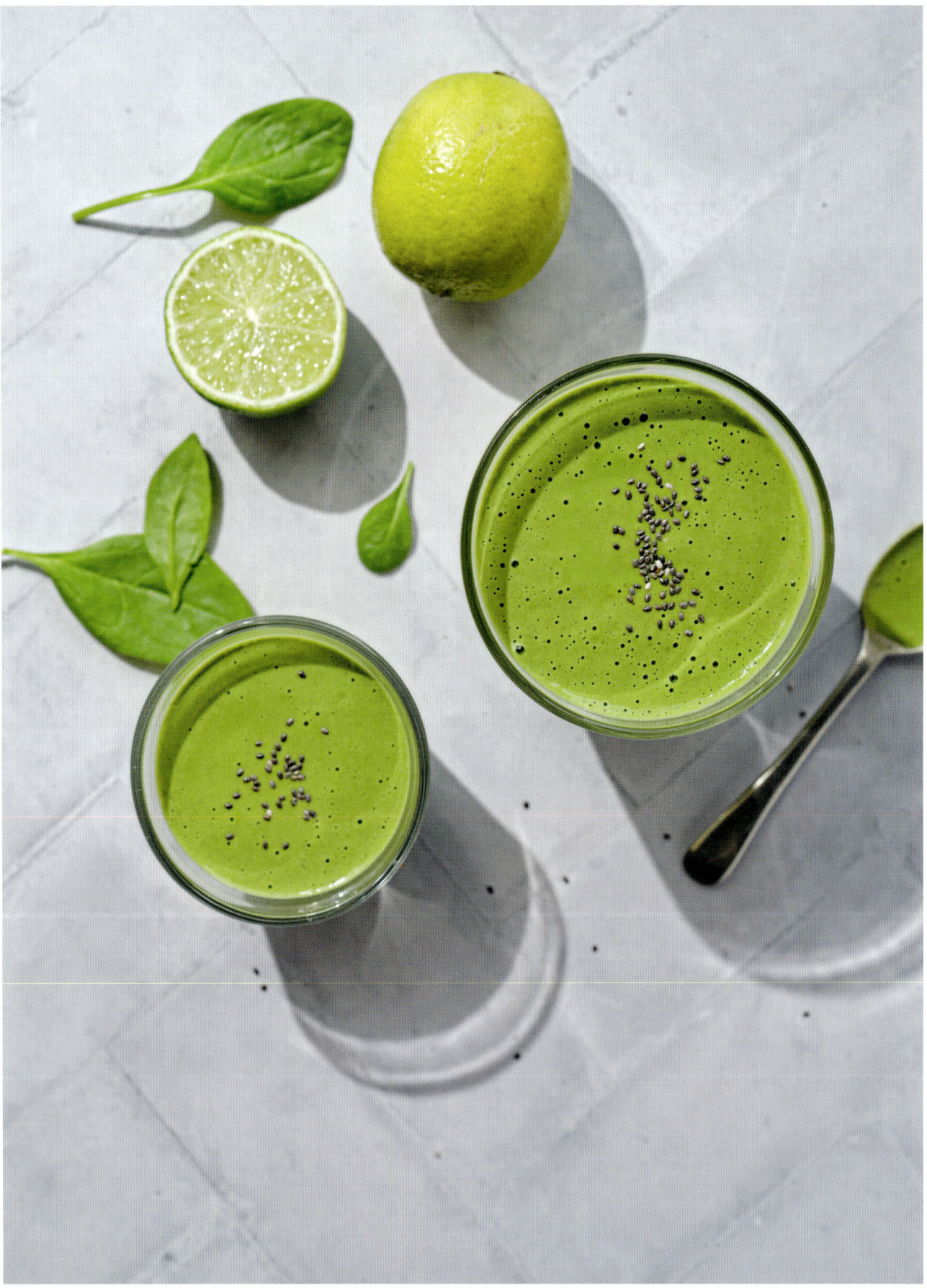

Probiotic Lime Green Smoothie

½ frozen or fresh banana

handful of organic spinach leaves

1½ tbsp pumpkin seeds

1 Medjool date, pitted

1 scoop vanilla pea protein

zest and juice of 2 limes

100ml water, kefir or kombucha, or the contents of 1 probiotic capsule

100ml organic soya milk, or 200ml if using the probiotic capsule

MAKES: 2 GLASSES

All the benefits of a smoothie – with that extra probiotic hit for your gut health. This is great in the morning with some sweet potato and apple breakfast cookies (see p110) or as a mid-afternoon snack.

1. Place all the ingredients in a blender and blitz on high until smooth. Enjoy it straight away.

Tip: Frozen bananas add chilled creaminess to your smoothies. If you are going to freeze a banana, peel it before placing it in a freezer bag. If you don't have any frozen bananas, just proceed with a room-temperature banana.

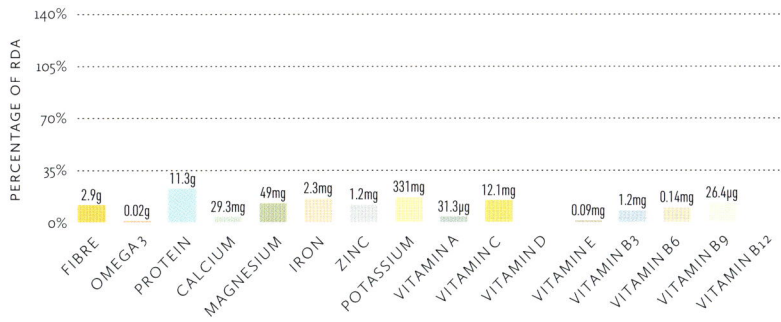

Frozen Yoghurt Bark

500ml live probiotic yoghurt (Greek-style, if possible)

1 tbsp vanilla bean paste or essence

1 tbsp maple syrup

2 capsules of everyday probiotics

2 tbsp pecan cinnamon granola (see p107)

4 ripe strawberries, finely sliced

10 raspberries, whole

10 blueberries, whole

15g dark chocolate (85% cocoa solids), chopped up small

MAKES: 10+ PORTIONS

Try this for a refreshing warm-weather treat! I have used a combination of my favourite berries, dark chocolate and granola, but you can choose whatever toppings you like. The addition of probiotics increases the amount of beneficial bacteria.

1. Pour the yoghurt into a mixing bowl and add the vanilla bean paste (or essence) and the maple syrup. Mix well.
2. Add the contents of the probiotic capsules and stir well.
3. Line a medium-sized (22cm) baking tray with parchment paper.
4. Pour the yoghurt mix into the lined tray and sprinkle the granola on top.
5. Start adding your selection of berries and chocolate on top.
6. Wrap in cling film and place in the freezer for at least 5 hours or overnight.
7. Remove from the freezer, cut into chunks and enjoy straight away.

PER 75G PORTION

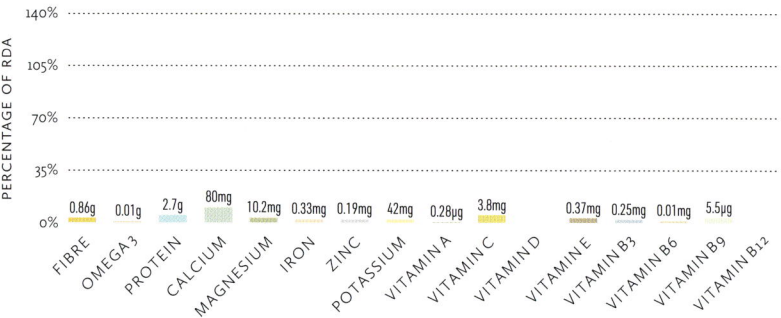

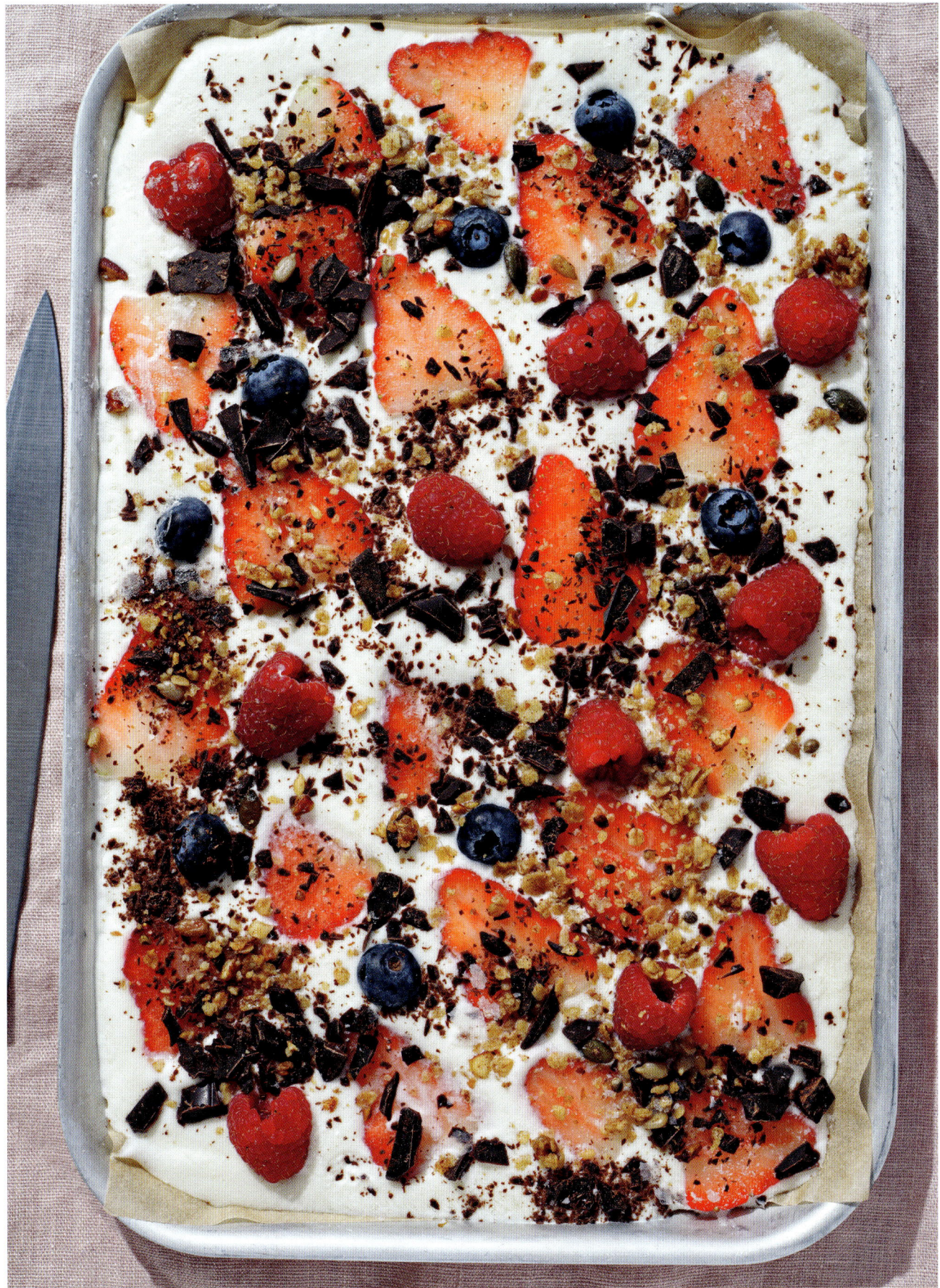

8. Brassicas

Brassicas are a family of vegetables that includes broccoli, cauliflower, kale and cabbage. They contain more phytochemicals with researched anti-cancer benefits than any other vegetable family. They're a good source of fibre and B vitamins and minerals, all of which support women's hormone balancing, along with a host of other benefits.

Brassicas are also budget-friendly, without compromising on taste. The cauliflower pea mash is a delicious low-carb and low-starch substitute for potatoes, while cauliflower rice is a quick, simple and healthy option for the middle of a busy week.

Steamed Cauliflower Rice

1 medium-sized cauliflower, broken into florets

pink Himalayan salt and pepper, to taste

fresh parsley, chopped

SERVES: 4

Home-made cauliflower rice tastes far better than the frozen shop-bought variety, and it can be flavoured in many ways. This is the basic recipe, which you can use to accompany any of the curries in this book, as part of a stir-fry or as filling for an omelette.

1. Put the cauliflower florets in a food processor, and blitz until they are broken down into small crumbs resembling rice.
2. Add the cauliflower crumbs to a colander, put a lid over the top and place over a simmering pot of boiling water.
3. Allow to steam for 10–12 minutes. When soft, remove and set aside, keeping it warm if needed.
4. Season with salt, pepper and some fresh parsley (or other herbs of choice) before serving.
5. This can also be prepped in advance and reheated when needed.

PER 60G PORTION

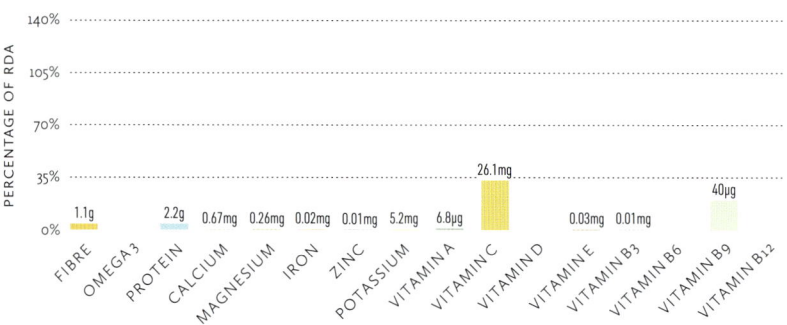

Roasted Cauliflower, Chickpea and Sweet Potato Salad

This is a tasty, make-ahead salad. Packed with vitamin C and fibre, and best served at room temperature, it's the perfect addition to a summer party or barbecue.

1 large sweet potato, peeled and diced

1 small cauliflower, chopped into bite-sized pieces (keep some of the smaller outer leaves for decoration)

2 yellow bell peppers, diced to a similar size as the rest of the veg

400g tinned chickpeas, rinsed and drained

2 tbsp extra virgin olive oil

pink Himalayan salt, to taste

2 cloves of garlic

1 tbsp toasted flaked almonds

large handful of fresh coriander, chopped

4 spring onions, finely sliced

seeds of ¼ pomegranate

DRESSING

3 tbsp extra virgin olive oil

zest and juice of 1 lemon

1 clove of garlic

1 tbsp maple syrup

½ tsp smoked paprika

½ tsp cumin

pink Himalayan salt, to taste

SERVES: 4+ (AS A SIDE)

1. Preheat the oven to 180°C.
2. Put the sweet potato, cauliflower pieces, yellow peppers and chickpeas in a large mixing bowl with the olive oil and salt. Mix well.
3. Grate the garlic over the mix and toss to combine again.
4. Move the mix to a roasting tray and place in the oven for 30 minutes, or until golden and slightly charred.
5. Add the small outer cauliflower leaves to the tray for the last 15 minutes of cooking time.
6. Meanwhile, make the dressing by putting all the ingredients in a jar and mixing well. Alternatively, place in a blender and blitz for a few seconds.
7. Check the veg: if the chickpeas are starting to crisp and the veg are soft and nicely browned, they are ready.
8. Remove from the oven and transfer to a large salad bowl. Add the dressing while the veg are still warm to absorb the flavours. Retain a little dressing for the end.
9. Top the salad with the almonds, coriander, spring onions and pomegranate seeds and drizzle over the last of the dressing. Decorate with the roasted cauliflower leaves.

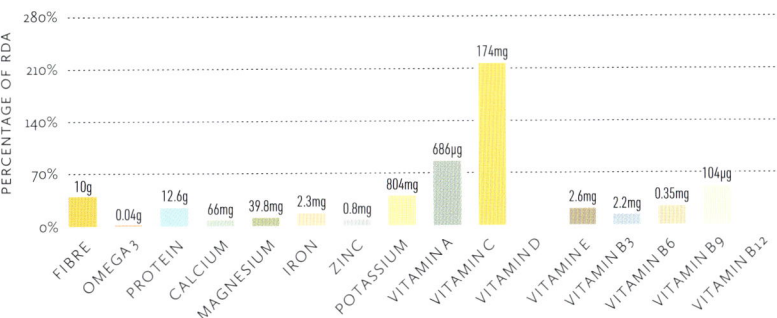

Cauliflower Pea Mash

with pan-fried leeks

1 medium-sized cauliflower, broken into florets

100g frozen peas

2–3 tbsp olive oil

1 large leek, finely sliced

1 clove of garlic, minced

pink Himalayan salt and pepper, to taste

MAKES: 4 PORTIONS

A very tasty alternative to mashed potatoes, this can be prepped in advance and reheated when needed. It is delicious served with pan-fried fish, roast chicken or a simple fried egg.

1. Put the cauliflower florets in a colander over a pot of simmering water and allow to steam until nearly tender.
2. Add the peas and cook for 2–3 minutes.
3. Heat the olive oil in a pan, and gently fry the leeks until soft.
4. Drain the cauliflower and peas into a bowl, and mash well together using a hand mixer or food processor.
5. Season with garlic, salt and pepper, plus a little extra olive oil.
6. Add most of the leeks to the cauliflower pea mash and mix well to combine.
7. Top with the remaining leeks and serve.

PER 180G PORTION

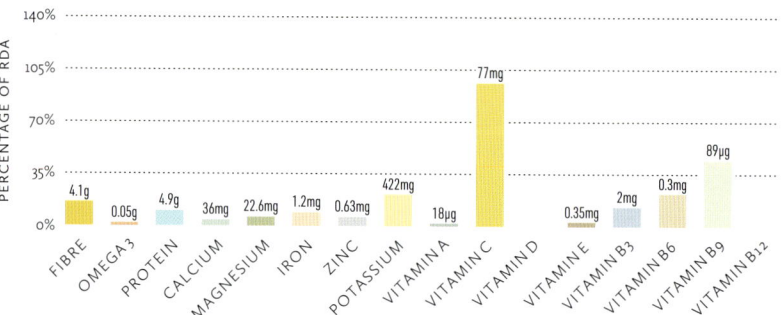

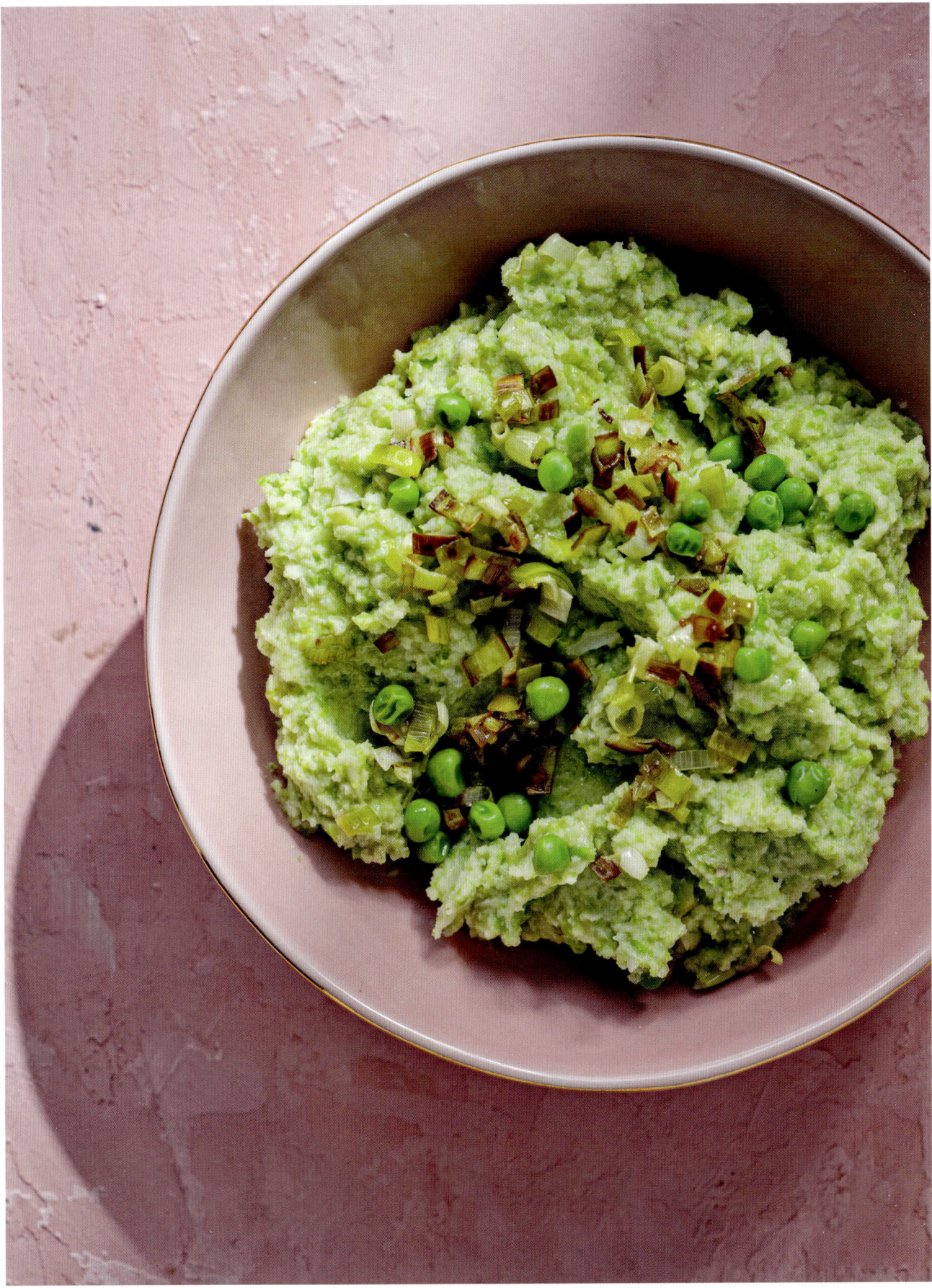

Rocket, Pine Nut and Parmesan Salad

150g rocket leaves (or a mix of rocket, radicchio, spinach etc), washed and dried

8–10 cherry vine tomatoes, halved

1 medium red onion, finely sliced

2–3 tbsp balsamic dressing (see p144)

25g pine nuts, toasted

25g Parmesan cheese, shaved

SERVES: 4

Great for the whole family, this is the ideal recipe to throw together when you are short of time and want to add a delicious side salad to a meal.

1. Put the leaves in a large salad bowl.
2. Add the cherry tomatoes and red onions.
3. Drizzle over the dressing, then toss the salad.
4. Sprinkle the pine nuts on top, followed by the shaved Parmesan (and another tablespoon of dressing, if needed).

PER 133G PORTION

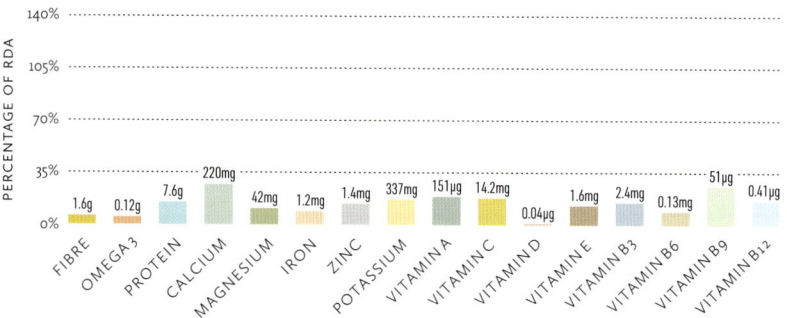

268 NOURISH FOR MENOPAUSE

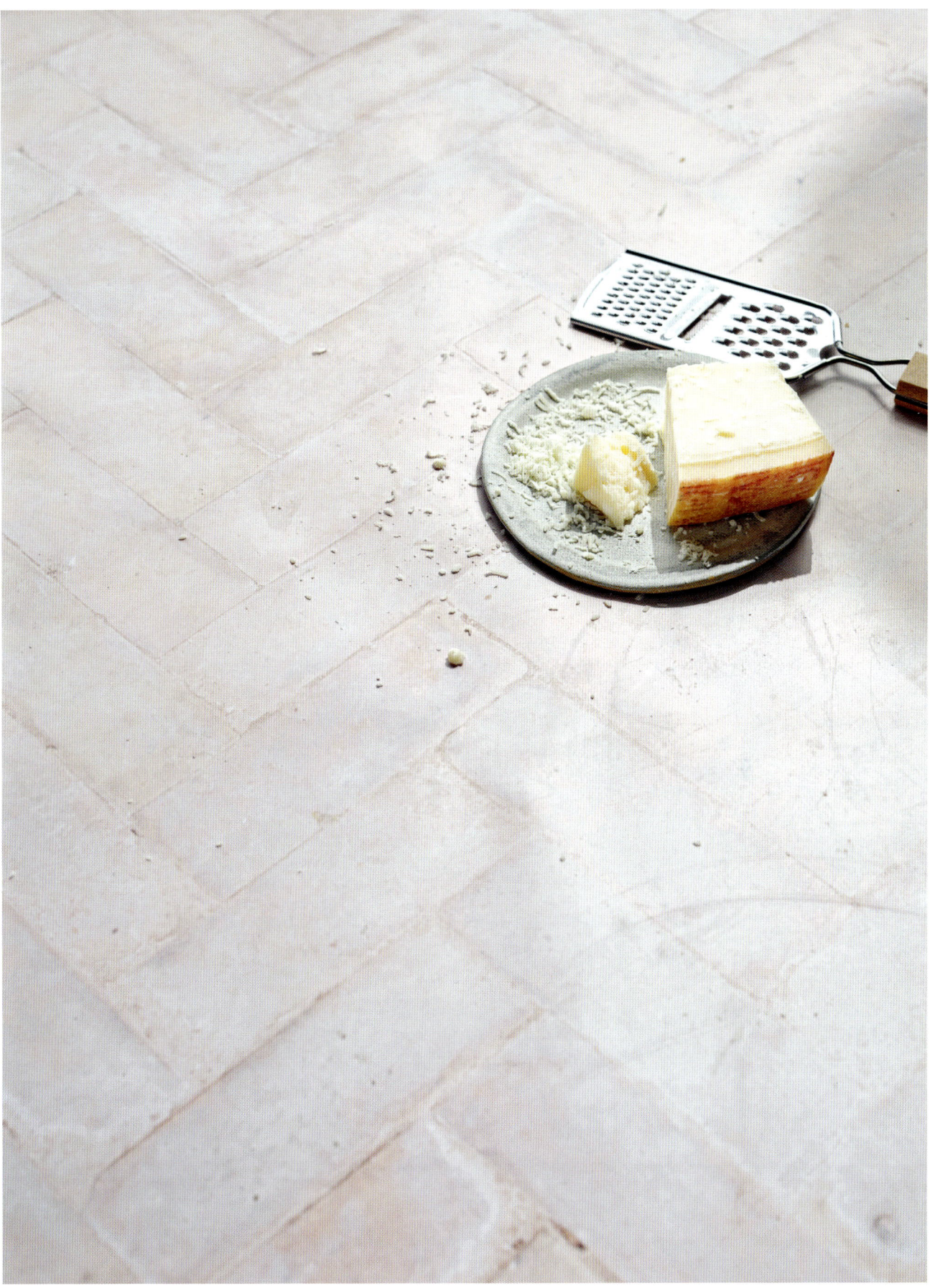

Balsamic Roasted Brussels Sprouts

with garlic, thyme and olive oil

450g Brussels sprouts, washed and dried, stalks removed

3 tbsp olive oil

1 clove of garlic, minced

leaves of 3 sprigs of fresh thyme

1 tsp pink Himalayan salt

1 tbsp balsamic glaze

SERVES: 4

Squashed and roasted with fresh thyme, garlic and olive oil, these caramelised Brussels sprouts are so tasty. Serve them as a side dish with grilled fish or add them to a salad.

1. Preheat the oven to 200°C.
2. Put the Brussels sprouts in a colander over a pot of boiling water with a lid on, and steam for 8–10 minutes.
3. Add the sprouts to a mixing bowl with olive oil, garlic and fresh thyme leaves, and season with salt.
4. Spread the sprouts and the marinade out on a lined baking tray.
5. Using a potato masher, press down on the sprouts to flatten them.
6. Put them in the oven for 20 minutes, then reduce the heat to 180°C and drizzle on a little balsamic glaze.
7. Roast for a further 10 minutes, until the sprouts are browned and caramelised.

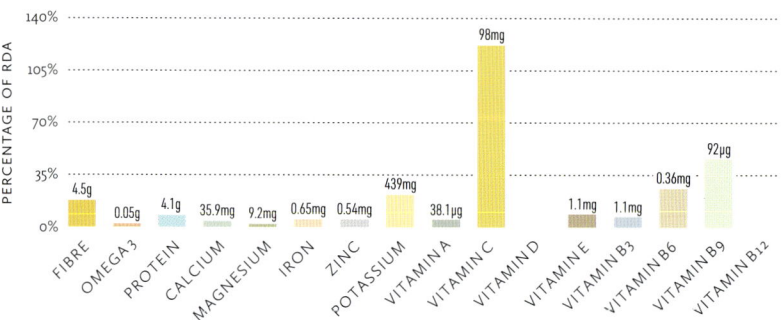

PER 125G PORTION

Flash-Cooked Tender Stem Broccoli

with garlic, chilli and olive oil

350g tender stem broccoli, trimmed and rinsed

2 tbsp olive oil

1 fat clove of garlic, minced

½ tsp dried chillies (optional)

1 tsp pink Himalayan salt

handful of toasted flaked almonds

SERVES: 4

A tasty side dish that is fast to prepare, this can be served with grilled fish or as an addition to a simple green salad with feta cheese.

1. Place the broccoli in a colander over a pot of simmering water with the lid on, and steam for 3–4 minutes (and up to 6 minutes if you don't like it al dente).
2. Put the olive oil, garlic, chillies (if using) and salt in a wok, and warm over a low heat, but don't allow the garlic to brown. Remove from the heat once it starts to sizzle.
3. When the broccoli is ready, plunge it into ice-cold water to stop the cooking process and maintain the vibrant green colour.
4. Add the broccoli to the wok and toss it in the garlic chilli oil mix until warmed through. Serve immediately, topped with the toasted flaked almonds.

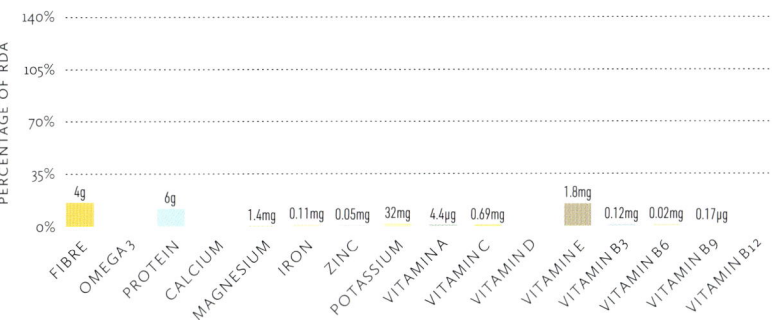

PER 110G PORTION

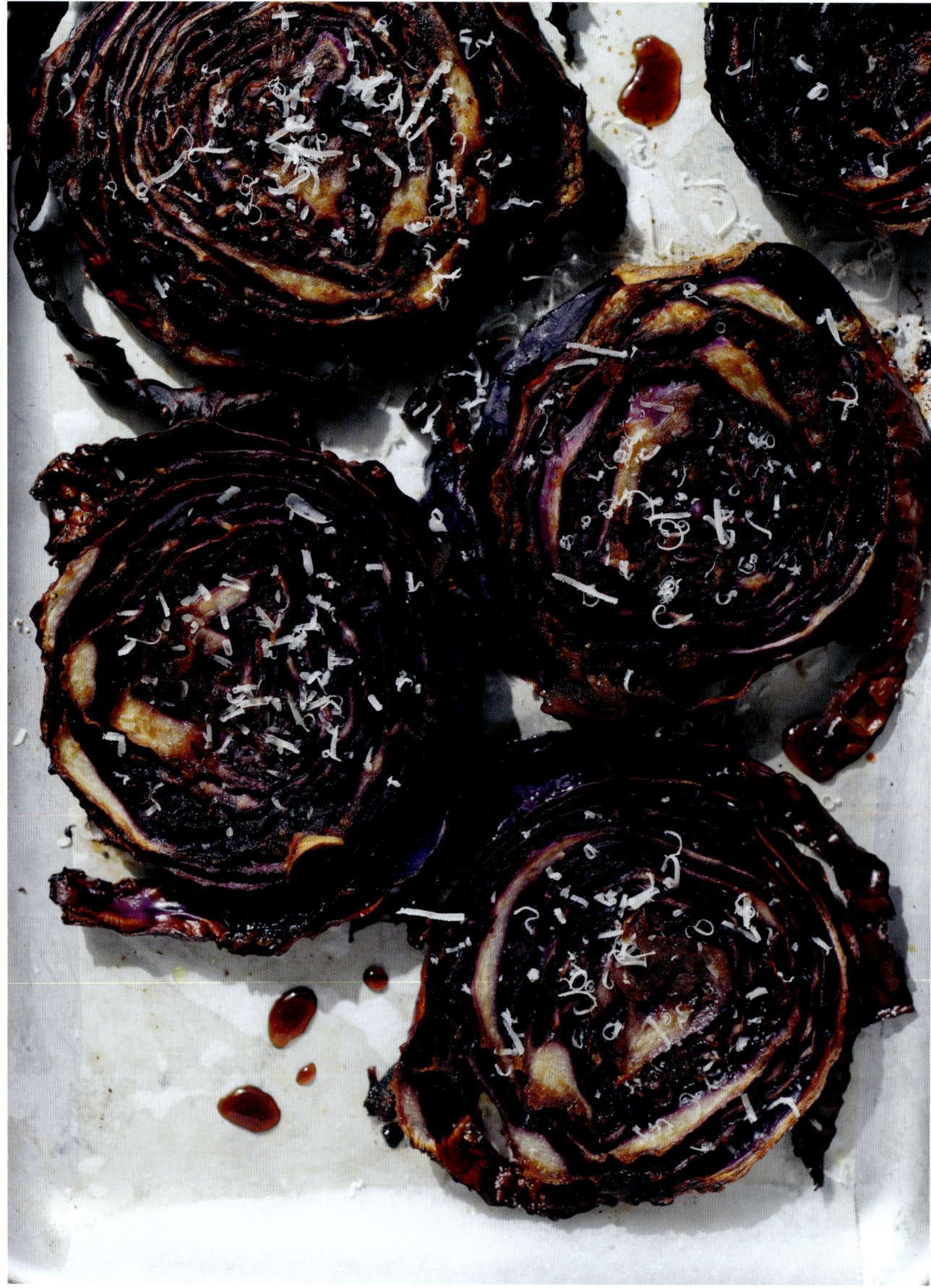

Balsamic Roasted Cabbage Steaks

1 large red cabbage, de-stemmed and with outer leaves removed

3 tbsp olive oil

1 fat clove of garlic, minced

leaves of 2 sprigs of fresh rosemary, finely chopped

1 tsp pink Himalayan salt

1 tbsp honey

2 tbsp balsamic vinegar

2 tbsp Parmesan cheese, grated

pinch of red pepper flakes (optional)

SERVES: 4

These are really delicious and could lead to a whole new appreciation of cabbage! Your digestive system will thank you for it; cabbage is a rich source of vitamin C, vitamin B6, calcium and magnesium.

1. Preheat the oven to 200°C.
2. Slice the cabbage into four thick slices with a sharp knife.
3. Place each slice on a roasting tray lined with parchment paper.
4. Mix the olive oil, garlic, rosemary and salt in a small bowl, and brush on to the cabbage slices with a pastry brush.
5. Place in the oven for 15 minutes, then reduce the temperature to 180°C for another 15 minutes.
6. Brush the cabbage slices with some honey and the balsamic vinegar and put them back in the oven for another 5–8 minutes.
7. Once ready, remove from the oven, sprinkle the Parmesan cheese on top and a pinch of red pepper flakes (if available).

PER 250G PORTION

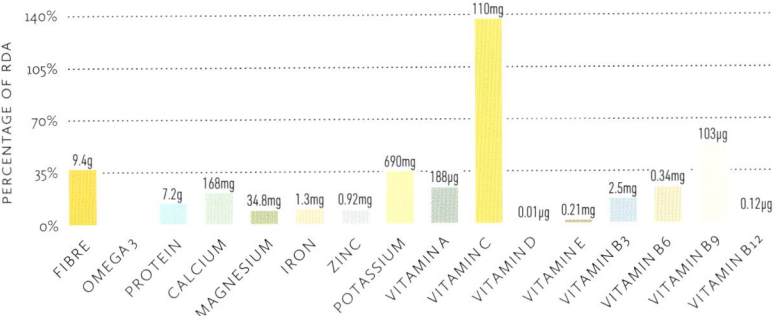

Cauliflower Chickpea Lemon Curry

with apple and dates

1 small cauliflower, chopped into bite-sized florets

½ courgette, chopped

400g wholegrain rice

1 tbsp olive oil

1 yellow onion, finely diced

1 tsp madras curry powder

1 tsp ground cumin

½ tsp cinnamon

1 tbsp turmeric

400ml light coconut milk

2 cloves of garlic, minced

1 thumb-sized piece of ginger, grated

1 tsp pink Himalayan salt

400g chickpeas, drained

1 apple, cored and grated

2 Medjool dates, stone removed and chopped small

large handful of baby spinach leaves

zest of 1½ lemons

juice of ½ lemon (optional)

SERVES: 4

This creamy, aromatic vegan curry is packed full of plant fibre and protein. The apple and dates provide a little sweetness – perfect comfort food for a cosy night in!

1 Preheat the oven to 200°C.
2 Put the cauliflower florets and courgette pieces in a lined baking tray, and roast for 30 minutes, until golden brown and tender.
3 Cook the rice according to the instructions on the packet and keep warm until ready to serve.
4 Heat the olive oil in a large skillet pan. Add the onions and dried spices, and allow to gently sweat with the lid on for 8–10 minutes.
5 Add the coconut milk, garlic, ginger and a pinch of salt. Mix to combine.
6 When the cauliflower and courgette are ready, add them to the pan, along with the chickpeas, grated apple, chopped dates and baby spinach leaves.
7 Stir to combine and cook gently for a few minutes. Add the lemon zest to the pan. If you want to intensify the lemon flavour, also add the juice from half a lemon, and stir well.
8 To serve, plate up 100g of rice per person and portion the curry. If I have any to hand, I like to top with some microgreens and toasted flaked almonds.

PER 550G PORTION (INCL. 100G OF RICE)

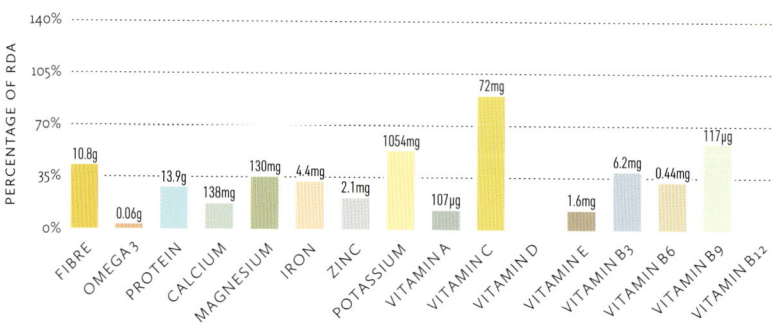

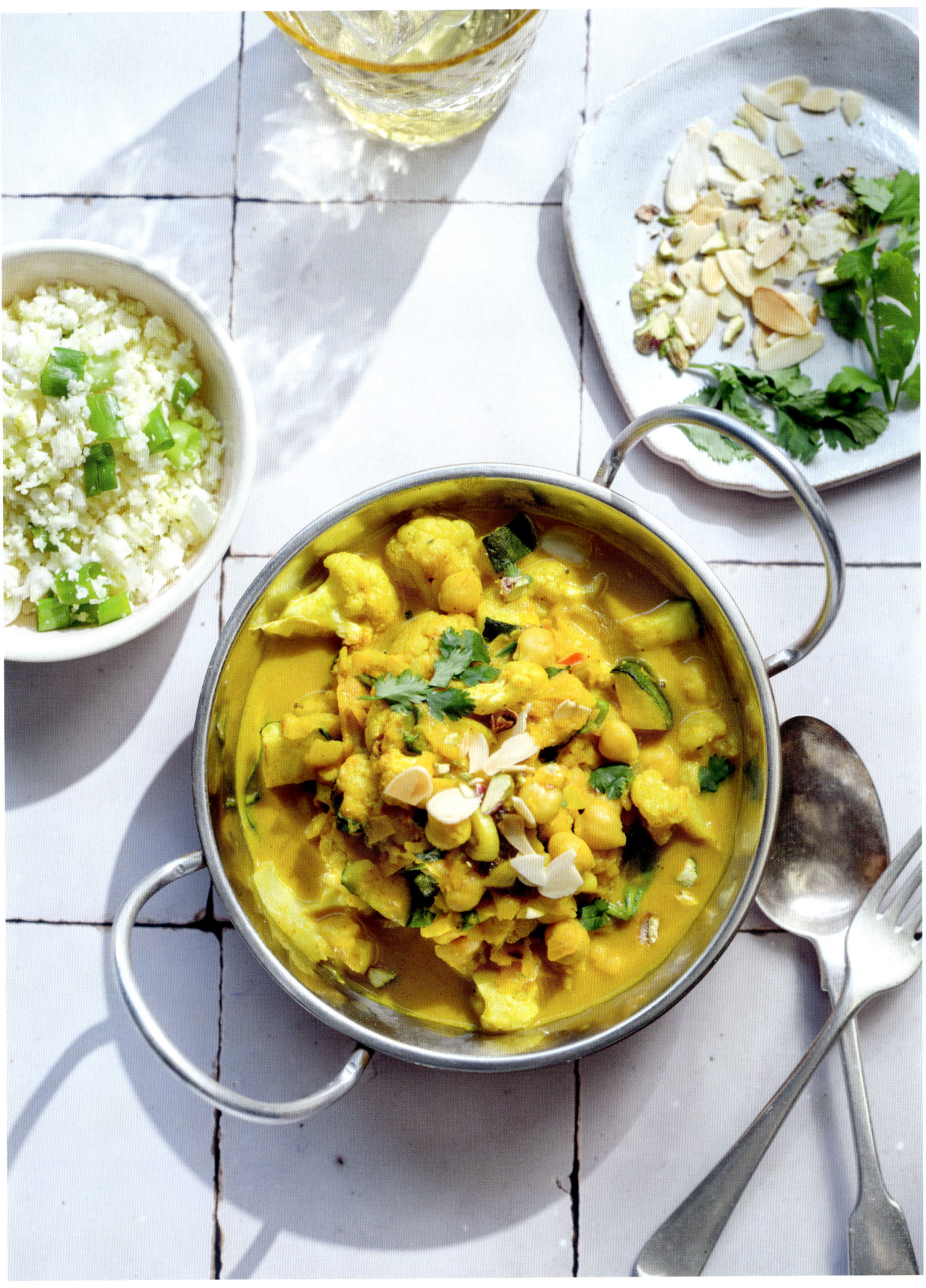

Kale Salad

with feta, pomegranate and roasted aubergine crisps

100g fresh kale, de-stemmed and chopped

3 tbsp balsamic dressing (see p144)

1 aubergine, finely sliced into rounds

1 tbsp olive oil

sprinkling of pink Himalayan salt

1 red onion, finely sliced

100g feta cheese, crumbled

seeds of 1 pomegranate

45g flaked almonds, toasted

SERVES: 4

Part of the cruciferous veg family, kale is one of nature's true superfoods. It's known for its anti-cancer benefits, and for being loaded with vitamin C, antioxidants (in particular vitamin A), iron and calcium.

1. Preheat the oven to 180°C.
2. Place the kale in a bowl with the dressing. Mix well and set aside until the leaves soften.
3. Place the aubergine slices on a large lined baking tray. Brush with olive oil and sprinkle with a little salt, then roast in the oven for 15–20 minutes, or until brown and toasted.
4. Time to assemble the salad. Top your kale with the onions and crumbled feta cheese. Using salad servers, mix until well combined.
5. Add the roasted aubergine slices, then top with pomegranate seeds, toasted flaked almonds and any remaining slices of aubergine. Feel free to drizzle over a little more dressing.

PER 200G PORTION

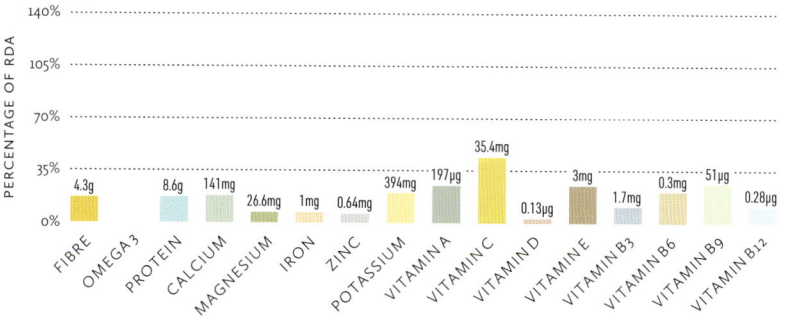

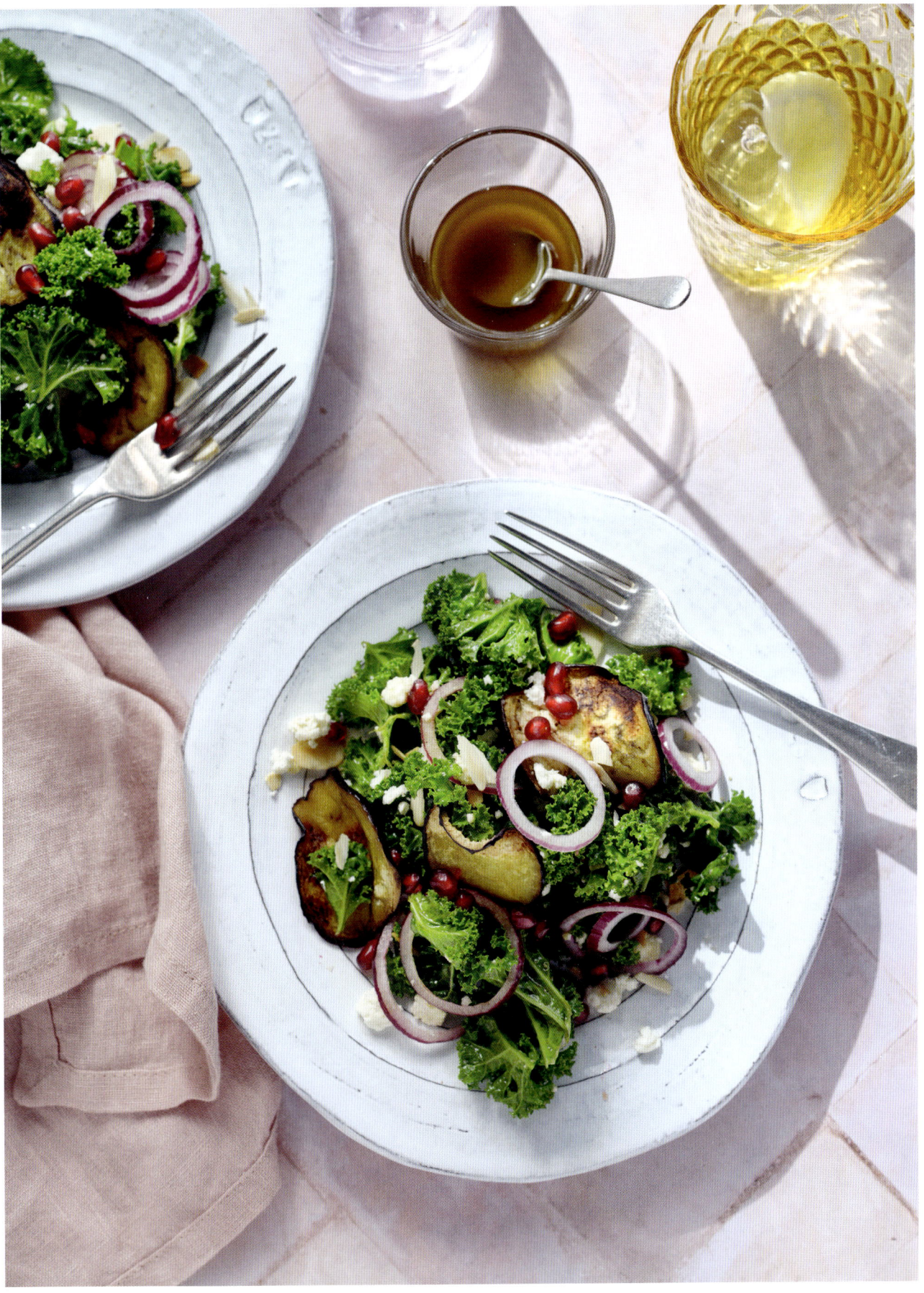

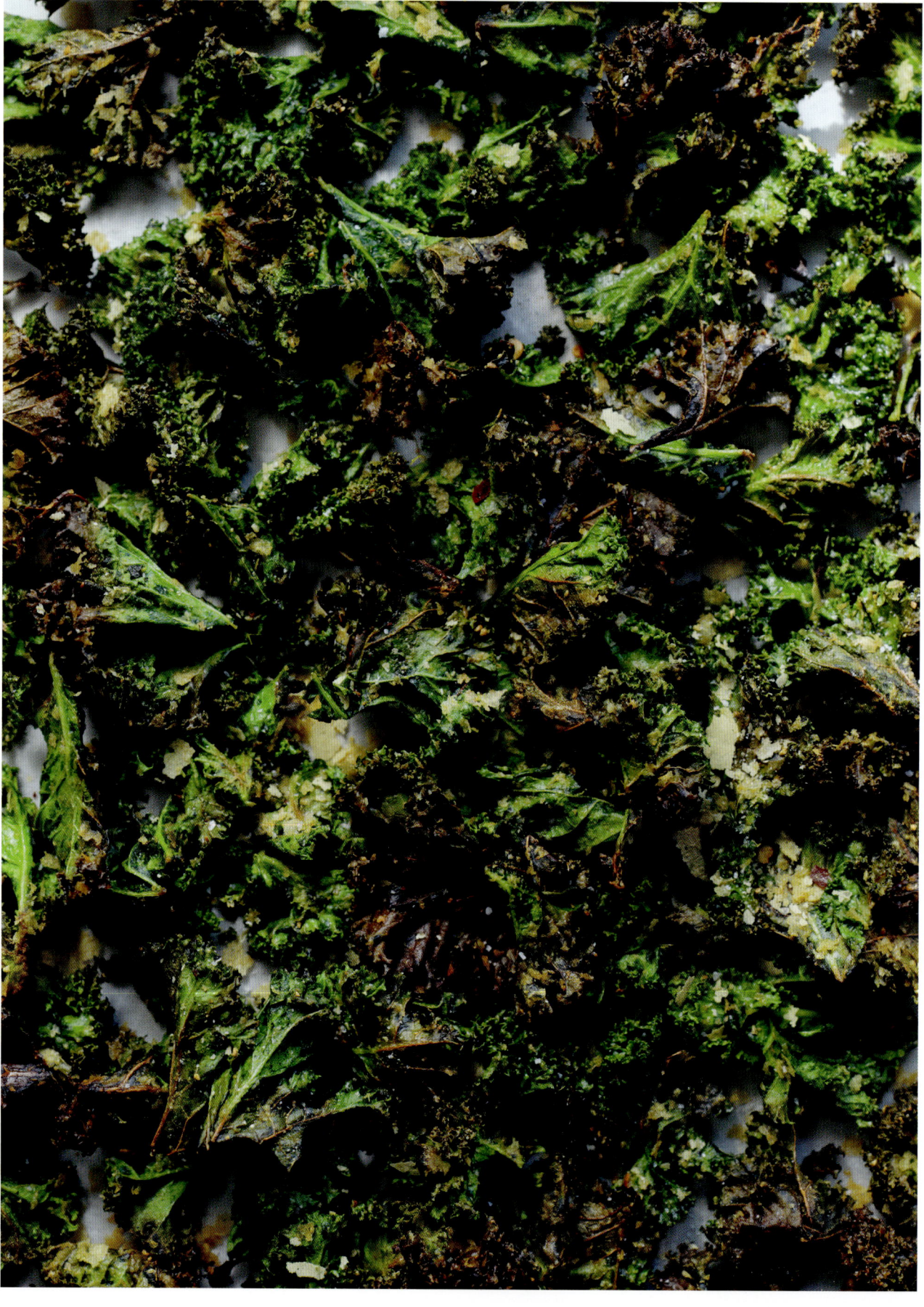

Cheesy Kale Chips

100g fresh kale (finished weight), de-stemmed and torn into small pieces

1 tbsp walnut oil

3 tbsp nutritional yeast

½ tsp pink Himalayan salt

1 tsp garlic powder

chilli flakes (optional)

SERVES: 2+

Kale contains a wealth of valuable nutrients, including antioxidants and minerals which are essential for cell repair. These easy-to-make chips are just the thing to satisfy that savoury craving, or you can add them as toppings to a salad.

1. Preheat the oven to 160°C.
2. Wash the kale and spin-dry it in a salad spinner. Then dry any excess with a paper towel. Place it in a bowl, drizzle with walnut oil and massage well.
3. Add the other ingredients to the bowl and mix well to coat all the leaves.
4. Put the leaves on a lined baking tray and bake in the oven for 12–15 minutes.
5. Remove from the oven and leave to cool for a few minutes to crisp up.
6. Tip into a dry bowl and serve, or store in an airtight container.

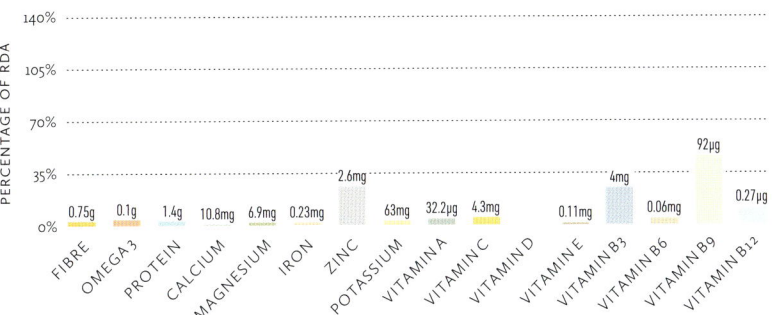

Resources

In this resources section, I want to share some of my favourite brands and places to shop. I use many of these brands daily myself because they prioritise high-quality, nutrient-dense ingredients that align with my values of supporting optimal health and wellness using the best resources I can find. These are my favourites, but you may like to experiment to see which ones work best for your cooking!

WHERE TO SHOP

Asia Market or other ethnic supermarkets

Ethnic supermarkets are an amazing treasure trove for hard-to-find ingredients from all corners of the globe, which can really enhance a recipe! It's particularly worthwhile to try and get your tahini here, as the quality and consistency is far superior to that which you might find in a regular supermarket. You'll be able to stock up on store cupboard staples as well as some unusual fruit and vegetables. You can also shop online at asiamarket.ie.

Below are some items I regularly buy at my local ethnic supermarket:
- Frozen lime leaves
- Frozen edamame beans (shelled)
- Medjool dates
- Nori seaweed sheets
- Lemongrass stalks
- Tahini (runny)
- Spices

Stocking up on nuts and seeds

Bulk-buying nuts and seeds is a cheaper option if you're regularly making nut butter, granola and more. For an extensive supplier of nuts, seeds, dried fruits, herbs and spices in Ireland, you can shop online at nutsinbulk.ie.

Sourdough starter

To start making sourdough bread, all you'll need is a starter culture. You can find a simple tutorial to make your own on my website, or dehydrated sourdough starter is available to purchase there (rachelgraham.ie/shop/sourdough-starter). I can ship nationwide and beyond, and it's complete with instructions to rehydrate and activate.

Probiotics

I often use probiotics in the preparation of fermented foods or to add to smoothies. Some of my favourites are:
- BioAcidophilus beneficial bacteria (LAB4 live strains)
- Optibac for Women (targeted strains to support women's genito-urinary health)

Fresh fruit, veg and other items

Green Door Market
This indoor food market in Dublin sells mostly organic, ethically sourced and locally grown plant-based foods. It's a fabulous place to shop and well worth the trip; you can find more information at thegreendoor.ie.

Drummond House garlic and asparagus
This home-grown heritage garlic hails from Baltray, Co. Meath. It's rich in medicinal properties (such as sulphur-containing allicin) and is now available in Tesco and Dunnes supermarkets nationwide.

McNally Family Farm
This certified organic farm in Balrickard, Co. Dublin, has been in operation since 1998. They grow a large variety of vegetables, herbs, salads, roots and fruits, and you can buy from the farm shop, Temple Bar Market or online at www.mcnallyfamilyfarm.ie.

ALTERNATIVES TO SUGAR

Chicory root syrup
This is a delicious, low-sugar syrup that is extracted from fresh chicory roots. It won't cause a spike in blood sugar and it's high in gut-healthy prebiotic fibre which supports our gut microbiome – try it drizzled on porridge or yoghurt. I like to buy my chicory root syrup from Homespun, an independent Irish company.

Organic blackstrap molasses
This nutrient-dense type of molasses offers a versatile alternative to refined sugar in cooking. I get mine from Meridian, a natural health food brand.

MY GO-TO BRANDS

Clearspring
This producer makes award-winning Japanese specialities and organic fine foods. I like to buy:
- Agar flakes (marine algae), a tasteless, odourless product for thickening sauces
- Organic oils such as toasted sesame seed or walnut oil for high-temperature frying
- Tofu (silken), which is ideal for desserts and miso soup
- White miso paste – perfect for dressings and marinades

Linwoods Health Foods
Linwoods makes high-quality pouches of cold-milled flaxseed and flaxseed blends that are an essential nutrient for hormone balancing and long-term health. I use these every day. Some of my favourites are: Menoligna – sprouted milled flaxseed and milled chia seeds with added Lignans. This is part of Linwood's functional range and specifically developed for menopause and hormone balancing.
- Flaxseed – organic cold-milled flaxseed that goes perfectly with porridge, yoghurt, smoothies and cereals.
- Chia seeds – organic milled chia seeds are also available blended with flaxseed and hemp.
- Shelled hemp seeds – these are a great source of protein to add to porridge or overnight oats.

Marigold
- Marigold vegetable bouillon is a convenient, additive-free and, in some cases, low-sodium option to flavour your soups and stews. My favourite products from Marigold are:
- Vegetable bouillon – you can choose from original, vegan and low-sodium. All are gluten free and contain no MSG.
- Engevita nutritional yeast flakes, which are fortified with vitamin B12, or in a variety of blends with protein, fibre, etc.

Nuzest
For plant-based protein powder, I like to use Nuzest products. My favourite, which I've used throughout the recipe section, is Clean Lean Protein Powder, derived from pea protein, in Vanilla Flavour.

Sunwarrior
This brand offers another of my favourite protein powders – I like their Classic Plus Protein Powder. It's a vanilla-flavoured rice protein with chia seeds, quinoa and amaranth, and is ideal for adding to smoothies, overnight oats and protein balls.

Synergy Spirulina
I head here for their Natural Organic Spirulina Powder – it's an energizing, whole food supplement that is rich in iron, protein and vitamin B12. I like to add it to smoothies or use it in recipes.

Vivo Life Perform Raw Plant Protein & BCAA
A blend of plant protein, BCAAs, turmeric and digestive enzymes to help you train harder and recover faster. Particularly beneficial for women lifting heavy weights or doing HIIT training. I like the Madagascan vanilla flavour. Available at www.pureandnatural.ie.

Acknowledgements

This opportunity feels like a dream come true! I am so incredibly grateful to Nicki Howard and Sarah Liddy from Gill Books for their unwavering support and excitement for my original self-published book, and for then helping to elevate it to a whole new level! While doing so, I have had the privilege to work with their extremely talented and professional team. I would like to give a special mention to Rachel Thompson, who worked tirelessly with me on all the copy edits. I truly appreciate her professional experience and keen eye for detail to ensure that everything was just right.

I would also like to acknowledge Jo Murphy, Orla Neligan and Ciara Fennessy for their invaluable contributions to the book. Our week-long photoshoot cooking, styling and photographing the recipes was an absolute joy, and their enthusiasm and passion for the project were just heart-warming. Jo's beautiful photography perfectly captures the essence of each recipe, and I am in awe of her ability to make every dish look so irresistible. Orla's styling skills are second to none, and it was a privilege to learn from her during the shoot. Ciara's tireless efforts in helping me to prepare and cook every recipe were truly appreciated. Overall, I am so grateful to everyone in Gill who played their part in bringing my book to life. It has been an incredible journey – a dream come true, and I am so excited to finally share it with you!

I also want to say a heartfelt thank you...
... to my incredible husband, Victor, for taste-testing almost every recipe and offering honest, constructive feedback – even though you're not my typical target audience! Your unwavering support for my dream of writing this book and your ability to lend an ear when I needed it has been invaluable.

Thank you for your impeccable timing when there was a sink-load of pots to wash, and for your daily humour, which kept me laughing. You truly lightened the load and it's these little things that really are the big things in the end ... you're the best and I love you so much!

... to all my friends, family and acquaintances who showed a big interest in my progress while writing this book – thank you so much! You have no idea how good it felt to hear your interest and words of encouragement on days when I was struggling with the sheer volume of work and doubting myself!
... to the generous brands that have supplied me with their unique products and superfoods: thank you! Your contributions have allowed me to develop the recipes that make this book what it is.

... to the wonderful women who have completed my programme or are part of my private Facebook group, Back To Life: thank you for being part of my community. The insights and shared experiences you've provided have been instrumental in shaping the content of this book.

And lastly, to you, the reader holding this book in your hands: thank you from the bottom of my heart for supporting my work and passion for healthy food! I'm thrilled to finally share my recipes with you, and I hope they bring you as much joy and feel-good benefits as they have for me.

My goal in writing this book was to bridge the gap between evidence-based information and delicious-tasting food, with benefits beyond basic nutrition. This is the kind of information that will enable you to navigate this life stage like a pro! Eating this way is good for both your body and mind; it is the blueprint I hope you will use and love to support your hormone health, and will give you the tools you need to take action in the kitchen, to future-proof your health and to live your best life!

Rachel x

Endnotes

PART ONE: UNDERSTANDING MENOPAUSE

1. Bingham, Sheila. 'High-Meat Diets and Cancer Risk.' *Proceedings of the Nutrition Society* 58, no. 2 (1 May 1999): 243–48. https://doi.org/10.1017/s0029665199000336.

2. Thomas L. Halton et al. 'Low-Carbohydrate-Diet Score and the Risk of Coronary Heart Disease in Women.' *The New England Journal of Medicine* 355, no. 19 (9 November 2006): 1991–2002, https://doi.org/10.1056/nejmoa055317.

3. Jama, J. Warsama, L.J. Launer, J.C.M. Witteman, J.H. Den Breeijen, Monique M.B. Breteler, D.E. Grobbee and Albert Hofman. 'Dietary Antioxidants and Cognitive Function in a Population-Based Sample of Older Persons: The Rotterdam Study.' *American Journal of Epidemiology* 144, no. 3 (1 August 1996): 275–80. https://doi.org/10.1093/oxfordjournals.aje.a008922.

4. Wium-Andersen, Ida Kim, Jørgen Rungby, Marit E. Jørgensen, A Sandbæk, Merete Osler and Marie Kim Wium-Andersen. 'Risk of Dementia and Cognitive Dysfunction in Individuals with Diabetes or Elevated Blood Glucose.' *Epidemiology and Psychiatric Sciences* 29 (1 January 2020). https://doi.org/10.1017/s2045796019000374.

PART TWO: FUTURE-PROOFING YOUR HEALTH

Bone health

5. Willett, Walter C. and David S. Ludwig. 'Milk and Health.' *The New England Journal of Medicine* 382, no. 7 (12 February 2020): 644–54. https://doi.org/10.1056/nejmra1903547.

Brain health

6. Gravesteijn, Elske, Ronald P. Mensink and Jogchum Plat. 'Effects of Nutritional Interventions on BDNF Concentrations in Humans: A Systematic Review.' *Nutritional Neuroscience* 25, no. 7 (10 January 2021): 1425–36. https://doi.org/10.1080/1028415x.2020.1865758.

7. Grosso, Giuseppe, Fabio Galvano, Stefano Marventano, Michele Malaguarnera, Claudio Bucolo, Filippo Drago and Filippo Caraci. 'Omega-3 Fatty Acids and Depression: Scientific Evidence and Biological Mechanisms.' *Oxidative Medicine and Cellular Longevity* 2014 (18 March 2014): 1–16. https://doi.org/10.1155/2014/313570.

8. Pochwat, Bartłomiej, Magdalena Sowa-Kućma, Katarzyna Kotarska, Paulina Misztak, Gabriel Nowak and Bernadeta Szewczyk. 'Antidepressant-like Activity of Magnesium in the Olfactory Bulbectomy Model Is Associated with the AMPA/BDNF Pathway.' *Psychopharmacology* 232, no. 2 (1 January 2015): 355–67. https://doi.org/10.1007/s00213-014-3671-6.

9. Bathina, Siresha and Undurti N. Das. 'Brain-Derived Neurotrophic Factor and Its Clinical Implications.' *Archives of Medical Science* 6 (10 December 2015): 1164–78. https://doi.org/10.5114/aoms.2015.56342.

Heart health

10. Harcombe, Zoë, David Baker, Stephen Cooper, Bruce Davies, Nicholas Sculthorpe, James J. DiNicolantonio and Fergal M. Grace. 'Evidence from Randomised Controlled Trials Did Not Support the Introduction of Dietary Fat Guidelines in 1977 and 1983: A Systematic Review and Meta-Analysis.' *Open Heart* 2, no. 1 (1 January 2015) https://doi.org/10.1136/openhrt-2014-000196.

11. Ripsin, Cynthia M. and Joseph M. Keenan. 'The Effects of Dietary Oat Products on Blood Cholesterol.' *Trends in Food Science and Technology* (1 January 1992). https://doi.org/10.1016/0924-2244(92)90167-u.

The truth about sugar

12. Nickerson, Kourtney P., Rachael B. Chanin and Christine F. McDonald. 'Deregulation of Intestinal Anti-Microbial Defense by the Dietary Additive, Maltodextrin.' *Gut Microbes* 6, no. 1 (4 March 2015): 78–83. https://doi.org/10.1080/19490976.2015.1005477.

13. Goran, Michael I., Stanley J. Ulijaszek and Emily E. Ventura. 'High Fructose Corn Syrup and Diabetes Prevalence: A Global Perspective.' *Global Public Health* 8, no. 1 (31 January 2013): 55–64. https://doi.org/10.1080/17441692.2012.736257.

PART THREE: THE MENO 8

Phytoestrogens

14. Knight, David W. and John A. Eden. 'A Review of the Clinical Effects of Phytoestrogens.' *Obstetrics & Gynecology* 87, no. 5 Pt 2 (1 January, 1996): 897–904.

15. Lucas, Edralin A., Robert A. Wild, Lisa A. Hammond, Dania A. Khalil, Shanil Juma, Bruce P. Daggy, Barbara J. Stoecker and Bahram H. Arjmandi. 'Flaxseed Improves Lipid Profile without Altering Biomarkers of Bone Metabolism in Postmenopausal Women.' *The Journal of Clinical Endocrinology and Metabolism* 87, no. 4 (1 April 2002): 1527–32. https://doi.org/10.1210/jcem.87.4.8374.

16. Thompson, Lilian U., Jian Chen, Tong Li, Kathrin Strasser-Weippl and Paul E. Goss. 'Dietary Flaxseed Alters Tumor Biological Markers in Postmenopausal Breast Cancer.' *Clinical Cancer Research* 11, no. 10 (15 May 2005): 3828–35. https://doi.org/10.1158/1078-0432.ccr-04-2326.

17. Horn-Ross, Pamela L., Katherine J. Hoggatt and Marion M. Lee. 'Phytoestrogens and Thyroid Cancer Risk: The San

Francisco Bay Area Thyroid Cancer Study.' *Cancer Epidemiology, Biomarkers & Prevention* 11, no. 1 (1 January 2002): 43–49.

Fibre

18 Gigleux, Iris, David J.A. Jenkins et al. 'Comparison of a Dietary Portfolio Diet of Cholesterol-Lowering Foods and a Statin on LDL Particle Size Phenotype in Hypercholesterolaemic Participants.' *British Journal of Nutrition* 98, no. 6 (December 2007): 1229–36. https://doi.org/10.1017/S0007114507781461.

19 https://www.researchgate.net/profile/William-Grant-6/publication/264121252_Grant_Alzheimer_1997/links/53ceed560cf2fd75bc59ac4d/Grant-Alzheimer-1997.pdf

Omega-3

20 Sacchetti, Stefano, Francesca Gelfo and Laura Petrosini. 'N-3 PUFA Improve Emotion and Cognition during Menopause: A Systematic Review.' *Nutrients* 14, no. 9 (9 May 2022): 1982. https://doi.org/10.3390/nu14091982.

Calcium and magnesium

21 Kritchevsky, Stephen B. 'ß-Carotene, Carotenoids and the Prevention of Coronary Heart Disease.' *Journal of Nutrition* 129, no. 1 (1 January 1999): 5–8. https://doi.org/10.1093/jn/129.1.5.

22 Joseph, James A., Barbara Shukitt-Hale, Natalia Denisova, Donna F. Bielinski, Antonio M. Martin, John J. McEwen and Paula C. Bickford. 'Reversals of Age-Related Declines in Neuronal Signal Transduction, Cognitive, and Motor Behavioral Deficits with Blueberry, Spinach, or Strawberry Dietary Supplementation.' *The Journal of Neuroscience* 19, no. 18 (15 September 1999): 8114–21. https://doi.org/10.1523/jneurosci.19-18-08114.1999.

23 Hannum, Sandra M., Harold H. Schmitz and Carl L. Keen. 'Chocolate: A Heart-Healthy Food? Show Me the Science!' *Nutrition Today* 37, no. 3 (1 May 2002): 103–9. https://doi.org/10.1097/00017285-200205000-00004.

24 Nakachi, Kei, Satoru Matsuyama, Satoshi Miyake, Masami Suganuma and Kazue Imai. 'Preventive Effects of Drinking Green Tea on Cancer and Cardiovascular Disease: Epidemiological Evidence for Multiple Targeting Prevention.' *Biofactors* 13, no. 1–4 (1 January 2000): 49–54. https://doi.org/10.1002/biof.5520130109.

25 Nakachi, Kei, Kimito Suemasu, Kenji Suga, Takeshi Takeo, Kazue Imai and Yasuhiro Higashi. 'Influence of Drinking Green Tea on Breast Cancer Malignancy among Japanese Patients.' *Japanese Journal of Cancer Research* 89, no. 3 (1 March 1998): 254–61. https://doi.org/10.1111/j.1349-7006.1998.tb00556.x.

Protein

26 Hu, Frank B., Meir J. Stampfer, Eric B. Rimm, JoAnn E. Manson, Alberto Ascherio, Graham A. Colditz, Bernard Rosner et al. 'A Prospective Study of Egg Consumption and Risk of Cardiovascular Disease in Men and Women.' *JAMA* 281, no. 15 (21 April 1999): 1387. https://doi.org/10.1001/jama.281.15.1387.

27 Hu, Frank B., Leslie Bronner, Walter C. Willett, Meir J. Stampfer, Kathryn M. Rexrode, Christine M. Albert, David J. Hunter and JoAnn E. Manson. 'Fish and Omega-3 Fatty Acid Intake and Risk of Coronary Heart Disease in Women.' *JAMA* 287, no. 14 (10 April 2002): 1815–21. https://doi.org/10.1001/jama.287.14.1815.

28 De Oliveira e Silva, E.R., Christine E. Seidman, J.J. Tian, Lisa C. Hudgins, Frank M. Sacks and Jan L. Breslow. 'Effects of Shrimp Consumption on Plasma Lipoproteins.' *The American Journal of Clinical Nutrition* 64, no. 5 (1 November 1996): 712–17. https://doi.org/10.1093/ajcn/64.5.712.

Brassicas

29 Van Poppel, G., D.T.H. Verhoeven, Hence J.M. Verhagen and R.A. Goldbohm. 'Brassica Vegetables and Cancer Prevention.' *Advances in Experimental Medicine and Biology* (1 January 1999): 159–68. https://doi.org/10.1007/978-1-4757-3230-6_14.

30 Michnovicz, Jon J. and H. Leon Bradlow. 'Altered Estrogen Metabolism and Excretion in Humans Following Consumption of Indole-3-carbinol.' *Nutrition and Cancer* 16, no. 1 (1 January 1991): 59–66. https://doi.org/10.1080/01635589109514141.

31 Nestle, Marion. 'Broccoli Sprouts as Inducers of Carcinogen-Detoxifying Enzyme Systems: Clinical, Dietary, and Policy Implications.' *Proceedings of the National Academy of Sciences of the United States of America* 94, no. 21 (14 October 1997): 11149–51. https://doi.org/10.1073/pnas.94.21.11149.

32 Steinkellner, Hans, Sylvie Rabot, Christian Freywald, Eva Nobis, Gerlinde Scharf, Monika Chabicovsky, Siegfried Knasmüller and Fekadu Kassie. 'Effects of Cruciferous Vegetables and Their Constituents on Drug Metabolizing Enzymes Involved in the Bioactivation of DNA-Reactive Dietary Carcinogens.' *Mutation Research: Fundamental and Molecular Mechanisms of Mutagenesis* 480–481 (1 September 2001): 285–97. https://doi.org/10.1016/s0027-5107(01)00188-9.

33 Cheney, Garnett. 'Rapid Healing of Peptic Ulcers in Patients Receiving Fresh Cabbage Juice.' *California Medicine* 70, no. 1 (1 January 1949): 10–15.

Index

5:2 diet, 31

açai berries, 59
acetylcholine, 42
ADHD (attention deficit hyperactivity disorder), 66
adrenaline, 23, 31, 66
agar flakes, 281
alcohol, 11, 21, 47, 50, 55
alfalfa seeds, 40, 42
allicins, 58
almond butter, 17, 56, 170–1, 215
almond milk, 173
almonds, 13, 46, 66, 177
alpha-carotene, 58
alpha-linolenic acid, 49, 50
Alzheimer's Disease, 7, 9, 16, 17, 21, 23, 29, 50–1, 57, 61
American Association of Cancer Research, 42
American Journal of Gastroenterology, 19
amino acids, 12, 14, 28, 64, 66, 70, 235
animal protein, 33, 34, 64, 65–6
anthocyanins, 57, 59, 61
antibiotics, 5, 47, 65, 69
anti-cancer phytochemicals, 58–60, 61–3
antioxidants, 2, 3, 4, 5, 9, 13, 16, 22, 28, 39, 40, 45, 50, 52, 54, 57–63, 65, 66, 71, 124, 179, 247, 279
anxiety, 7, 9, 14, 16, 17, 51, 54, 55, 133, 249
apple cider vinegar, 69–70, 249, 255
apple doughnuts, 114
apples, 28, 33, 34, 39, 47, 48, 61, 250, 274
arachidonic acid, 4–5
arginine, 61
aromatase, 29
arteries, 4, 8, 20, 51, 61
arthritis, 18, 70
artichokes, 17, 44, 45
artificial sweeteners, 23, 26
Asia Market, 280
asparagus, 17, 45, 58, 167–8, 219
atherosclerosis, 20, 58
aubergines, 57, 207–9
  aubergine crisps, 211–12, 276
  roasted aubergine involtini, 85–6
autoimmune diseases, 17, 18
avocados, 44, 96, 222
  avocado, papaya and mint salsa, 140
  avonaise, 120
avonaise, 120

baby gem caesar salad, 164
baked goods, 51
baked Moroccan eggs, 220
balsamic dressing, 144
balsamic roasted Brussels sprouts, 270
banana nice-cream, 215
banana sambal, 90
barley, 22
basil pesto, 196
BDNF (brain-derived neurotrophic factor), 16, 17
bean stew, 161
beans, 5, 14, 22, 34, 64, 66
beetroot, ginger and fennel juice, 180
beetroot ketchup, 121, 222, 223
berries, 28, 33, 34, 44, 58, 59, 237, 253
beta-carotene, 183, 190, 204
beta-carotenes, 57, 58, 59, 62
beta-glucan, 22
Bifidobacterium, 68
Bircher muesli, 237
blackstrap molasses, 281
blood
  glucose, 4, 8, 9
  pressure, 8, 16, 20, 50, 53, 54, 56, 59, 61, 64, 70, 101, 157, 180
  sugar, 4, 8, 20, 22, 23, 24, 26, 28, 30, 31, 35, 36, 43, 45, 47, 70, 101
blue zones, 21, 22
blueberries, 59, 61
blueberry compote, 105
bok choi, 13
Bolognese, 217, 231
bones, 8–9, 11–13, 40, 43, 54, 56, 79, 157, 217, 283
bouillabaisse, 133, 138
BPAs, 5
brain, 9, 13–14, 16–18, 45, 52, 54, 65, 66, 133, 283

brain fog, 1, 17, 55
brassicas, 2, 3, 33, 34, 58, 71–4, 263, 284
breads, 19, 24, 35, 50, 65, 280
  brown, 24
  naan, 244
  packaged, 24
  porridge, 37, 45, 80, 102, 220
  rye, 34
  sourdough, 69, 249, 256, 280
  white, 4, 20, 70
  wholegrain, 43
breakfast, 37
breast cancer, 29, 40, 42, 50, 52, 62, 71, 72
British Journal of Nutrition, 46
broccoli, 13, 14, 30, 37, 44, 46, 54, 57, 58, 63, 66, 71, 72, 271
broccoli sprouts, 66, 72
brown bread, 24
brownies, 177
Brussels sprouts, 40, 44, 58, 270
burgers, 228–9
butter, 7
  almond, 17, 55 170–1, 215
  cocoa, 61
  maple almond, 215
  nut, 157
butyrate, 19, 48

cabbage, 73
cabbage steaks, 273
cacao, 17, 174, 177, 240
Caesar salad, 164
caffeine, 30, 55, 62, 238
calcium, 2, 3, 8, 11, 12, 13, 19, 28, 35, 53–4, 64, 72, 73, 117, 157, 174, 273, 276, 284
calories, 33, 36, 50
cancer, 5, 18, 23, 29, 39, 40, 42, 45, 48, 53, 57, 58–9, 61, 62, 63, 64, 68, 70, 71, 72, 79, 217, 263, 276
cannellini beans, 146, 161
carbohydrates, 4, 5, 8, 13, 20, 22–3, 30, 31, 35–6, 49, 50, 54
cardiovascular disease, 7, 8, 16, 21, 26, 29, 39, 40, 59
carotenes, 59, 71
carotenoids, 57, 58

carrots, 28, 44, 57, 58, 59
    carrot, ginger and celery soup, 199
    carrot, red pepper, orange and ginger juice, 183
    carrot cake squares, 129–31
cashew cream, 113
cauliflower
    cauliflower chickpea lemon curry, 274
    cauliflower pea mash, 263, 266
    characteristics, 71–2
    roasted cauliflower, chickpea and sweet potato salad, 265
    steamed cauliflower rice, 263, 264
celery, 39
celery, carrot and ginger soup, 199
cell membranes, 14, 42, 49, 51, 62, 65
cellulose, 45
central adiposity, 9, 29, 49
cereals, 24
cerebral cortex, 14
cheese, 13
cheesy kale chips, 279
chemicals, 5
Cheney, Garnett, 73
chia pudding, 133–4
chia seeds, 5, 16, 19, 22, 44, 49, 53, 180, 237, 238, 281
chicken, 65, 190
    chicken bone broth, 161, 235
    chicken breast, 243
    chicken salad, 190
    chicken tagine, 225
chickpeas, 265, 274
    chickpea pancakes, 244
chicory
    chicory and smashed avo with orange and miso dressing, 96
    chicory root syrup, 28, 280
chips, kale, 279
chlorophyll, 52
chocolate, 33, 34, 61, 253
chocolate tahini bliss balls, 174
cholesterol, 4, 8, 13, 16, 19, 20, 21–2, 23, 24, 39, 40, 42, 45, 46, 48, 51, 52, 54, 61, 64, 65, 66, 101
chondroitin sulphates, 235
citrus fruits, 47, 48, 63
cleaning products, 7
Clearspring, 281
clotting, 20, 53, 57
cocoa butter, 61
coconut sugar, 28

coconut yoghurt, 253
coeliac disease, 11
co-factor nutrients, 14, 17, 66
coffee, 238
coleslaw, 74, 92
collagen, 63, 235
compotes
    blueberry, 105
    rhubarb, apple and pear, 108, 128, 240
concentration, 1, 5, 7, 9, 13, 14, 16
constipation, 19, 42, 43, 45, 55
cookies, 110
copper, 14, 40, 42, 66, 73
coronary heart disease, 66
corn oil, 5
cortisol, 9, 22, 23, 31–2
courgette rolls, 219
courgette tortillas, 222
crackers, 143
CRP (c-reactive protein) levels, 20
cruciferous vegetables *see* brassicas
curcumin (turmeric), 17
curries
    cauliflower chickpea lemon curry, 274
    lemongrass curry, 90
    Thai red curry, 83–4

dahl, 244
daidzein, 40, 42
daily dahl, 244
dairy products, 4, 11, 12, 13, 14, 23, 64
dates, 28, 280
    cauliflower chickpea lemon curry, 274
    date and ginger caramel, 124
    pear tart with date and ginger caramel, 125–6
    sage and date hummus, 118
delta-6 desaturase, 50
dementia, 7, 9, 16, 17, 18, 21, 26, 29, 50–1, 52
depression, 9, 16, 17, 31, 51, 54, 66, 133, 249
detoxification, 2, 4, 7, 18, 20–1, 45, 68, 71, 72, 96
DEXA scan, 12
diabetes, 7, 8, 21, 23, 24, 26, 29, 42, 45, 49, 53, 54, 63, 70, 101
    see also type 2 diabetes
diarrhoea, 26, 42, 45
digestive health, 18–19
dinner, 37
dopamine, 23, 26, 66

doughnuts, 114
dressings, 24, 28, 35, 70, 73
    balsamic, 144
    ginger miso, 96, 150
    for grilled baby gem Caesar salad, 164
    miso, ginger and chilli dressing, 190
drinks, 24, 26, 27
Drummond House garlic and asparagus, 280
dysbiosis, 18

edamame beans
    edamame and sesame rainbow slaw, 92
    edamame bean hummus, 91
EGCG (epigallocatechin gallate), 62
eggs, 7, 14, 31, 34, 51, 65, 66, 68, 220
elimination, 45, 68
enoki mushrooms, 169
enteric system, 17
enzymes, 53, 54, 64, 68, 70, 71
essential fats *see* omega-3 fats
ethnic supermarkets, 280
exercise, 3, 4, 7, 9, 11, 12, 13, 18, 21, 27, 30, 32
extra virgin olive oil, 16, 52–3

faecal weight, 45
falafel wrap with avocado and beetroot ketchup, 223
falafels, 99
fasting, 31
fats, 5, 13, 14, 16, 19, 20, 30, 31, 32, 35, 36, 40, 42, 49, 50, 51, 54
    see also monounsaturated fats; omega-3 fats; saturated fats; short-chain fatty acids; trans fats
fennel, 39, 192, 250
    fennel, beetroot and ginger juice, 180
fermented foods, 68–70, 249, 250, 280
feta, 276
fibre, 2, 3, 5, 8, 13, 14, 17, 18, 19, 22, 23, 24, 28, 30, 35, 42, 43–8, 54, 61, 91, 101, 284
    see also insoluble fibre; soluble fibre
fight or flight response, 32
fish, 16, 31, 34, 49–50, 51, 53, 63, 64, 65–6
    see also mackerel; salmon; sardines

flash-cooked tender stem broccoli, 271
flavonoids, 58, 59, 61, 62
flaxseed, 105
flaxseed crackers, 143
flaxseeds, 5, 16, 17, 19, 22, 39, 42, 44, 49, 50, 53, 79, 238, 281
folic acid/folate, 14, 40, 45, 66, 73, 190
food labels, 23–4
food pyramid, 33–4
formononetin, 42
four-seed rye sourdough bread, 249, 256
free radicals, 40, 52, 59, 63
frittata, 218
frozen yoghurt bark, 260
fructooligosaccharides, 68
fruit, 5, 7, 21, 28, 33, 34, 53, 57, 61, 63, 280
fruit juice, 28

garlic, 17, 22, 58, 80
genistein, 40, 42
ghrelin, 30
ginger, 124
ginger miso dressing, 92, 96, 150, 169
glaucoma, 61
Glow Bowl, 200
glucomannan, 45, 46, 47
glucosamine, 235
glucose, 23, 24, 26, 28, 30, 31, 32, 35, 45, 47
glucose spikes, 8
glucosinolates, 71, 72, 73
glycaemic index, 24, 28
glycaemic load, 22–3
glycosylation, 8
gnocchi, 204, 206
Goss, Paul, 42
grains, 5, 14, 24, 44, 53, 55, 64, 66, 68
   see also wholegrains
granola
   pecan cinnamon, 107
   savoury, 122
green banana sambal, 90
Green Door Market, 280
green juice, 184
green tea, 59, 62
gut bacteria, 5, 14, 16, 17, 18–19, 28, 45, 47–8, 68, 249, 256

harissa charred salmon, 140
Harvard School of Public Health, 8

harvest pressing dates, 52
hazelnut butter brownies, 177
HDL cholesterol, 20, 40, 66
heart
   disease, 4, 5, 7, 8, 18, 19, 20, 21, 23, 24, 39, 50, 51, 53, 58, 59, 61, 62, 63, 64, 70, 79, 157, 217
   health, 4, 5, 7, 16, 20–3, 43, 51, 56, 57, 59, 157, 180
   see also cardiovascular disease
Helicobacter pylori, 72
hemp protein, 65
hemp seed, 108
hemp seeds, 19, 108, 183, 189
herbs, 55
high-fructose corn syrup, 24, 26
high-GL foods, 8, 30, 35
highly processed sugars, 24, 26
hip fractures, 11
HMG-CoA reductase, 48
Homespun, 28
homocysteine, 20–1
honey, 28, 34
hormones, 2, 3, 4, 5, 9, 13, 19, 30–3, 49, 64, 68, 73, 133, 189, 235, 263
hotpot, red lentil, turmeric and kale, 162
HRT (hormone replacement therapy), 43
hummus
   edamame bean, 91, 219
   roasted carrot and yellow pepper, 117, 243
   sage and date, 118
hydration, 7
hypercholesterolaemia, 21
hypertension, 26

IBS (irritable bowel syndrome), 26, 28
ice-cream, 215
Indole-3-carbinole, 71, 72
inflammation, 4–5, 9, 16, 17, 19, 20–1, 23, 24, 28, 29, 31, 39, 47–8, 51, 52, 59, 62, 79, 124, 179
inflammatory bowel disease, 24
insoluble fibre, 19, 43–4, 45, 48, 68
insulin, 4, 8, 9, 20, 24, 26, 28, 29, 31, 35, 42, 45, 47, 49, 70
insulin resistance, 9, 29, 30, 49
intermittent fasting, 31
International Osteoporosis Foundation, 12
intrinsic factor, 17
inulin, 28, 68
involtini, roasted aubergine, 85–6

iodine, 169
iron, 13, 19, 35, 42, 54, 64, 65, 66, 73, 276, 281
isoflavones, 39, 40, 42, 43, 91, 92
   see also phytoestrogens
isothiocyanates, 57–8

The Journal of Neuroscience, 61
juices
   beetroot, ginger and fennel, 180
   carrot, red pepper, orange and ginger, 183
   life-giving green, 184
juicing, 53

kale, 13, 17, 40, 58, 62, 71, 72–3, 162
   kale chips, 279
   kale quinoa wraps, 163
   kale salad, 276
kedgeree, 154
kefir, 13
ketchup, 121, 222, 223
kidneys, 8, 23, 56, 64, 70
kombucha, 70–1

Lactobacillus, 47, 68, 69
lacto-fermentation, 69, 70
lasagne, 207–9
LDL cholesterol, 8, 40, 46, 66
lecithin, 42
leeks, 17, 45, 58, 266
legumes, 5, 13, 22, 40, 46, 48, 54, 64–5, 68
lemon cashew cream, 129–31
lentils, 5, 22, 34, 43, 44, 64, 65, 90
   lentil and mushroom burgers, 228–9
   lentil Bolognese, 217, 231
leptin, 30
life-giving green juice, 184
lignans, 40, 42, 44, 50
lime chia pudding, 133–4
lime green smoothie, 259
linseed *see* flaxseeds
Linwoods Health Foods, 19, 50, 281
lit-from-within chicken salad, 190
liver, 7, 26, 32, 40, 46, 48, 62, 68, 96, 169
longevity, 18, 21, 63
low-GL diet, 4, 22–3, 34, 35–6
lunch, 5, 27, 37
lycopene, 57, 58

mackerel
   mackerel niçoise salad, 149

smoked mackerel pâté, 146
magnesium, 2, 3, 8, 17, 19, 35, 40, 42, 53, 54–6, 64, 72, 73, 157, 273, 284
magnesium citrate, 56
magnesium oxide, 55
maltodextrin, 24
manganese, 28, 42, 73
mango, turmeric and hemp seed smoothie, 189
maple almond butter, 215
maple syrup, 28
Marigold, 281
mash
    cauliflower pea, 263, 266
    root vegetables, 232–4
matcha, 62
McNally Family Farm, 280
meal plans, 36, 37
meat, 4–5, 23, 37, 53, 64, 68
Med veg tofu, 85–6
Mediterranean seafood bouillabaisse, 133, 138
Mediterranean vegetable frittata, 218
Mediterranean vegetable lasagne, 207–9
Mediterrean vegetables, 197, 207–9, 218
melatonin, 66
memory, 1, 5, 7, 9, 11, 14, 16, 52, 133
meno food pyramid, 33–4
Meno 8, 2, 3, 4, 38–74, 283–4
Menoligna, 50, 281
meno-middle, 29–32
Menopause Charity, 2
metabolic syndrome, 26
methionine, 64
methylation, 66
microbiome, 16, 17, 18, 70, 71, 256
microgreens *see* broccoli sprouts
milk, 7, 11, 12–13, 54, 62
milks
    almond milk, 173
    organic soy golden milk, 17, 95
minerals, 5, 9, 19, 50, 55, 59, 65, 138, 228–9, 263, 279
minestrone bean stew, 161
miso dressings, 92, 96, 150, 169, 190
molasses, 281
monounsaturated fats, 5, 16, 22, 52, 53, 59, 120, 144
Moroccan eggs, 220
Moroccan quinoa, 219, 226, 243
Moroccan spiced chicken tagine, 225

Mosconi, Lisa, 9
muesli, 237
Multiboost Organic Milled Hemp Seeds, 19
muscle, 30, 31, 54
mushroom and lentil shepherd's pie, 232–4
mushrooms, 80, 169, 211–12, 228–9, 232–4
    see also Shitake mushrooms

naan bread, 244
natural killer cells, 40
neuroplasticity, 16
neurotransmitters, 14, 17, 49, 55, 64, 66
The New England Journal of Medicine, 12–13
niacin, 169
niçoise salad, 149
nitric oxide, 59, 61, 180
non-alcoholic fatty liver disease, 26
nori seaweed hand roll with prawns and enoki mushrooms, 169
nut butter, 157
nutrient powerhouse smoothie bowl, 137
nuts, 5, 22, 33, 34, 39, 44, 46, 53, 54, 55, 63, 68, 79, 196, 280
nutsinbulk.ie., 280
Nuzest, 281

oat bran, 43, 45, 46
oats, 22, 23, 24, 31, 43, 44
    mocha chia protein overnight oats, 238
    oat and flaxseed porridge with blueberry compote, 105
    oat and hemp seed porridge, 108
    over parfait, 240
    porridge bread, 102
    spirulina, lime and mint overnight oats, 104
    see also overnight oats; porridge oats
obesity, 20, 21, 26, 49
oestrogen, 3, 8, 9, 20, 39, 40, 42, 43, 50, 68, 71, 72, 79
oestrogen dominance, 29
okra, 13
oleic acid, 52, 59
oligosaccharides, 48, 65
olive oil, 5, 16, 22, 52–3
omega-3 fats, 2, 3, 5, 14, 16, 22, 35, 45, 49–53, 65, 66, 133, 180, 189, 284

omega-6 fats, 5, 13, 14, 16, 17, 22, 35, 45, 49–51
onions, 19, 45, 57, 58, 61
Open Heart, 20
ORAC (oxygen radical absorbency capacity) units, 4, 58
oranges, 57, 96, 183, 250
organic blackstrap molasses, 281
organic coconut sugar, 28
organic food, 7, 14
organic maple syrup, 28
organic soy golden milk, 17, 95
osteoblasts, 11
osteoclasts, 11
osteopenia, 12
osteoporosis, 7, 8–9, 11–13, 39, 40, 54, 64, 72
Osteoporosis Foundation, 54
overnight oats, 19, 45, 104, 237, 238, 240, 281
overnight oats parfait, 240
oxidative load, 5, 7
oxidative stress, 20, 52, 59, 63, 74

packaged bread, 24
pancakes, 244
papaya, mint and avocado, 140
parsley, 39, 46, 54
parsley gremolata, 195, 199, 211
pâté, smoked mackerel, 146
PCBs, 5
pears, 28, 34, 59
    pear tart with date and ginger caramel, 125–6
    pear-a-misu, 240
    poached pears, 240
peas, 43, 44, 46, 54, 57, 58
pecan cinnamon granola, 107
pectin, 47
peptic ulcers, 73
pesto, 196
phenols, 52
phospholipid bilayer, 49
phospholipids, 14
phosphorus, 72, 169
photo-oxidation, 52
phthalates, 5
phytochemicals, 57–60, 61–3, 71, 263
phytoestrogens, 2, 3, 5, 39–43, 79, 283–4
phytonutrients, 16, 179, 184
phytosterols, 42
pine nuts, 268
pistachios, 226
plant oils, 5

plant protein, 33, 34, 64–5, 217, 228–9
plant sterols, 46–7, 61
plants, 5, 37
poached pears, 240
polyphenols, 16, 28, 52, 59, 61, 62, 70
polyunsaturated (PUFA) fats, 16
pomegranate, 59, 276
porcini mushroom risotto, 211–12
porridge bread, 37, 45, 80, 102, 220
porridge oats, 34, 46
    oat and flaxseed porridge with blueberry compote, 105
    oat and hemp seed porridge, 108
    porridge bread, 102
portion sizes, 36
potassium, 35, 42, 53, 71, 72
prawns, 66, 150, 167–8, 169
prebiotic fibre, 19, 28, 45, 256
prebiotics, 14, 17, 68, 454
pro-anthocyanins, 61
probiotic lime green smoothie, 259
probiotics, 2, 3, 50, 68–70, 125–6, 237, 249, 253, 280
processed fats, 51
processed foods, 53
processed meats, 5, 22, 47
propionate, 48
prostate cancer, 40, 62, 71
protein, 2, 3, 4, 5, 9, 12, 14, 19, 23, 30, 31, 33, 34, 35, 36, 40, 44, 64–7, 189, 217, 281, 284
    protein bars, 24
    protein powders, 281
    Thrive protein balls, 247
prunes, 45
psyllium husks, 45, 47

quinoa, 14, 31, 64, 66, 163, 226, 228–9

ramen bowl with crispy tofu and miso, 88
raspberry mousse, 134
recommended daily amounts, 2, 3, 34
recovery-boosting salad in a jar, 158
red lentil, turmeric and kale hotpot, 162
red pepper, 46, 63, 183, 204, 206, 207, 209, 243
rhubarb, pear and apple compote, 108
ricotta cheese, 207–9
risotto
    porcini mushroom, 211–12
    spinach, pea and mint, 167–8

roasted aubergine involtini, 85–6
roasted Brussels sprouts, 270
roasted cabbage steaks, 273
roasted carrot and yellow pepper hummus, 117
roasted cauliflower, chickpea and sweet potato salad, 265
roasted chicken breast, 243
roasted Mediterranean vegetable frittata, 218
roasted Mediterranean vegetable lasagne, 207–9
roasted Mediterranean vegetables, 197
roasted red pepper and tomato sauce, 204, 206, 207
roasted root vegetable mash, 232–4
rocket salad, 37, 58, 268
root vegetable mash, 232–4
root vegetables, 33, 34
rye bread, 34

sage and date hummus, 118
salads
    edamame and sesame rainbow slaw, 92
    grilled baby gem Caesar, 164
    kale, 276
    lit-from-within chicken, 190
    mackerel niçoise, 149
    recovery-boosting salad in a jar, 158
    roasted cauliflower, chickpea and sweet potato, 265
    rocket, pine nut and parmesan, 268
salmon, 16, 22, 34, 49–50, 65–6, 222
    harissa charred salmon, 140
    salmon kedgeree, 154
salsa, 140
salt, 21, 50
sambal, 90
saponins, 40
sardines, 13, 16, 22, 50
saturated fats, 21, 22, 23, 49, 50, 53, 61
sauces, 27, 35
    bottled, 24
    pasta, 24, 73
    roasted red pepper and tomato, 204, 206, 207, 209
sauerkraut, 70, 74, 250–2
savoury granola, 122
seafood bouillabaisse, 133, 138
seaweed, 47, 54, 55, 88

seaweed hand roll, 169
seeds, 5, 14, 33, 34, 44, 46, 53, 54, 55, 63, 68, 237, 280
selenium, 45, 65, 66
serotonin, 66
serving size, 23–4
sesame rainbow slaw, 92
Shakshuka, 220
shepherd's pie, 232–4
shitake mushrooms, 14, 66, 90, 232–4
shopping, 280
short-chain fatty acids, 19, 47–8, 68
skin, 62, 69–70, 179, 235
Slavich, George, 21
slaw, 74, 92
sleep, 1, 17, 18, 30, 32, 54, 55, 157
smoked mackerel pâté, 146
smoking, 11, 21, 63
smoothies
    fountain-of youth smoothie bowl, 202
    glow bowl, 200
    mango, turmeric and hemp seed smoothie, 189
    nutrient powerhouse smoothie bowl, 137
    probiotic lime green smoothie, 259
snacks, 24
soluble fibre, 43–4, 45, 46, 47
soups
    carrot, ginger and celery soup, 199
    red lentil, turmeric and kale hotpot, 162
    tomato, chilli and fennel soup, 192
sourdough bread, 69, 249, 256, 280
soy beans, 5, 14, 39, 40, 42, 79, 91
soy milk, 40
soy products, 64
spiced chicken tagine, 225
spinach, 13, 17, 62, 80, 207–9
spinach, pea and mint risotto with roasted asparagus and prawns, 167–8
spirulina, 14, 104, 281
spirulina, lime and mint overnight oats, 104
statin therapy, 21, 46
steamed cauliflower rice, 263, 264
stevia, 26
stress, 17, 18, 21, 23, 30, 31–2, 55, 57
stroke, 9, 53, 62

sugar, 20, 23-4, 26-9, 32, 49, 53, 280-1, 283
sulphur-containing foods, 68
sulphurophane, 57-8, 71, 72
summer rolls, 150
Sunwarrior, 281
sweet potatoes, 22, 31, 37, 58, 204, 206, 265
    sweet potato and apple breakfast cookies, 110
    sweet potato gnocchi, 204, 206
    sweet potato, lentil, shitake, tofu and lemongrass curry, 90
    sweet potato sauce, 85-6
    sweet potato toast, 186
sweeteners, 23, 26
symbiotic culture of bacteria and yeast (SCOBY), 70
Synergy Spirulina, 281

tagine, 225
tahini, 280
tarts, 125-6
teas, 27
tempeh, 5, 14, 40, 66
tender stem broccoli, 190, 271
Thai red curry, 83-4
Thrive protein balls, 247
thyroid, 169
thyroid cancer, 42
toasted pistachios, 226
tofu, 5, 23, 31, 34, 40, 46, 50, 64, 66, 79, 88, 281
tofu dishes
    crispy tofu Thai red curry, 83-4
    Med veg tofu, 85-6
    sweet potato, lentil, shitake, tofu and lemongrass curry, 90
    tofu scramble with spinach, garlic and mushrooms, 80, 222
tomato, chilli and fennel soup, 192
toxins, 5, 45, 57, 63, 68
trans fats, 5, 16, 53
transit time, 43, 45, 49, 55
triglycerides, 19, 20, 35, 42, 46, 51, 70
tryptophan, 64, 66
T-scores, 12
turmeric, 9, 17, 22
turmeric roasted chicken breast, 243
type 2 diabetes, 7, 8, 26, 29, 70, 101
    see also diabetes
tyrosine, 66

University of California, 21
urinary tract infections, 61

vagina, 42, 249
vagus nerve, 17
vegan power bowl, 113
vegetable bouillon, 281
vegetable frittata, 218
vegetable lasagne, 207-9
vegetables, 5, 7, 13, 21, 36, 46, 53, 54, 57, 61, 63, 197, 280
vinegar, 255
vision, 59, 61, 62
vitamins
    A, 35, 53, 57, 58, 59, 62, 183, 276
    B, 5, 9, 14, 21, 28, 35, 40, 45, 59, 64, 65, 66, 70, 71, 73, 113, 263, 273
    B6, 35, 65, 73, 273
    B12, 17, 35, 65, 66, 281
    C, 14, 35, 40, 57, 59, 61, 63, 66, 70, 71, 72-3, 74, 138, 169, 183, 190, 265, 273, 276
    D, 8, 12, 13, 35, 65
    E, 35, 45, 57, 62-3, 73
    K, 59, 65, 71

water, 7, 48, 49
weight, 3, 4, 11, 23, 24, 26, 29, 30-2, 47, 48, 101
wheat bran, 43, 45, 46, 55
white bread, 4, 20, 70
whole foods, 30-1
wholegrain breads, 43
wholegrains, 5, 8, 22, 33, 34, 39, 46, 63, 79
    see also grains
wine, 33, 34
World Health Organization (WHO), 5, 26
wraps, 74, 117
    falafel, 37, 223
    kale quinoa, 163, 223

The XX Brain, 9
xylitol, 26

yeast flakes, 281
yoghurt, 13, 24, 50, 125-6, 237
    coconut yoghurt, 253
    frozen yoghurt bark, 260

zinc, 9, 14, 28, 35, 40, 53, 64, 66, 169

Notes